THE SUPERMEDS

ALSO BY ROCHELLE JONES

The Other Generation: The New Power of Older People

The Big Switch: New Careers, New Lives after 35

The Private World of Congress (coauthor)

THE SUPERMEDS

•

How the Big Business of Medicine Is Endangering Our Health Care

•

ROCHELLE JONES

Charles Scribner's Sons NEW YORK

Charles Scribner's Sons
Macmillan Publishing Company
866 Third Avenue, New York, NY 10022
Collier Macmillan Canada, Inc.

Library of Congress Cataloging-in-Publication data
Jones, Rochelle.
The supermeds : how the big business of medicine
is endangering our health care / Rochelle
Jones.
p. cm.
Bibliography: p.
Includes index.
ISBN 0-684-18695-0
1. Medical corporations—United States. 2. Medical care—United States. 3. Medical care, Cost of—United States. I. Title.
R728.2.J66 1988
362.1'0973—dc19 87-21755
CIP

Macmillan books are available at special discounts for bulk purchases for sales promotions, premiums, fund-raising, or educational use.
For details, contact:

Special Sales Director
Macmillan Publishing Company
866 Third Avenue
New York, NY 10022

10 9 8 7 6 5 4 3 2 1

Designed by Jack Meserole

PRINTED IN THE UNITED STATES OF AMERICA

For my father,

CHARLES PEABODY JONES

CONTENTS

ACKNOWLEDGMENTS

First, a caveat. In *The Supermeds* I am writing about social and economic trends and the health care corporations that helped to create them. I am writing, too, about the nature of investor-owned corporations. I have questioned their ability to deliver high-quality, affordable health care to consumers, and my research has confirmed those doubts. I have met some supermed officials who seem single-mindedly dedicated to the profit motive, but I have also met others who are dedicated and compassionate, who are aware of these problems and worry about them daily even as they seek to increase company profits and in the process price health care beyond the reach of many Americans. At times I saw them as victims of their own corporations—although they are unlikely to agree—and even more of the insatiable demands for higher profits that are placed on all publicly held corporations. I know, too, that not all doctors pursue profits to their patients' detriment. Yet I have concluded that the medical profession has changed, and too many physicians have come to see their practices in profit-and-loss terms.

Many people helped to shape this book. I owe a debt of deep gratitude to my agent, Gail Ross of Goldfarb & Singer, who always believed in the book and my ability to write it. Her faith supported me throughout. All writers should have such an understanding agent. Erika Goldman of Charles Scribner's Sons was enormously helpful in preparing the manuscript for publication.

I also appreciate the help of a number of friends. Ken Cummins of the *Fort Lauderdale News/Sun-Sentinel* was consistently ahead of other reporters on the International Medical Centers story. He graciously shared his research and insights with me. Carolyn Weaver read parts of the manuscript and offered valuable criticisms. Her friendship helped to sustain me. I am indebted to Peter Woll, who helped me to understand the regulatory process and the relationship between regulation and politics. I want to thank Dudley Marsteller for his continued assistance. Dudley supplied essential information about the supermeds and helped to keep my research up to date. I am grateful, too, for his encouragement and interest.

ROCHELLE JONES
Washington, D.C.

THE SUPERMEDS

CHAPTER ONE

•

The Medical Marketplace

WHEN HUMANA, INC., a diversified health care company, opened its new corporate headquarters in Louisville in 1985, the building shook the city and started a controversy about its design that has raged undiminished ever since. Residents who once argued heatedly about horse bloodlines and Bourbon blends discovered that architectural design could also send pulses racing. Humana headquarters soars twenty-seven stories above the banks of the Ohio River one block away. Although a twenty-seven-story-tall building is a major skyscraper in Kentucky, it was not the building's height that stunned residents; next door on Main Street the First National Tower rises forty stories tall, but it is an unassuming steel and glass tower. Humana headquarters is a building that steps out with bravado. It exerts a nearly magnetic force, and since the ribbon-cutting ceremony almost all of Louisville has come to stare at this instant landmark. There is a lot to see. Two-inch-thick pink granite slabs, quarried in Finland, cling to the walls with maroon, green, gray, and black granite trim imported from four continents. Six waterfalls tumble fifty feet down the exterior on either side of massive bronze doors. Above them gold letters spell out H-U-M-A-N-A, while gold-leafed fluting edges thirty-foot pillars. Over forty-five thousand square feet of hand-cut marble decorates the lobby, while bird's-eye maple and mahogany panel the elevators. Despite the wonder this inspires, or perhaps because of it, Louisville residents leave the site profoundly uneasy. The significance of its design or the splendor of its execution is beside the point. The building is a monument to corporate power and riches. And to the Louisville elite who huddle in the unassuming confines of the extremely wealthy and very exclusive Pendennis Club, the building represents an upstart corporation's drive for power.

David A. Jones, the founder of Humana, didn't necessarily intend to stir up such uneasiness when he decided to build a corporate headquarters. Humana's five thousand employees were working in rented offices scattered throughout Louisville and needed to be brought together under one roof. Jones, the son of a self-employed Louisville contractor, believed a building would be a sound investment. At the same time he tackled the project with a splashy abandon that suggests a desire to make an enduring mark on his hometown. Jones grew up in an unpretentious neighborhood and distinguished himself from numerous other working-class children with his surefootedness in the boxing ring. His family was too poor to send him to college, but Jones was ambitious even then, and after high-school graduation he swept floors in North Carolina tobacco markets for a year to help pay his tuition at the University of Louisville. Now, as chairman of the board and chief executive officer of Humana, Jones runs the corporation from a corner office that looks out not on the broad Ohio River but on the modest working-class neighborhood of his childhood.

While it might have been logical to use the city's own resources to build a corporate headquarters, Jones decided not even to consider local architects for the commission, and that, too, suggests he was motived by more than merely financial considerations. Humana executives didn't believe that Louisville architects could design a building that now has architectural critics from as far away as Italy juggling plane schedules to Louisville. Instead, Jones announced an international competition and invited five world-famous architects to submit designs that would generate excitement and capture the public's imagination. Humana set up a jury to select the winning design, and it chose the work of Michael Graves, an internationally renowned architect based in Princeton, New Jersey. Humana spent three years and $60 million to fulfill his compelling

Post-Modernist vision. Jones got his wish. Humana and Graves' building are perfectly matched. The building has been called a turning point in twentieth-century architecture, a perfect setting for a corporation that is a turning point in twentieth-century health care. Just as its headquarters seized control of the Louisville skyline, so Humana is fighting to control the future of health care in the United States. Humana is moving boldly and aggressively to establish a health care system that seeks to wrest profits from sickness, a corporate strategy that troubles the medical power structure as much as its headquarters disturbs the Kentucky Derby crowd. Humana is in the midst of transforming the delivery of medicine and, like most usurpers of power, it arouses smoldering passions. In its hometown and beyond it is envied, criticized, feared, and resented.

Humana is an example of a new kind of business, a health care corporation that delivers medical care to make a profit. These medical giants, the supermeds, didn't exist in the 1970s, but they are growing swiftly in the 1980s in both size and scope. From their origins in general hospitals the supermeds have expanded into virtually every health field—insurance, nursing homes, psychiatric care and rehabilitation centers—and may be the most influential force in the health care system for the rest of this century. They will shape the cost, quality, and kind of medical services that are offered consumers. In the end they will help determine the ability of Americans to get any health care at any price. The supermeds believe that medicine is a product to be bought and sold. Their corporate officers are making critical decisions that will affect patients, doctors, health care administrators, and workers. Many of these changes, however, are not well received by the medical establishment—the doctors, medical schools, and university hospitals—who have traditionally controlled medicine and who are unwilling to concede their authority without a fight. Behind the scenes a fierce competition is being waged, pitting doctor against doctor, hospital against hospital, doctor against hospital, and entrepreneurs against both. As Dr. David Rollo, Humana's senior vice president for medical affairs, said, "Rather than a revolution going on in health care, it's a civil war and if it keeps up, everybody is going to lose."

The date was November 25, 1984. The place was Humana Hospital-Audubon, a Humana-owned facility on the outskirts of Louisville, a modern 484-bed facility whose walls are graced by original John Audubon bird prints. Dr. William DeVries slipped his hands into the chest of William Schroeder and pressed an artificial heart into place. This is a story of a man, his doctors, a supermed, and the medical establishment.

William Schroeder was dying that fall. For two years the Jasper, Indiana, man had battled crippling heart disease. His doctors had succeeded in keeping him alive with a double heart bypass and the entire battery of modern medical technology. Yet, despite the care of leading cardiologists, he was losing the fight. He was suffering from the final stages of advanced cardiomyopathy, a chronic disease that weakens the heart muscle and restricts the flow of blood to the body. His ravaged heart could pump only one third of the normal flow of blood through his body. A year earlier he had been forced to retire from his job as a quality assurance specialist at Crane Army Ammunition Activity. By the time he arrived at Humana Hospital-Audubon on November 11, he was in almost constant pain. A heavy smoker for thirty years, Schroeder could barely walk twenty feet across his hospital room without gasping for breath. His wife of thirty-two years, Margaret, knew he was near death. She told his doctors, "I feel him fading from me."

Doctors gave Schroeder and his family few choices. At fifty-two he was considered two years too old for a heart transplant. Even if he'd met the age requirements, the operation would have been difficult. Aside from his heart disease, Schroeder was afflicted with other complicating ailments. He had diabetes that would be aggravated by the antirejection drugs needed after surgery. His kidneys were failing, and he was recovering from gall bladder surgery. At the Humana Heart Institute, located within Humana Hospital-Audubon, cardiologists presented only two alternatives: Schroeder could risk the experimental artificial heart implant, or he could die. The Schroeders grasped for hope and agreed to the artificial heart. By mid-November Schroeder was failing rapidly, and the heart implant operation was hastily rescheduled from Wednesday, November 28, to Sunday, November 25. DeVries and Dr. Allan M. Lansing, the director of Humana Heart Institute, had decided the operation could wait no longer. Without it Schroeder might not survive the weekend.

The operation began at 7:05 A.M. when Schroeder was wheeled into the second-floor surgical suite. Surrounding him was a team of five heart surgeons and eleven nurses. Dr. Robert Jarvik, the inventor of the artificial heart that bears his name, looked on. Margaret Schroeder and their six children, ranging in age from nineteen to thirty-one, waited for news of the operation's success or failure on the hospital's sixth floor with a Roman Catholic priest.

As the lilting strains of Vivaldi and Mendelssohn were piped into the operating room, DeVries began the seven-hour operation. DeVries was the only surgeon licensed by the federal government to perform the heart implant operation. He was a boyish-looking forty-year-old surgeon who wore tennis shoes with his surgical greens but whose unassuming Dr. Kildare exterior concealed enormous ambition. Schroeder was administered anesthesia, and two lines were inserted in his heart and tethered to a heart-lung machine that would keep his vital organs alive during the operation. At 10:00 A.M. the surgeons prepared for the actual implant. The diseased lower chambers or ventricles of Schroeder's heart were removed. The two upper chambers or atria were left in place and attached to white Dacron tubing to help hold the artificial heart in place. Similar tubes were sewn to the aortic and pulmonary arteries that pump blood to the body and lungs. Then the lower chambers of the artificial heart, two translucent yellow cups fashioned out of polyurethane and aluminum, each the size of a man's fist, were snapped in place. More tubes were threaded through Schroeder's upper abdomen, secured with additional Dacron, and connected to the external air compressor that powers the artificial heart. A key was turned to start up the 323-pound compressor, and a Compaq console computer began regulating the second-by-second flow of blood in and out of the heart. By 1:00 P.M. Schroeder's artificial heart was beating on its own. His chest was closed and he was taken to the intensive-care unit. At about 4:40 P.M. Schroeder opened his eyes and squeezed his surgeons' hands.

While DeVries remained with his patient, Lansing, a cardiovascular surgeon with a Cary Grant-style handsomeness, went to brief reporters. Humana had spent four months preparing for this moment, drilling its public-relations staff as thoroughly as race-horse owners train for the Kentucky Derby. Its preparations were so fastidious that critics wondered if Humana considered the press or the surgeons more important to the operation's success. In fact, according to Humana spokesman George Atkins, the operation was conceived from the very beginning as a joint project by "the surgical team, the hospital team, and the public-relations team." While the surgical team went through dress rehearsals in the operating room, the public-relations department staged its own practice sessions. Even before the Food and Drug Administration gave its final consent to Schroeder's operation, long months before the actual surgery, construction workers had begun transforming a classroom at Humana Hospital-Audubon into a press headquarters. While the surgical team flew to Utah to consult with the surgeons who had performed the first artificial-heart implant, Humana's public-relations director took two trips in the company jet to discuss media strategy with the University of Utah's public-affairs department.[1]

Hefty briefing books were printed; graphics and videotapes explaining the implant procedure were assembled for use by the print and electronic media. Two photographers were hired to accompany the surgical team into the operating room. At the last moment, as press calls came from as far away as Sydney, Australia, and as interest swelled, the press center was switched from the specially constructed room at Humana Hospital-Audubon to the convention center several miles away. Humana rented blocks of rooms for reporters at local hotels and installed thirty-five telephone lines for collect calls only at the convention center. Since reporters could walk to the convention center from downtown hotels, Humana canceled plans for shuttle buses to the hospital several miles away. A week before the operation over one hundred reporters had already descended on Louisville. David Jones, Robert Jarvik, Allan Lansing, and Humana's public-relations staff spent eight hours at a press briefing. The meticulous advance work paid off. By the time DeVries donned his surgical gloves, there were few things the press didn't know about Humana, Inc., and its role in artificial hearts. Humana managed two almost equally impossible feats simultaneously. It controlled all the news, and it was praised for its openness. Atkins, who was Humana's spokesman when Lansing was unavailable, recalled in his Kentucky drawl, "We did it all in the full glare of publicity and it worked. There was considerable downside risk. It worked because the operation was successful."

Over 234 news organizations sent reporters to Louisville. Television satellite dishes dotted the streets like flying saucers. *USA Today* sent two reporters and installed its own direct telephone line. Japanese and West German television crews tripped over the eighty thousand feet of cable that ABC News installed for its remote station. Reporters waited eagerly as Lansing arrived at the convention center to announce the outcome of the operation. "He knows he has survived but he really feels very little," Lansing told the press. "We'll be happier at this time tomorrow. But as of this moment, I would say he is just as well off as we could possibly hope he would be. The heart has functioned beautifully. The patient has responded well. His kidneys are functioning. His lung function is quite satisfactory. The heart function is excellent and he has awakened."

The success of Schroeder's operation, only the second artificial heart to be implanted in the United States, monopolized the news that day and for weeks to come. It contained all sure-fire elements of a major story—an important medical breakthrough and the drama of a man fighting for his life. The ABC, CBS, and NBC networks told the country about William Schroeder's operation at Humana Heart Institute on their Sunday night programs. The next morning *The Washington Post, The New York Times,* and other leading newspapers ran the story on their front pages. When Schroeder sat up and drank a Coors beer, when President Reagan called Humana Heart Institute with get-well wishes, headlines followed.

Almost before the public learned of the remarkable events at Humana Hospital-Audubon Sunday night, the medical powers that be were lashing out at the heart implant team and Humana. The backstabbing was vicious. Dr. Arnold Relman, editor of the *New England Journal of Medicine,* Harvard Medical School professor, and the epitome of the medical establishment, was especially critical. He told reporters, "Humana does no teaching and no research and they have never done clinical investigation. Humana has made no contribution to medical research at all. That, in my view, is not the best place to carry out this procedure." The president of the American Medical Association, Dr. Joseph E. Boyle, also attacked Humana. He called on the AMA to investigate heart implant surgery and adopt guidelines that would guard against "the apparent commercialization of this whole process by widespread publicity."

Dr. David I. Olch, a Los Angeles internist and member of the AMA ethical council, suggested that artificial-heart surgery should be prohibited if it was to take place only at for-profit hospitals. Olch said, "To the general public, Humana stands to acquire an aura of credibility that is undeserved in the sense that real credibility should come from service to people and from providing high-quality medical care and not from making headlines. . . . My concern is whether or not the artificial-heart program has been as well thought out on behalf of the patients as it has on the part of the investigators. Will the artificial heart benefit Schroeder as much as it benefits Dr. Jarvik, Humana, and the surgical team?" In a lengthy interview with the *American Medical News,* Olch accused the heart implant team of violating medical ethics, of putting their research and careers ahead of Schroeder's welfare. He said, "It's the wrong approach and the wrong setting." Olch's charges were serious, and by raising them in the *American Medical News,* published by the American Medical Association and circulated to its members, he guaranteed that they would receive widespread attention.[2]

Legitimate ethical and moral issues surround the artificial heart. In a sense the operation does use humans as guinea pigs, and the danger exists that potential recipients, dying men and women clutching at life, will not fully comprehend its experimental nature even when properly informed of the risks. Hope can conquer reality.

These issues would receive a proper airing when the National Institutes of Health held a public meeting on the artificial-heart-implant procedure. At that time, after a day-long hearing, Humana would be praised for its procedures. And the NIH would grant approval for further heart implants at Humana.

The medical establishment, represented by Relman and his colleagues, wasn't disturbed by issues of medical ethics alone. They were perturbed by something far more fundamental. The establishment was furious that such a significant breakthrough would occur outside their world of medical schools and academic teaching hospitals. They weren't just incensed, they were also profoundly afraid. Their attack would not have been so ferocious if the stakes had not been so high. With its heart implant and the ensuing publicity, Humana was altering the balance of power in the private world of medicine. As Olch warned his fellow physicians, "The infusion of proprietary dollars into clinical research has the potential to change the entire concept of how research is conducted and monitored." Moreover, Humana wasn't entering that world quietly; it walked in brazenly, and the world noticed. In terms of prestige and status, Humana, Inc.'s Audubon Hospital was no match for Harvard Medical School's Massachusetts General Hospital. But by reacting so violently, the medical establishment drew further attention to Humana's achievement. Ironically, they increased Humana's stature by their criticism; through their attacks they elevated Humana into a serious rival.

The attacks were proof that Humana had arrived. David Jones heard in them confirmation that Humana wasn't just another hospital corporation. Serious people were taking Humana seriously. In time Jones came to conclude that Arnold Relman needed Humana far more than Humana needed him. Relman sought to preserve the medical establishment's power through his attacks while Humana, ignoring his criticisms, continued to demolish its authority. In fact, Jones says of Relman, "This is a turf battle. It's a battle over power, and no one gives up power voluntarily. Arnold Relman's basic claim to fame seems to be criticism of investor-owned corporations. This is a nonissue. No person who goes about pontificating, as he does, can have true relevance. The moral high ground can't be gained by assertion as he tried to do."

Humana Heart Institute doctors, however, couldn't forget the criticism quite so easily. Years later they were still agitated by it. Dr. Richard Zinger, a Louisville cardiologist, has never forgotten—or forgiven. Zinger headed the medical panel that reviewed Schroeder's medical records and decided he would be the second person to receive the artificial heart. Zinger said, "In essence they said that we were bought off by Humana. They said we were inept. And not one of them, not Arnold Relman or any other of the critics, to this day has ever come here or contacted me. It is a total insult."

A lot hung on those seven hours in the operating room. The surgery held many risks, but the rewards, too, could be enormous. If the heart implant was successful, glory, fame, and riches lay ahead for Humana, Inc., the Humana Heart Institute, Humana Hospital-Audubon, DeVries, Lansing, and the surgical team. The triumph could be theirs. All they had to do was reach out and seize it. But the chain of events that would lead DeVries to Humana, and Humana to worldwide recognition, had a far more humble origin. Its beginnings lay in the cutthroat competition among Louisville hospitals, particularly in the rivalry between the Humana hospitals and Jewish Hospital. With 466 beds and a before-tax income of $3.2 million, Jewish Hospital was Louisville's number three hospital in both size and profitability. Its capacity was considerably smaller than Norton-Kosair Children's Hospital, the city's largest hospital with 613 beds, while its income was significantly less than Humana Hospital-Audubon, whose before-tax income of $12.3 million was Louisville's highest. Jewish Hospital lured patients throughout Kentucky largely because Dr. Allan Lansing was its highly esteemed chief of heart surgery. And Lansing and his eleven partners were a major source of income for Jewish Hospital.

Humana embarked on an extended courtship of Lansing, his partners, and their revenue-rich practice of two thousand surgical patients. Humana tried to entice the partnership by offering to appoint Lansing as director of its new heart institute. Lansing resisted that at first. He was well established at Jewish Hospital; he was content and he saw no compelling reason to relocate his practice. He worried, too, that the alliance could be dangerous, that medicine and money might not mix. But Humana kept coming back and dangling new lures. It promised to help the doctors expand their practices and attract new patients from around the country. And it offered to send Lansing to Salt Lake City, where he could study the artificial-heart-implant procedure under William DeVries. Finally Lansing reconsidered. "I'd been [at Jewish Hospital] twenty years and I couldn't see that ten years later things would be any different," he said. "I realized that Humana had enormous resources and maybe we could do together something that we couldn't do separately. I saw this becoming a leading educational, surgical, and technological research center which would also maintain a quality of touch and caring in treating patients, not just an aortic valve."

Jewish Hospital was stunned when Lansing and his partners announced their departure. The hospital administration was deeply distraught about the loss of revenue; moreover, try as they might, they could not comprehend that the doctors could leave nonprofit Jewish Hospital for profit-making Humana. The entire Louisville medical community was shocked. Even though the doctors would not be on Humana's payroll, it was as if they had traded in medicine for money. A partner of Lansing said, "They acted as if we had betrayed them. We were treated like outcasts in the community and, to some extent, we still are."

Meanwhile, DeVries was encountering trouble at the University of Utah, where he'd performed the world's first artificial-heart implant on Dr. Barney Clark, a Seattle dentist, on December 1, 1982. Clark survived 112 days, and a year had passed since then. DeVries was eager to operate again. He had been given permission by the federal government to perform seven artificial-heart operations, an arbitrarily set number, and he was still searching for his second candidate. But he was hindered by a lack of money. The university refused to support further research on the artificial heart. After demanding that DeVries raise money to cover Clark's $250,000 hospital bill, it was insisting that he produce $180,000 in advance for the second implant. DeVries was traveling the country, prospecting for funds instead of operating, and his frustration was mounting.

DeVries was in Durham, North Carolina, where he had once done research at Duke University Medical Center, still looking for funds, when he accepted an invitation to visit Lansing. It was a typical rainy spring weekend in Kentucky in 1984 that became a turning point for DeVries, Lansing, and Humana. DeVries complained bitterly to Lansing about the University of Utah's lack of support for his research. DeVries was thoroughly disgusted and Lansing sensed that with the right offer DeVries could be induced to move to Kentucky. That offer was quickly forthcoming. Humana had already realized the potential of the artificial heart, investing $1 million in Kolff Medical, the Utah manufacturer of the Jarvik-7 heart. It would make sense for Humana to invest in clinical trials of the heart at its own heart institute.* An appointment was easily arranged between DeVries and David Jones. When the two met, Jones asked for an estimate of the number of operations it would take to learn if the artificial heart was a practical procedure. DeVries estimated ten. "We'll do ten times ten if this will help you push the technology to its limits," Jones told him. "With one caveat—that scientific progress is being made." For DeVries, still struggling to raise the $180,000 for his second operation, the offer was stunning. The University of Utah could not possibly match it. Moreover, Lansing extended an invitation to DeVries to join his private medical practice.

Lansing recalled, "DeVries wasn't going anyplace at the University of Utah and we offered to support his research. This program could never have been undertaken at a university center. It would have been bankrupt. If the University of Louisville or Harvard Medical School had tried to support it, everybody else at the medical school would have been screaming. The federal government has cut off all funds. It is up to private business to pick up the support."

At the same time that DeVries was being lured to Louisville, Humana was beginning to market the "Humana" brand name, to make Humana to hospitals what Xerox was to photocopying machines. While rival supermed Hospital Corporation of America tried to deemphasize corporate control of its hospitals, creating a folksy image of local hospitals serving local people, Humana was busy stamping its name on hospitals and treatment centers. When it bought or managed a new hospital, the official blue and white

*Humana sold its interest in Kolff Medical before the first heart implant at Humana Hospital-Audubon.

Humana colors and the corporate "H" logo were tacked on and the name changed. For this marketing strategy to succeed, however, the Humana name had to stand for something. Its officers thought they had that "something" in their so-called Centers of Excellence at fourteen Humana hospitals around the country. These centers, combining the latest diagnostic equipment and clinical research, specialize in the treatment of diabetes, spinal cord and joint injuries, burns, and lung and cardiovascular disease, among other medical complaints. Humana expected that with the right kind of publicity the centers would attract new patients to all its hospitals. Humana vice president Neal Westermeyer, who switched from marketing commodities to selling health care, said later, "The Centers of Excellence, if marketed correctly, can be the kingpin of our entire strategy. If we use this properly, we can use it not just to build up our hospitals but also to sell health insurance. They are the added value that the people are looking for."

Humana was searching for new patients. The year before, Congress passed a new financing system for Medicare, and as a result admissions of elderly patients was dropping rapidly. In communities throughout the United States, hospital occupancy rates were falling. It shouldn't have been surprising. Health care experts had been warning for years that the country had too many hospital beds, but no one was listening. Now administrators looked at their vacant rooms and the ones across town and began to understand. Humana officials didn't even have to leave Louisville to observe this ominous trend. In their own hometown eleven hospitals, four of them owned or operated by Humana, were struggling to coax enough patients into their beds to survive. David Laird, the administrator of Humana's University of Louisville Hospital, said, "Five years ago hospitals were full and patients were waiting to get in. The hospital planners warned us but the hospital administrators in our wisdom would scratch our heads and say, 'If we're full, how can there be too many beds?' " But Laird said that local hospital administrators learned. With a countywide population of less than a million there were simply too many beds and not enough patients to go around. The hospital administrators looked at their vacant rooms and the census figures for other hospitals and finally believed. While Laird could be justifiably proud of a 75 percent occupancy rate, a substantial number of hospitals in Louisville were less than half full, and only a third could claim that they were actually attracting more patients. It was obvious by 1984 that only the most tenacious hospitals could stay in business. The others would either fold or merge with former competitors.

The artificial-heart operation was a priceless opportunity for Humana to publicize the Humana Heart Institute and its other Centers of Excellence. Shortly after the implant, Humana Hospital-Biscayne in Miami, Florida, and other Humana hospitals around the country issued press releases saying they would refer critical heart patients to DeVries for the artificial-heart implant. Very few of those patients, if any, however, were apt to pass the stringent guidelines set up by the federal government and become serious candidates for the operation. They were far more likely to stay at the hospital where they originally sought treatment. Optimism, however, could fill hospital beds that might otherwise lie empty.

Not all the hopes that surrounded the artificial-heart operation were fulfilled. Perhaps there was too much at stake; perhaps there were too many, too towering egos involved. DeVries and Humana siphoned off the biggest rewards for themselves. With the help of Humana's public-relations blitz DeVries became a media figure, overshadowing Lansing, his Humana mentor, in terms of public recognition. Lansing resents that. "I'm not the best [heart surgeon] in the world but I do think I'm probably the best in this region," he said in a slighting reference to DeVries, adding that the celebrity surgeon "may not understand as yet how much I accomplished and how much I did for him."[3] Humana, however, achieved its purpose. Overnight it became a household name, indelibly identified in the public consciousness with the artificial heart, the earlier operation at the University of Utah all but forgotten except by the medical establishment.

Tensions remain high at the Humana Heart Institute. Lansing's partners say that they were promised more patients if they went to Humana, and their expectations have yet to be realized. They complain that Lansing and DeVries were the only beneficiaries of the heart implant. They say that their practices have not expanded and their incomes have not increased. A surgeon said, "The potential advantage of the heart institute was that by being together with a big company which has arms all over the state, we would have a potentially large number of patients outside of the immediate surrounding area. It has not changed our lives much. So far, the patients haven't flocked to us. In fact, we've lost money."

The medical wars continue in Louisville. Humana hospitals and Jewish Hospital compete as intensely as ever. Jewish Hospital doctors performed the first heart transplant in Kentucky in 1984, beating out Humana Hospital-Audubon for the honor and some of the income that goes along. Then, in 1986, Lansing opened The Lipid Center at Humana Heart Institute to diagnose, treat, and prevent arteriosclerosis. "It's made a lot of doctors in the community furious," Lansing said. If The Lipid Center manages to prevent heart attacks, many cardiovascular surgeons could be standing in unemployment lines.

Four other artificial-heart implants have been performed since Schroeder was operated on. None of the patients survived as long as William Schroeder, who died of a stroke and respiratory problems on August 6, 1986, at the age of fifty-four, and none was nearly as important to Humana or to the medical establishment. As Lansing said, "I have no regrets about the operation. It was good for the press and the family; the only person it was bad for was Arnold Relman."

CHAPTER TWO

•

The Supermeds

IN THE EARLY 1980s health care was changing from a virtual cottage industry dominated by physicians and nonprofit hospitals into a nationwide network of for-profit corporations that run a variety of medical enterprises. Surveying this new world of health care, Virginia Hunt, administrator at Shands Hospital, the teaching facility for the University of Florida Medical School, said, "The fact of life is that health care is an industry like the steel industry and the hamburger industry."

The financial stakes are unbelievably high. In the first half of the 1980s the United States has tripled its health care spending. By 1987 Americans were spending over $1 billion a day on health care, $458 billion a year, compared to $248 billion in 1980. That figure represents a staggering per-capita increase from $1,049 to $1,837 annually. Nearly 60 percent of that amount is spent on hospital care and physician services. While individual Americans are spending more, the nation's health bill is rising, too. In 1986 health care consumed 10.9 percent of the gross national product, the nation's total output of goods and services, compared to 9.4 percent in 1980.

Numerous factors have contributed to medical bills that would make a Pentagon general blanch. Medical progress and technological advances have driven up the cost of care. A growing population and increasing numbers of senior citizens have also contributed, but a larger and frailer population utilizing the newest medical treatments is responsible for a relatively small fraction of this growth. By and large, Americans are spending more because they are being charged more. According to the Department of Health and Human Services, rising prices account for 64 percent of the increase in health care spending. Hospitals, physicians, and other medical providers raised charges at rates that far exceeded inflation. In 1986, for instance, when the overall inflation rate rose 1.9 percent, health care costs went up 7.5 percent. Americans spent 8.6 percent more on prescription drugs, 7.2 percent more for physician fees, and 6 percent more on hospital care in 1986. Moreover, the federal government projects that health care spending will triple again, to $1.5 trillion in the next twelve years. By the year 2000 health care is expected to grow to 15 percent of the gross national product while individuals can expect to pay an average of $5,551 a year on medical bills.[1]

Attracted by these rising expenditures and beckoning profits, corporations have rushed into health care. These corporations, the supermeds, are engaged in the marketing and delivery of health care throughout the United States. They own general and specialty hospitals, health maintenance organizations, ambulatory clinics and nursing homes. While they deliver care, many are involved, too, in the sale of health insurance to finance that care. These corporations built their medical empires on the hospital chains that continue to be their operational bases. Two companies, Charter Medical Corporation and Community Psychiatric Centers, operate only psychiatric facilities. In 1988 a total of twenty-four corporations each owned or managed more than ten hospitals in communities across the country, but just four investor-owned companies—Humana, Inc., Hospital Corporation of America, American Medical International, and National Medical Enterprises—dominated the industry.

In the 1980s supermeds have nearly doubled in size. According to the Federation of American Health Systems, in 1979 these companies owned 561 hospitals with 76,985 beds; in 1988 they operated 1,114 facilities with 139,508 beds. The big four companies ran almost 80 percent of those hospitals. Hospital companies operate 118 facilities with 15,153 beds in 19 foreign countries. Their expansion is continuing. Eighty-six for-profit hospitals with 8,722 beds were under construction in the United States and Puerto Rico in 1988. Supermeds control almost one in five of the nation's 7,000 hospitals. In certain sections, particularly the Sun Belt, they have captured an even heftier market share. They control, for example, 43 percent of the hospitals in Florida, 41 percent in Tennessee, 39 percent in Nevada, 36 percent in Texas, 34 percent in Louisiana, and 33 percent in California. In Houston they run over half of the hospitals. In St. Petersburg, Florida, they operate two-thirds of the facilities. Their growth has been particularly rapid in Florida, where they added 15 hospitals in 1986 alone, and the Hospital Corporation of America became the state's third largest employer. The supermeds are a rapidly expanding $14 billion-a-year industry. Already 20 to 25 percent of all health care dollars goes to for-profit corporations, and their share is expected to climb to 40 to 50 percent in the 1990s. By the twenty-first century the United States is expected to be the only country in the world with a medical system monopolized by large corporations that deliver health care to make a profit.

Arnold Relman first drew attention to these health care corporations in the *New England Journal of Medicine* in 1980 when he identified "the new medical-industrial complex" with "broad and potentially troubling implications for the future of our medical-care system." In Relman's terms the new medical-industrial complex is composed of corporations such as hospital and nursing home chains that deliver services for a profit while the old medical-industrial complex consisted of corporations such as pharmaceutical companies that made a profit by selling products. Relman warned that the new medical-industrial complex could rival the military-industrial complex in power. Repeating President Dwight Eisenhower's admonition about concentrated power, Relman wrote, "We must guard against unwarranted influence. We should not allow the medical-industrial complex to distort our health care system to its own entrepreneurial ends." Relman hoped that physicians would remain isolated from the medical-industrial complex and use their moral authority to restrain the commercialization of medicine: "As the visibility and importance of the private health-care industry grow, public confidence in the medical profession will depend on the public's perception of the doctor as an honest, disinterested trustee. That confidence is bound to be shaken by any financial association between practicing physicians and the new medical-industrial complex."[2]

But Relman's hopes have not been realized. Doctors have been profoundly influenced by the corporatization of health care. Dr. James Boyle, former president of the American Medical Association, cautions that doctors are being forced to choose between the "business ethic or the medical ethic" and that the business ethic is gaining. And Richard J. Davidson, executive vice president of the Maryland Hospital Association, said, "I go to hospital meetings [and] the whole language has changed. You would think you were out there with twenty go-go entrepreneurial executives in plastics or the telecommunications field. You listen to the language of market share and marketing the strategic plans to maximize profits. . . . It seems to be out of sync. . . . I don't hear anybody talking about [curing and caring]." Young doctors are far less worried about the dangers of the medical-industrial complex than Relman would like. When the American Medical Association surveyed the attitudes of physicians over and under the age of forty, it found they differed substantially in a number of crucial areas. The doctors under forty, who represent nearly half of all practicing physicians, were more likely to favor the growth of for-profit hospitals and less likely to think that quality of care was affected by a hospital's ownership. They were also less likely to see a potential conflict of interest if they referred patients to facilities in which they had a financial interest. More doctors are likely to hold these attitudes as the number of medical students who are trained in supermed facilities grows. Since the mid-1980s the supermeds have expanded their interest in medical education. They operate the major teaching hospitals for the medical schools of universities such as Creighton University, the University of Mississippi, the University of Southern California, the University of Miami, the University of South Florida, the University of Florida, and the University of Medicine and Dentistry of New Jersey.

Before the advent of for-profit health care corporations, the hospital business was relatively straightforward: Patients walked in the door, were admitted, treated, and released. Supermeds, however, aren't content to wait passively for patients; they actively recruit them. By 1985 an astounding 40 percent of consumers reported that they had read, seen, or heard a hospital advertisement during the previous month. The hoopla and hype is a clear sign that health care has become big business, promoted as aggressively as McDonald's hamburgers. In 1981 only an estimated 5 or 10 percent of the nation's hospitals employed a marketing director. By 1984 approximately 50 to 60 percent of hospitals had at least one full-time professional to market their services. And while only two out of three hospitals advertised in 1985, nine out of ten did in 1986, according to SRI Gallup Hospital Market Research. Of the hospitals that used advertising, six-figure budgets were common, and among hospitals with more than 350 beds, advertising budgets averaged $176,900. Steven Steiber, SRI's president for research and development, noted that the nature of advertising has changed markedly, too. In 1984 hospital marketing executives reported that their primary function was public relations. But by 1986, he said, "A bottom-line orientation—revenues—is beginning to dominate. U.S. hospitals now conduct market research to identify consumer demand, then modify their advertising accordingly."

Hospitals are one of the fastest-growing and most important sources of local television advertising revenues as the industry discovers the media's ability to deliver new consumers. Hospitals spent an estimated $1 billion on advertising in 1985, nearly double the 1984 figure. Spending on television ads alone topped $125 million in 1985, a rise of $36 million or 40 percent over 1984, according to the Television Bureau of Advertising. The dollars—and number of commercials—are bound to grow, says Jay Lewis, president of Market Scope, a Miami, Florida, firm specializing in health care research, since the industry is discovering that more consumers choose the hospitals they will use themselves, instead of relying on their doctor's recommendation. Lewis says that in 1986 an estimated 41 percent of patients made that decision compared to 6 percent in 1980. "Those hospitals that encourage promotion have the best chance of survival in the twenty-first century," he said.

Supermeds mastered that lesson early. Richard K. Eamer, chairman and chief executive officer of National Medical Enterprises, told stockholders at its 1984 annual meeting that the company would be hustling its services in the coming year. "It is not enough to be a leader in developing new health care services and alternative treatment settings," he said. "In today's consumer-driven market, we need to market our services aggressively—and we will. The emphasis will be on improving market share in the communities we serve. We plan to direct our advertising to the consumer because individual patients will be making more decisions concerning which facilities they go to for care."

The supermeds are promoting their services with a variety of sophisticated techniques ranging from soft- to hard-core advertising. Humana's Sunrise Hospital in Las Vegas staged a lottery for patients who checked in on weekends, a typically slack time at hospitals. The grand prize was a cruise for two. The promotion was so successful that occupancy rates soared by 60 percent in eighteen months. Hospital Corporation of America blitzed Houston residents for a month with its slogan "We Care for America. We Care for You." The message was nearly inescapable. When they turned on their televisions, Houston viewers saw a picture of a blissful mother and her newborn baby that slowly dissolved into a scene of a physical therapist teaching his patient to walk again. An off-camera voice said, "There's a whole world of caring at Houston's fourteen HCA hospitals." Listening to the radio or reading their daily newspapers, residents also learned that HCA cared for them. They also found the message tucked into their mailboxes on flyers. And mired in traffic jams during their daily commute, they were confronted by billboards emblazoned with the same "We Care for America. We Care for You" message.

The supermeds, however, aren't just courting patients who need to be hospitalized and must decide where to go. They are also trying to convince consumers to purchase services they were previously unaware they needed. Republic Health Corporation, a Dallas-based supermed, studied Ritz crackers and learned to convert surgical procedures into product lines, then marketed them directly to consumers under distinctive brand names. "Health care is a commodity but most people don't think of it that way. We modeled ourselves after other consumer goods," said Michelle Salazar, director of product management. "Nabisco, for example, doesn't advertise the Nabisco name, it advertises Ritz crackers. So we pulled out five or six surgical specialties and began marketing those as products." The product lines include "You're Becoming," cosmetic surgery that can be financed through Republic-arranged bank loans, and "The Gift of Sight," cataract surgery promoted in publications appealing to the elderly. Republic also offers foot surgery in "Step Lively" and maternity services in "Miracle Moments." Republic found that marketing surgery like crackers worked. At its Decatur Hospital outside Atlanta, plastic surgeons performed 49 operations in 1983, but 10 months after the advertising campaign was launched, they performed 540 operations; a year later they operated on 725 patients. Republic credits the unusual marketing strategy with the abrupt turnabout at its Beverly Hills Medical Center. Under Hospital Corporation of America's ownership the hospital was losing $2 million a year; but a year after its purchase by Republic, the hospital was earning a $2 million profit.

Supermeds have invested heavily in psychiatric hospitals and are spending substantial sums to upgrade their image. They hope to convince consumers that their mental health can improve if they check in for just a short stay. HCA is embarking on a multimillion-dollar campaign to promote its psychiatric facilities while Charter Medical Corporation spent millions to undo the *One Flew over the Cuckoo's Nest* image of psychiatric hospitals. The for-profit psychiatric hospitals ran ads that tried to reassure potential patients with slogans like, "If You Just Can't Cope Anymore, You're Not Alone" and "It's Not Easy Growing Up These Days." Richard Woodard, administrator of Charter's Westbrook Psychiatric Hospital in Richmond, Virginia, said, "Three years ago psychiatric hospitals had an image problem and we were trying TV to try to change that. Our ads [in the future] will be much heavier. Now we're advertising specific programs dealing with serious disorders such as schizophrenia and manic-depression." Charter markets to manic-depressives through ads that show two women on a merry-go-round. One woman laughs heartily and clutches a shiny brass pole while a second woman, whose mouth is pursed into a grimace, clings desperately to the mane of a horse that paws the floor.

Meanwhile, Humana's California hospitals market their services to the obese who are unhappy with dreary calorie-counting.

They are told, "The newest way for obese people to successfully take weight off is by eating less the Humana way. Believe it or not, air is the main ingredient in this program." The ads are aimed at people like "Ann, once a high-school cheerleader" who has ballooned from "big-boned" to "chubby" to "pleasingly plump." Ann can lose weight the Humana way, without dieting, if she visits one of their outpatient clinics and has a gastric bubble inserted in her stomach. The gastric bubble will occupy 25 percent of Ann's stomach so that she'll feel full even when her stomach isn't. Humana's brochure concludes, "One-tenth of an ounce of prevention can be worth 75 pounds of cure. Ann stopped making excuses and now her obesity is disappearing into thin air without surgery, without drugs, without a fad diet, and without an overnight stay in the hospital."

Although all the health care corporations accelerated their marketing activities throughout the 1980s, Humana, with its singular flair for self-promotion, far outdistanced its competitors in 1986 when it became the first supermed to employ a corporate officer whose mission was to create a single theme for all its products, from hospitals to health care insurance to walk-in clinics. Neal Westermeyer was the person hired to fill the newly created position of vice president for advertising. Westermeyer knew nothing about health care before he joined Humana, but that didn't faze top management. He possessed boundless energy and enthusiasm and, most important, he knew how to sell. At Ralston Purina, his previous marketing position, Westermeyer had convinced millions of dog owners that their puppies, like their babies, required special diets. He was the promotional genius behind Puppy Chow.

Westermeyer created a $20 million campaign for Humana that was simple and straightforward. It was the first nationwide advertising campaign for a supermed, and it sent Humana's competitors like Hospital Corporation of America scurrying to catch up. Humana spent millions just to produce the spots, hiring acclaimed cinematographer Sven Nykvist, famous for his work on Ingmar Bergman's films, to shoot the softly focused television commercials with their flattering lights and swelling, romantic music. In "The Healing Touch of a Doctor's Hands" a physician's gnarled fingers reach out to touch his patient's unwrinkled hands. In soft focus the commercial recalls Michelangelo's famous fresco in the Sistine Chapel where God's outstretched hand reaches to touch the finger of Adam and give him life. In "Humana: Bringing the Human Being in Need into the Hands of a Doctor," a Norman Rockwell-type physician ministers to apple-cheeked children and wizened but attractive senior citizens. It was a Madison Avenue version of American medicine, and by 1988, with the help of supermeds like Humana, that ideal was rapidly disappearing.

Westermeyer said, "The health care industry is well behind every other industry in terms of its marketing. What I'm trying to do is to add value to the Humana name, to make Humana the most trusted name in health care so when people think of health care, they think of Humana, of its quality and affordability. We're building this whole imagery for Humana. We have this strategy, the structure inside the company and commitment on the part of management to do what no one has ever done before. I think attitudinally we're positioning Humana as a compassionate and caring entity. We're not just a blank face by a name like some of our competitors. This allows us to preempt the marketplace. We're using a marketing strategy that gives us a preemptive position. Our competitors will never be able to catch up."

Westermeyer devised new marketing outlets for Humana. While other supermeds were still thinking in terms of television and print campaigns, Humana was moving in entirely new directions. Westermeyer dreamed of a world where consumers would think about Humana all the time, not just when they are sick, and he set about creating it. Toward that goal Humana and HEB, a Texas supermarket chain, teamed up to market National Diabetes Month. Humana distributed special menus for diabetics with their slogan, "Bringing the Human Being in Need into the Hands of the Doctor" printed on the bottom, and HEB earmarked the aisles on which the products could be found. Westermeyer hoped the recipe cards would beam Humana's message onto thousands of kitchen bulletin boards and refrigerators across Texas. Westermeyer said, "This isn't just advertising; it's recruiting. We think it has a cumulative effect. The more information we distribute, the more we're being thought of."

Intense battles are being waged over local market share between supermeds and community hospitals. As Seth Shaw, a hospital administrator turned Wall Street analyst says, "They're all killing each other to get patients." In the hotly contested South Florida market, for instance, where hospitals are battling for $2.5 billion in health care spending, marketing personnel strain to come up with new gimmicks. Health care professionals are still envious of the publicity Baptist Hospital received when it held a splashy open house for its new emergency facilities. The hospital managed to recruit *Miami Vice* star Philip Michael Thomas and eight members of the Miami Dolphins football team, who drew major media coverage, and a crush of Miamians who usually spent their Sunday afternoons at the beach. Baptist won the publicity prize, but other South Florida hospitals profit from tried and true marketing strategies. American Medical International's Parkway Regional Medical Center spent $500,000 in a year to promote its arthritis center and its eating disorders program, which requires a minimum hospital stay of forty days at prices ranging up to $375 a day. At South Miami Hospital's Stork Club new mothers and fathers celebrate with a steak and champagne dinner served by tuxedoed waiters. The hospital also markets a Weekend Guest Program "Because sometimes you both can use a weekend off" to adult children who care for elderly parents. It is a $100-a-day escape for children who can check their parents into South Miami from 3:00 P.M. Friday to 8:00 A.M. Monday. "A nice long weekend," the hospital advertises. Patients leave South Florida hospitals with more than just the bill as a memento of their stay. They cart home collections of toiletries, coffee mugs, teddy bears, Frisbees, T-shirts, bumper stickers, pens, and pillows. Former South Miami patients receive a regular newsletter. Doctors Hospital of Hollywood, operated by the Universal Health Services chain, provides transportation to and from its facility. If Mount Sinai patients in Miami Beach, Florida, become enamored of its chicken soup, they may purchase a can from the gift shop. AMI's Southeastern Medical Center advertises a flat rate for maternity services, promising prospective parents, "The Bottom Line Is: Having a Baby Doesn't Have to Be Expensive."

Baptist and South Miami hospitals are nonprofit facilities competing vigorously in the free-for-all patient sweepstakes in South

Florida. Without the supermeds' brand names or promotional budgets, they must use their limited resources audaciously to stay in business. South Miami executive director Merrill Crews said, "We don't have the luxury of being able to fall back on tax subsidies like public hospitals, nor can we ask for help from corporate headquarters if we get into trouble, as an investor-owned hospital can. We don't have any sugar daddies. We fall back on operations to run this hospital." South Miami Hospital intends to be one of the survivors when the last commercial is lobbed onto television screens and a truce finally declared. To succeed, Crews says that the hospital has to be "lean and mean and more aggressive." If nonprofit hospital administrators like Crews seem to share the sentiments of NME's Eamer or Humana's Westermeyer, it is a sign that supermeds are nipping at their heels. They are beginning to think and talk like their business managers. Humana, Inc., and Kaiser Permanente, a California-based nonprofit health maintenance organization famous for its low-cost medical care, appear to be as far apart philosophically as they are geographically, but when their top executives talk, for instance, about health care for the poor, they sound remarkably similar. Both agree that the responsibility for such care does not lie with them. David Jones says, "I think we've done our homework. We've taken on the most complex, difficult problems and now we're applying that learning to the people who can afford to pay." James Vohs, chief executive officer of Kaiser Foundation Health Plan, believes "Our health plan members should not bear a disproportionate share of the [indigent care] burden. Indeed, we see this as a problem for our society as a whole and do not see the logic in looking to health insurers and health care providers as the sole or primary source of financing the solution. This problem should be addressed in the political arena."[3]

The supermeds are creating an upheaval in medicine that is changing health care from a social service to a business. They are destroying what health care analyst Kenneth Abramowitz of Sanford C. Bernstein & Co. calls the Dr. Kildare Syndrome, a condition caused by the popular television program. Abramowitz says, "[W]e've been lulled into believing that all physicians spend all their time selflessly saving people's lives in hospitals that similarly selflessly help these benevolent physicians produce miraculous recoveries in patients. And, in return, the doctors get a smile and a kiss and a hug from the patient. We don't see physicians and hospitals in a business sense. We don't see them as a normal supplier of a normal product." That day is near, however. Many health care observers believe that the supermeds will lead to medical product lines sharply differentiated by price. Consumers will have to select, on the basis of price, the type and quality of health care they can afford. Roger Rusley, a Denver-based medical practice consultant, believes that health care will be broken down into three classes, just as airline fares are. First class will be limited to affluent Americans who put "the quality, comfort, and convenience of their health care above cost considerations"; a second class will offer no-frills prepaid care primarily to middle-class Americans, "patients who consider cost first," and a third class will provide government-subsidized care to the elderly and the poor.

All the health care corporations are in medicine to make money, but some, like the Big Four supermeds, also need to produce profits to satisfy stockholders. In the 1980s institutional investors, owners of major blocks of supermed stocks, have become involved in health care. These investors are not always noted for their patience. In their quarterly reports they need to show a profit, and if their holdings are not advancing in price, they can have a strong incentive to sell. Late in 1985 they sold, and the consequences were far-reaching.

The selling began when Hospital Corporation of America announced that its earnings were likely to be flat in 1986. HCA didn't suggest that the company was losing money. In fact, earnings weren't even declining. The company estimated that it would earn 10 percent in 1986, a return that had previously elated investors. But investors are an avaricious lot, easily dissatisfied and always wanting more. They rushed to dump HCA stock, pushing the price down by more than 20 percent, from $39.00 to $31.25 a share in one day's frantic trading. Other supermed stocks faltered, too. Humana stock fell 12 percent; National Medical Enterprises' stock dropped 10 percent, although at its annual meeting only days before, management announced that earnings were expected to grow by 15 percent in the coming year. Later in the week American Medical International announced its earnings would suffer, too, and its stock plummeted 20 percent. Wall Street analysts estimated that the supermeds lost over $1.5 billion in market value within days.

While the selling rocked the industry, the for-profits corporations immediately plunged into a flurry of new activity. The supermeds feverishly bought and sold, exchanging marginal properties for promising new ones. The Federation of American Health Systems reported that for-profits bought 62 specialty hospitals in 1986, bringing their total to 469 facilities and 41,223 beds. It noted, "Specialization continued to increase as an effective marketing strategy and appears to play a needed role in many areas." It found that for-profits were expanding their offerings of inpatient and outpatient services. The supermeds reorganized and pruned unnecessary managers.

As this restructuring continues, Edward M. Kerschner, chairman of Paine Webber's investment policy committee, believes that five or ten supermeds will emerge to dominate the health care industry. Kerschner says that corporations underwent a similar consolidation between 1898 and 1903. At the turn of the century financiers combined dozens of medium-sized companies and created giant trusts like U.S. Steel and DuPont that controlled 50 to 90 percent of their industry. But Kerschner also believes that while the current restructuring will strengthen individual companies, it may weaken the powers of their managers. "The Great Restructuring of the 1980s is actually reversing the evolutionary effects of trustification . . . and shifting financial power from professional managers to investors and financiers," he says.[4]

Meet the Big Four of the supermeds.

Humana: The Money-Makers

If Wyatt, Grafton & Sloss, a Louisville law firm, had paid its associates higher salaries, Humana, Inc., might not exist. Two of its associates, David Jones and Wendell Cherry, now Humana's president, were struggling to raise families on their salaries in the 1960s when they heard that another young Louisville attorney was prospering in the nursing home business. The rumors were enough to spur their imagination. During a weekend golf game they mulled over the financial pros and cons and decided. With confidence born of total ignorance, Jones borrowed $1,000 from Household Finance Corporation, Cherry chipped in $1,000, and they opened a nursing home. They figured if there was money to be made in long-term care, they would find a way to make it, and they did. They earned more than they ever imagined possible that day at the Harmony Landing golf course. Jones would be one of the United States' highest-paid corporate officers, earning over $18 million a year. Cherry, the son of a Horse Cave, Kentucky, grocer, would assemble a private art collection that includes a $5.3 million Picasso self-portrait and a $2.8 million Edvard Munch. When *Art & Antiques* listed the collection among the one hundred best in the United States, Cherry reportedly said buying masterpieces beat playing checkers at the Horse Cave gas station.

Their company, Extendicare, succeeded beyond their fantasies. In 1963 they were opening one facility a year and Extendicare was becoming one of the country's largest nursing home chains. Then a flu epidemic hit New Haven, Connecticut, and transformed the company. After a hospital administrator sent flu patients to Extendicare, Jones and Cherry discovered that hospitals earned more than nursing homes. Within a year Extendicare built its first hospital in Huntsville, Alabama. The partners were still cautious, however. Almost nine years elapsed before Jones felt secure enough to quit Wyatt, Grafton and devote full time to Extendicare. In 1969 the company's previously respectable rate of expansion accelerated. For three years they bought a hospital a month. Next they went on a building binge, constructing twenty-seven hospitals in three years. Sometimes they spent half their revenues on new acquisitions. When there wasn't enough money, they borrowed. They borrowed up to their credit limit of $304 million in 1978, then struck with dazzling ferocity at hospital rival American Medicorp. When Medicorp chairman Alan Miller agreed to be acquired, the nation's third-largest for-profit chain swallowed up the second-largest. The company was rechristened Humana. By 1980 Wall Street analyst Michael LeConey was saying, "No company in this country has accomplished more and come further with less than Humana." In Louisville Jones and Cherry were being called "the Gold Dust Twins."

Humana was the third largest supermed in 1987 after Hospital Corporation of America and American Medical International. It operated eighty-seven hospitals in twenty-two predominantly Southern states and abroad in Switzerland and England, where the gift shop sells diamond and ruby necklaces to rich Arab patients. Among the supermeds it is known for its unusual combination of rat terrier aggressiveness, dashing creativity, and, throughout most of its history, its profits. During the 1980s Humana was called "the company that didn't disappoint" by Wall Street analysts. The Gold Dust Twins raked in profits as easily as their hospitals took in patients. Revenues doubled from $1.1 billion in 1980 to $2.2 billion in 1985, while pretax profits soared from 10.7 percent to 17.5 percent. Investors were happy, too. Their per-share earnings climbed from $0.64 to $2.19, and between 1981 and 1986 return on equity averaged 30 percent.

Humana was always ahead. When rival supermeds were still buying up hospitals in the 1980s, Humana stopped shopping and concentrated on filling its 17,700 beds. It pioneered new products, opening a network of walk-in medical centers called MedFirst, and selling group health insurance policies under the Care Plus brand name.

Henry J. Werronen, head of Humana's group health division, says the company was forced into the insurance business. "Hospitals need patients," he said. "The sharp decline in hospital utilization over the last two years has left most hospitals with substantial unused capacity, often as much as 30 percent to 50 percent. Just like a manufacturing plant with idle machines or a hotel with empty rooms, hospitals must find uses for this unused capacity or their long-term economic viability will be threatened. This is not a passing phenomenon—it is a matter of survival."

Suddenly, in 1986, the company that couldn't fail was doing a lot of fixing. The MedFirst clinics began demanding heavy infusions of cash, Care Plus started hemorrhaging, and Humana reported its first quarterly earnings drop in fifteen years. Humana sold 70 unprofitable MedFirst clinics, retaining 100, and canceled 20,000 Care Plus policies in 11 small markets, continuing to operate in 22 areas. But Care Plus problems went deeper.

In four years Humana signed up over 600,000 Care Plus members, but that wasn't enough to produce profits. In 1986 Humana lost $70 million on its operation. Care Plus premiums were based on the assumption that 75 percent of the policyholders who needed to be hospitalized would choose Humana hospitals when, in fact, only 40 percent did. As a result, Humana was paying substantial sums to hospitalize Care Plus patients at competing facilities. Some patients were being referred to those hospitals by doctors who didn't like for-profit health care. In San Antonio oncologist Stephen C. Cohen urged doctors to boycott Humana and other for-profit facilities. "They're looking to cut costs. We look at the well-being of the patient," he said. Other doctors reportedly helped patients to avoid the stiff deductibles that were required when Humana hospitals weren't used. David Jones said that doctors were so suspicious of Humana that they retaliated by claiming incorrectly that admissions were emergencies. Humana conceded that the situation hadn't been handled well. Humana vice president John H. Morse said, "Basically, we did not include doctors in the design of the product. We basically went right to the customer." The company set about soothing fragile physician egos even while corporate controls were being tightened. Before patients were hospitalized, doctors were told to contact a Care Plus representative who would select the appropriate Humana hospital. Doctors who didn't follow this procedure wouldn't be paid for their services.

Despite its continuing losses Humana continued to have high expectations for Care Plus and so did Wall Street analysts. Salomon Brothers advised clients, "Humana, in our view, has the best strategy of vertical integration in the industry." On the strength of such reports, investors bid Humana stock to a new high in the summer of 1987, paying $29 a share for a stock then earning only 2.8 percent. The price-to-earnings ratio of 106 reflected extraordinary confidence in Humana's future.

American Medical International: Back to Basics

American Medical International officials looked at hospitals in the 1950s and perceived profits where less imaginative corporate managers saw merely beds. AMI was a small medical laboratory company based in Beverly Hills, California, when it began buying up West Coast hospitals in 1957. AMI went public in 1960, launching the investor-owned hospital business and transforming the health care industry. With the arrival of Medicare and the California population boom, profits sprinted ahead. A decade later AMI hired Royce Diener, the investment banker who handled its initial public offering, to run the company. Diener had an unusual background for a supermed official. Growing up in Baltimore in the depths of the Depression, he had been taught that money and medicine didn't mix. His father, Louis, was a doctor who was frequently paid for his services with bottles of olive oil, red wine, Italian sausage, and produce. Dr. Diener repeatedly warned Royce that medicine was an unprofitable career. Royce listened and learned. At Harvard University he studied philosophy, which he believed was a practical major because it taught students to focus on problems. Then he went into finance. When he took over AMI in 1973, it was a $150-million-a-year company. Over the next decade he proved his father wrong. Money and medicine could have a strong affinity. Diener oversaw rapid growth that produced a twentyfold increase in revenues. By 1986 AMI was taking in $2.8 billion a year in revenues.

Behind that growth was a corporate strategy that his competitors would adopt and ultimately employ more successfully. "We're not just hospital management," Diener told *The Executive* in 1985. "We're in the field of health care services, and that's not just a difference in semantics. From the time I became CEO we scratched ourselves from the 'bed derby' and became interested only in how many services we could deliver to generate revenues and thereby spread our fixed costs investments." Under Diener's direction AMI developed new products. AMI repackaged hospital services and marketed them to outpatients through its ambulatory clinics. AMI developed free-standing, single-day surgery centers where 750 medical procedures such as cataract lens replacement could be performed. It realized the promotional possibilities in affiliations with prestigious medical schools before other for-profit companies. Touting old-fashioned convenience and service, it staffed mobile vans with doctors who were on call twenty-four hours a day, seven days a week. AMI Doctors House Calls were sent to homes, offices, and hotels, and to ships docked in the Gulf of Mexico.

AMI was one of the first for-profit companies to begin marketing group health insurance through its AMICARE policies. In its announcement of AMI's decision to enter the insurance business in 1984, Diener said, "Doctors have been the gateway to hospitals. Now doctors are being influenced by their patients." AMICARE subscribers who used AMI-approved doctors and AMI facilities would be reimbursed for 90 percent of their costs. If they also used its preadmission and discharge planning services, all their expenses were paid. But AMICARE proved to be ill conceived. Although AMI hospitals were less than half full, with occupancy rates around 42.8 percent, executives were promising Wall Street analysts that AMICARE could reduce hospital services by a minimum of 33 percent. Under those circumstances AMI would be able to open bowling alleys in the empty corridors. At the same time that AMICARE executives were suggesting that one third to one half of hospital services were used inappropriately, its hospital executives were relying on those facilities to produce 92 percent of AMI's profits.

AMICARE was an early sign that despite its initial innovations, AMI was a troubled company. Instead of concentrating on filling its American hospital beds, it expanded internationally with facilities in Saudi Arabia, Spain, Switzerland, Australia, and Scotland. It ignored the thriving business in psychiatric and specialty hospitals until long after other supermeds were gathering in their profits. Analyst Kenneth Abramowitz of Sanford C. Bernstein & Co. said, "The lack of a highly focused, centralized management appears to have stymied the sense of urgency needed for bold, creative action."

In 1985 Deiner stepped down as chief executive officer and Walter Weisman, who had risen to president in his sixteen years with AMI, took over. In a subsequent interview with *Modern Healthcare* Weisman, an avid Los Angeles Dodgers fan, says he is the "kind of guy who sits around and calculates [baseball] averages."[5] Weisman had looked at AMI's figures, too, and knew that the company desperately needed a new strategy to survive. "We are not managing our costs effectively," he admitted. In fact, AMI was partially losing control because it was providing too much care to people who couldn't afford to pay. "Only in hindsight can you get the sense that we weren't conservative enough," said Weisman. He added that patients were having trouble paying bills because of cuts in government programs and insurance benefits. Many AMI facilities were located in Texas, which was in the midst of a severe oil and gas recession. AMI's annual report noted in 1985 that its hospitals were caring for an increasing number of indigent patients. The company was forced to reserve an additional $28 million, a 20 percent increase, in 1986 to cover its expected bad debts.

After his promotion Weisman hefted his machete. The blow fell first on AMICARE, which had lost $25 million in 1986 and was projecting additional losses of $100 million in 1987. "[Group Health Service's] profitability proved illusory," Weisman said in understatement. AMI's Brookside Recovery Centers, eleven alcohol and substance abuse treatment facilities, were sold to Parkside Medical Services Corporation for over $30 million. During the first half of 1986 AMI cut nearly two thousand employees from its management staff. Weisman marked his first anniversary by announcing a far-reaching corporate restructuring. AMI would slash capital spending by $500 million in 1987, eliminate six regional offices, divest unprofitable facilities, and lay off more corporate employees. When the reorganization ended, AMI was back to basics. It kept a few health maintenance organizations, psychiatric centers, and other medical services, representing about 5 percent of revenues, but AMI had refocused its operations on eighty-six acute-care hospitals, primarily in California, Texas, and Florida, and twenty-two overseas facilities.

AMI's reorganization made it a considerably tighter company but also a more vulnerable takeover target. Many Wall Street observers thought that AMI would be the first victim of the supermed winnowing envisioned by Paine Webber's Edward Kerschner. Throughout 1985 and 1986 AMI stock rose or sank as takeover rumors floated through financial markets. Among those said to be interested were Equitable Life Assurance, Universal Health, Aetna Life & Casualty, General Motors, and Bass Brothers Enterprises. Early in 1987 Pesch & Co., a little-known diversified health care firm, offered $1.74 billion in a takeover bid. The Chicago-based company announced it intended to acquire roughly 86.9 million outstanding shares of AMI common stock through its wholly-owned subsidiary Alpha Health Systems. AMI directors said the offer was "seriously inadequate" and rejected Pesch's proposed bid summarily.

Company officials insisted that AMI would refuse other takeover bids, too. Rebecca Kupper, federal-relations director, said, "Any company that would make an offer would just want to reap the benefits of all the hard work we've undertaken. I don't believe that is going to happen."

National Medical Enterprises: Club Supermed

Directly west of downtown Delray Beach, Florida, where the new town-house developments start to disappear into the saw grass, is a snapshot of medicine's past and future.

On one side of a busy highway is the Palm Beach County Community Mental Health Center, slowly fading from modest to shabby. It is housed in a low-slung building with all the architectural distinction of a drab green shoe box. It is set back only a few feet from the asphalt, with few trees or shrubs to soften the sharp cement edges. It could easily be mistaken for a discount tire store. The Community Mental Health Center was a product of noble objectives and the Community Mental Health Act. Starting in the late 1960's, legislation provided federal funds to mental health centers when few private insurance policies covered psychiatric care. With the government subsidies the community centers could offer help on a sliding-fee schedule to patients who needed help but couldn't spend $50 an hour for sessions with psychiatrists. In deference to Congressman Paul Rogers, Democrat of Florida, who helped write the law, Palm Beach County received some of the first funds to become available. The community mental health centers flourished until insurance companies started to increase mental-health benefits and middle-class Americans could afford to be treated by private practitioners. When they fled, the clinics were left with only the poor and uninsured who could pay the least for their treatment.

On the other side of the highway is National Medical Enterprises' lavish $50 million medical campus. It includes Fair Oaks Psychiatric Hospital, which is typical of the boom in specialty hospitals. In fact, NME has set up two subsidiaries, Psychiatric Institutes of America and Recovery Centers of America, to operate psychiatric and substance-abuse hospitals. Almost 20,000 patients spend roughly $246.9 million a year to be treated at its facilities. Fair Oaks Psychiatric Hospital now draws many of the patients who used to be treated at Palm Beach County Community Mental Health Center, and it is scarcely surprising they cross the street. Except for its sign the hospital might be a luxury hotel. The white stucco building is tucked well back from the intersection in the midst of forty tastefully landscaped acres. Its rooms overlook a tranquil lake where underground fountains send jets of water leaping forth and an occasional leaf darts across the surface like a tiny green fish. Nearby, linked together by broad plazas and serpentine roads, are other NME facilities: the 160-bed Delray Community Hospital, a rehabilitation facility; a medical office building; and a $3.2 million, 120-bed nursing home, Hillhaven Convalescent Center. A shopping center houses a pizza parlor, optician, branch bank, and travel agency. Altogether the campus has the flavor of a medical Club Med.

NME is developing these medical campuses throughout the United States. At Los Angeles' University of Southern California NME is building a $100 million center that features a 75-room hotel for outpatients and relatives and a 1,600-space parking garage. At Tucson's Villa Campana, NME designed a medical Club Med for the elderly with specially equipped retirement apartments; a skilled-nursing facility; and home care services. The campus is next to a large community hospital and several medical office buildings. By combining services and locating facilities together, NME is hoping for automatic referrals. At Delray Community Hospital, for instance, approximately 80 percent of the patients are elderly; many could be discharged directly to the Hillhaven Convalescent Center next door. NME chairman Richard Eamer said, "We have enormous potential to bring about closer integration between our several lines of business, and we will exploit this to the maximum. The most obvious benefit is a greater number of patient referrals from one facility to another. Our medical campus developments are an expression [of this]."

NME's strategy is succeeding. Although the company is not the largest supermed, it is clearly the most diversified. Perhaps it has done so well because the company's founder knew why some hospitals succeeded and others failed. In the 1960s Eamer was a young California lawyer and public accountant whose clients included a large number of ailing nonprofit hospitals. He became absorbed by hospital finance and the bottom-line difference between efficiently run and poorly managed hospitals. When Eamer believed that he knew enough to succeed in the hospital business, he recruited a law school classmate, John C. Bedrosian, and a law partner, Leonard Cohen, and formed National Medical Enterprises in 1969. The three founders still run the company. Unlike some supermed officials, Eamer cultivates a homespun, "aw, shucks" style. NME has made Eamer—and his original partners—wealthy men, but despite a keen fascination with racehorses, he would never be considered flamboyant. He resides in the same house in suburban Los Angeles where he has lived for the past twenty years.

Eamer's low-key approach has served NME well. NME outmaneuvered Humana to buy New Orleans-based Westbank Medical Center Ltd. because its executives didn't feel comfortable with Humana's hard-chargers. Wall Street analyst Michael LeConey explained, "Humana pulled out all the stops but Westbank felt more comfortable with the 'just plain folks' of NME." Eamer's outward diffidence masks an incisive intellect, however. Long before his competitors, Eamer saw that hospital costs needed to be trimmed and instituted tough personnel cuts. NME's hospitals reduced the number of registered nurses on staff from 40 to 25 percent of the work force. Even more important, Eamer recognized that companies like NME couldn't survive on hospital beds alone. NME was the first hospital company to begin restructuring. It moved into the right markets at the right time through a series of strategic acquisitions at reasonable prices. Over the years NME bought out Rehab Hospital Services Corporation, the nation's largest provider of rehabilitative services, and Hillhaven Convalescent Centers, the second-largest nursing home chain with 323 facilities and nearly 40,000 beds. It started up Recovery Centers of America, specializing in drug and alcohol treatment, and National Medical Homecare and CuraCare to supply a variety of services to hospitals and patients. The strategy has paid off. NME has steadily reduced its reliance on its acute care facilities. These hospitals contributed only about half its earnings in 1987, down from 58 percent in 1985. Its psychiatric and rehabilitation facilities supplied approximately one third of earnings in 1987, up dramatically from 12.6 percent in 1985. Nursing homes, health products, and services make up the remainder.

But NME has its share of problems, too. It has been accused of bribing officials in New Mexico, trading campaign contributions for political favors, to expand its operations in the state. NME is a codefendant in a $50 million lawsuit that has been brought by nonprofit Memorial General Hospital, the only facility in Las Cruces. The other defendants include state officials, several state agencies, and the former chairman of the state's Democratic Party. According to documents filed in U.S. District Court by Memorial General, NME allegedly contributed $18,750 to New Mexico Democrats to gain approval to construct a $28.3 million hospital in Las Cruces in violation of the state health plan. The proposed 145-bed hospital would compete directly with Memorial General.

The court documents purport to trace a pattern of contacts between NME executives and party officials, including Governor Toney Anaya, over an eighteen-month period. National Medical Enterprises allegedly began its contributions to state politicians on June 16, 1982, when it donated $3,000 to Anaya's election campaign. The next day, June 17, Michael R. Farien, NME's vice president for legislative and regulatory affairs, wrote a letter to Anaya requesting a meeting where he and senior vice president Steve Dominguez could discuss expansion in the state. NME also gave $2,000 to a fundraising dinner for Santa Fe mayor Louis Montano, who supported NME's efforts to acquire the city's St. Vincent Hospital. An internal NME memorandum stated, "New Mexico is an intensely political state. HCA has attempted to acquire St. Vincent and failed due to lack of political support and inside information sources." NME submitted its application to build the Las Cruces facility in 1983. On December 1 the application was still pending when Dominguez sent a memo to John Bedrosian, recommending that the company contribute $5,000 to the Democratic Presidential Campaign Committee. Dominguez wrote, "If we can gain the inside track on these two projects [Las Cruces and St. Vincent], the cost savings would be tremendous." On December 20 NME gave $2,500 to the Democratic Party of New Mexico. In a memo to Bedrosian from Patti Archuletta, assistant director for government relations, the check was called "an investment in the Las Cruces project."

Despite the "investments," the project was turned down in January 1984. State planners said the facility would create a surplus of hospital beds and violate the state health plan. NME continued to make political donations, however. It donated $10,000 to a Democratic Party fundraiser in June 1984. One month later the state reversed itself and approved NME's application. NME would get its Las Cruces hospital—and the lawsuit. In a court brief NME asserted that the suit was without legal standing. "Neither the Constitution nor the federal statutes and regulations implicated by the Section 1122 process [Medicare and Medicaid reimbursement for capital costs] recognizes Memorial's interest in being free from competition," the brief read. Moreover, Bedrosian told the press, "Our lawyers have investigated and say we're clean." The suit is still pending.[6]

Hospital Corporation of America: The One to Beat

Thomas F. Frist, Jr., president and chief executive officer of Hospital Corporation of America, is an avid private pilot, frequently seizing controls of the corporate jet during shopping trips around the United States. In the late 1960s, according to corporate lore, when the lean and lanky Frist spied a promising-looking hospital, he would settle the plane down in a nearby cornfield and buy it. The legend may or may not be true, but it does reflect HCA's acquiring style. Frist created the world's largest supermed by buying just about everything he saw. Given the corporation's background, perhaps that's understandable. Frist, a surgeon, founded HCA with his father, Thomas, Sr., and Jack Massey, the financial genius behind the Kentucky Fried Chicken chain. Massey saw in medicine the same entrepreneurial opportunities that he once spied in chicken legs. If the Kentucky colonel could sell fried chicken, Massey reasoned, then Nashville-based HCA could sell health care.

HCA illustrates the rapacious growth that has marked the hospital chains. It is big, rich, diverse, and extremely hungry. It is the largest and most regionally diversified supermed. By 1970 HCA, already the country's largest for-profit chain, owned or managed 367 facilities throughout the United States with a daily patient population of 7.5 million and 40,000 physicians on staff. Although some corporations might have paused and consolidated, HCA kept on growing. By 1987 HCA owned or managed 477 hospitals with over 40,000 beds in 390 communities in the United States and abroad. During those years Frist also ventured into different types of hospitals. He bought 40 specialized psychiatric hospitals with over 5,000 beds and an expanding network of research and teaching facilities. When hospital occupancy rates declined in the mid-1980s, HCA announced that it was revising its previously announced expansion. But HCA meant only that it would expand at a declining rate. Its scaled-down expansion would have represented substantial growth for many major corporations. HCA said that it would chop the $1.4 billion, originally budgeted for expansion in 1986, to $700 million and then to $400 or $500 million in 1987. HCA expected to own or manage 80,000 hospital beds by the 1990s.

By the mid-1980s, however, Frist was becoming increasingly selective about the hospitals that bore the HCA name. It bought fewer facilities in the medium-sized communities, once so eagerly sought after, that fueled its early growth. Humana had its heart research; now HCA was searching for renown and found it could be bought. In a major corporate coup HCA convinced five teaching hospitals affiliated with medical schools and research centers to become its affiliates. The medical schools included the University of Kansas, the University of Miami, the University of Florida, Vanderbilt University, and the University of Mississippi. Typical of these new partnerships was the arrangement between HCA and the nonprofit Scripps Clinic in LaJolla, California. After extensive discussions the Scripps Clinic leased its Green Hospital to HCA and became one of its major worldwide referral centers for its sickest patients. The arrangement was extremely lucrative in terms of profits and prestige. The Scripps Clinic is an internationally known medical research center that attracts 400,000 patients a year. Its 158-bed Green Hospital is almost always filled to capacity. It is the acute care and major surgery center for the clinic, its research institute, 14 regional clinics, and the 300 physicians who comprise the Scripps Clinic Medical Group. Although hospital occupancy rates are dropping, the number of operations has been doubling annually at Green Hospital. HCA was so impressed by its partnership with the Scripps Clinic that it devoted two pages to it in its 1984 annual report.

HCA could be discriminating because, like other supermeds, it was diversifying. HCA was one of the first hospital chains to have aspirations beyond a network of hospitals. HCA wanted to create a total health care system. HCA would be to the health care business what General Motors is to the automobile industry. In corporate lingo this is called vertical integration. General Motors does more than manufacture cars. It also produces and supplies their parts, controls the outlets that sell and repair them, and finances their purchase. HCA would consolidate a variety of medical services capable of supplying birth-to-grave health care under its corporate logo and market them to the public.

To launch this new strategy, HCA created two new subsidiaries in 1984. HCA Capital Corporation pursued investments in the high-tech health care industry. During its first year HCA Capital invested over $10 million in a diverse group of companies that were developing filmless X-ray systems, fiberoptic sensing systems for testing body chemicals, and equipment to extend the life of medical electronic components. By investing early, HCA believed that it might steal an advantage from its competitors. Meanwhile, HCA's Business Development Group began running a variety of hospital-related businesses, including clinical laboratories in Chattanooga, San Diego, and Salt Lake City; ambulance companies in New Orleans, Spokane, Tacoma, and Seattle; and TransMed home health care services in Houston, Long Beach, and three Tennessee cities.

HCA went on a buying spree in 1984 and 1985 that was unmatched in the health care industry. It spent $20.4 million to buy a 26.7 percent interest in Scientific Leasing, Inc., a Farmington, Connecticut, company that rents medical equipment. It acquired a major share of Beverly Enterprises, a nursing home chain, which was later sold. Then it bought outright Johnson & Johnson's home health care business; Hill-Richards & Co., an insurance claims processing firm that handles over 300,000 claims a year; and E. F. Hutton Life Insurance Company's marketing rights in thirty-four states. And finally, within the span of a few months, HCA acquired:

- The 760-bed Wesley Medical Center in Wichita, Kansas, which would become the largest hospital in the HCA chain, for $265 million; and the 407-bed Presbyterian Hospital in Oklahoma City, Oklahoma, for more than $100 million.
- An 80 percent interest in the 235-bed Lovelace Medical Center in Albuquerque, New Mexico, a major teaching facility for the University of New Mexico Medical School, and its 5 affiliated clinics for $63 million. Along with the medical center came 5 walk-in Urgent Care Centers, a 50,000-member health maintenance organization, and the group practice of 126 physicians.
- New Century Life, licensed to sell insurance in 35 states, for $7 million. Through its purchase HCA would be able to market traditional indemnity as well as prepaid health insurance.
- Forum Group, a chain of 9 psychiatric and 5 general hospitals, for an undisclosed amount.
- Three health maintenance organizations—Los Angeles-based Healthgroup International for $24 million; United Medical Plan, operating in Houston and Richmond, Virginia, for $24 million;

and Health Care Plus, Inc., with 59,000 members throughout Kansas and Oklahoma City, for an undisclosed amount.

With its HMO acquisitions HCA struck out in a new direction. It had operated a 675,000-member HMO in Brazil for years; now it was bravely entering a United States insurance market that was rapidly becoming overcrowded. It started up PriMed, similar to AMI's AMICARE, which offered substantial discounts to policyholders who used HCA hospitals and affiliated doctors. During the first 12 months HCA enrolled 500,000 subscribers, including all 65,000 employees of the Winn-Dixie Food Corporation. It asked 34 states for permission to market health insurance policies. It expanded its prepaid plans to a dozen markets, signed up 650,000 enrollees, and was approaching $100 million to $120 million a year in revenues. HCA said it expected to write 1 million insurance policies by 1990. Fourteen months later its strategy was switched abruptly. Instead of forging ahead on its own, HCA formed a joint venture, called Equicor, with The Equitable Life Assurance Society of the United States, the nation's third-largest life insurance company, in 1986. Stock market analysts were dubious about Equicor. HCA was new to the health insurance business, and while Equitable was experienced, it was more with failure than success. Randall Kuyser, a health care analyst with San Francisco's Montgomery Securities, observed, "It's hard to turn an elephant on a dime. Equitable is so large and it's been so unprofitable in the health care business that HCA's going to have its work cut out." But there was promise, too. Equitable brought 15 million policyholders to Equicor, and if even a small fraction could be induced to stay at HCA hospitals, they could fill a large number of vacant beds.

HCA was hoping that in the future it would have far fewer beds to fill. In 1987 Frist announced that HCA would sell about 100 hospitals, worth approximately $1.5 billion to $1.8 billion, to a new employee-owned company to be headed by a top HCA official. HCA would maintain a 20 percent ownership in the new company. It would keep 80 of its largest hospitals and some 50 psychiatric centers with a high growth potential. The spin-off was a radical effort to trim the $4.9 billion company and boost earnings. Frist said that the sale proceeds would be used to buy back stock and reduce its $3 billion debt. It was a dramatic move, but it immediately won Wall Street's version of a standing ovation. HCA stock hit a new 52-week high.

CHAPTER THREE

•

The Rise of the Supermeds

THE SUPERMEDS owe a sweeping debt of gratitude to the federal government; without its generosity the health care industry would not exist. The federal government has magnified their profits and subsidized their expansion. It has promoted a health care system driven by profit and increasingly dominated by large corporations. By underwriting the supermeds' growth, the federal government is reversing a half century of effort by the medical profession to banish for-profit enterprises from health care. And in doing so the federal government is helping to diminish the medical profession's power over health care.

It happened this way. As the twentieth century began, medicine was a tightly controlled cartel. The medical elite derived their power from their ability to grant staff privileges at their not-for-profit hospitals. By closely guarding their sole right to admit patients, they managed to monopolize medicine and all but eliminate competition. Only 2 percent of the doctors in the United States were able to admit patients to the nation's hospitals. Unable to hospitalize their patients, new medical school graduates found themselves effectively barred from the practice of medicine. In desperation, physicians began to establish their own hospitals. Unable to attract the endowments that supported the elite eastern hospitals, the doctors organized for-profit hospitals across the nation. Although many were poorly financed, they flourished in the South and West, where a growing population needed medical care but couldn't summon the private financial resources to create nonprofit hospitals.

Doctors had another motive to go into the hospital business. Research breakthroughs, particularly in surgical techniques, were pushing medical knowledge forward. For the first time doctors could do more than hold the hands of the dying. They could actually cure some patients. In addition, medical progress raised the prospect of profiting from treating the ill. Surgeons set up freestanding clinics catering to the rich and middle class who could afford their services. By 1910 about 56 percent of the nation's hospitals were for-profit enterprises.

Doctors didn't think it unusual to operate profit-making hospitals since many were educated in for-profit medical schools. These commercial schools, independent of universities and teaching hospitals, were common in the late nineteenth and early twentieth centuries. Their standards were slack; many students lacked even a high-school diploma. The doctors-to-be pursued a quixotic study schedule. They received no clinical training during their two-year program. Some never felt a pulsebeat until they examined their first paying patient. The major criterion for admission was the ability to pay the tuition; the major requirement for graduation was that the tuition had been paid. The publication of the revolutionary Flexner Report in 1910 changed all that. Abraham Flexner was a young educator who undertook an investigation of the commercial medical schools at the behest of the American Medical Association. Flexner was bitingly critical of the schools. Not surprisingly, since it condemned the competition, the university-based medical establishment rushed to embrace his report. Harvard University president Charles Eliot wrote, "So long as medical schools are conducted as private ventures for the benefit of a few physicians and surgeons who have united to form a corporation or a faculty, the community ought not to support them."

In truth, there was little difference in the quality of education between the commercial and university medical schools, but by inflicting such stinging criticism on the for-profit institutions, Flexner focused public attention on their deficiencies. They never recovered. With the exception of Philadelphia's Jefferson Medical College, the commercial schools slowly went bankrupt or merged with the university medical colleges. Flexner's report defined the medical power structure for the next sixty years and solidified the authority of the academic medical establishment. Through their control of medical school admissions, these doctors became a self-perpetuating elite.

As the Flexner Report banished for-profit medical schools, proprietary hospitals also began to disappear. By 1928 only 36 percent of the nation's hospitals were for-profit, down 20 percent from their peak in 1910. Their numbers continued to decline steadily, dropping to 27 percent in 1938 and 18 percent in 1946. For-profit hospitals controlled 6 percent of all hospital beds in 1934 but only 2.8 percent in 1944. Shunning conspicuous commercialism, doctors retreated from entrepreneurship, claiming that medicine wasn't a business but a service. They considered themselves free to earn substantial sums just as long as they didn't make a profit.[1]

The retreat from for-profit medicine lasted until the Great Depression. With an economy in collapse, many Americans could no longer afford medical care. Private enterprise found a solution: medical insurance. It was a life support system to hospitals that couldn't collect payment from bankrupt patients. Private insurance guaranteed that the middle class could afford to be hospitalized. As hospital revenues plummeted, insurance brought in new patients. Blue Cross, the first hospital insurance plan, was founded in 1929 when Baylor University Hospital agreed to provide 1,500 Dallas schoolteachers up to 21 days of care for a premium of $0.50 a month.

Health insurance found a ready market in the middle class. Only 12 million Americans had hospital insurance in 1940, but in the next decade coverage expanded to 76 million. Over 123 million Americans were insured in 1960 and 188 million by 1980. Insured families no longer worried that they would be devastated financially by an unexpected illness. Health insurance was paying a rising share of their medical bills. In 1950 Americans paid an average of 66 percent of their medical bills personally while insurance paid 9 percent. During the next decade, as two thirds of all families bought coverage, insurance paid more of the total. Americans were paying 52 percent, barely half of their health costs, and insurance was covering 24 percent in 1965. Insurance coverage and benefits reached an all-time high in the early 1980s, when Americans were reimbursed for one third of their medical expenses.

Along with the growth in health insurance came a rapid expansion of the medical system. After World War II the U.S. government turned its attention to neglected domestic needs, including health care. In 1946 members of Congress, always eager to speed the flow of federal funds to their districts, passed the Hill-Burton Act. Named after its chief Senate sponsors, Lister Hill and Harold H. Burton, the legislation launched one of the most ambitious construction programs ever undertaken by the federal government. Initially it provided $3 million for planning and $75 million a year for five years to aid hospital construction. With this federal stimulus new hospitals began to dot the landscape. During the next 30 years over $5.9 billion were spent to construct an estimated 350,000 hospital beds. Almost one third of the United States' community hospitals were financed through Hill-Burton funds.

Despite a building boom and growing competition, health insurance enabled these hospitals to attract enough new patients. Insurance companies were willing to pay far more to hospitalize seriously ill patients than they were to cover the costs of preventive care to keep them well. Thus insurance companies steadily expanded the hospital market. In the process they furthered the institutionalization of medical care and the rise of the hospital industry. Between 1950 and 1970 the number of health care workers more than tripled, from 1.2 to 3.9 million, while health care spending leaped from $4 billion in 1950 to $425 billion in 1985.*

The health care system seemed to be working well. Insurance companies kept selling policies. Hospitals filled their beds. Doctors hospitalized their patients gladly, since insurance companies frequently paid more for their services when they were rendered in hospitals than in their offices. Aside from their monthly insurance premium, middle-class consumers paid relatively little for their health care.

In the 1950s the middle class continued to be the primary beneficiaries of this explosive growth. Most of the Hill-Burton hos-

*By contrast, the United States spent a grand total of $289 billion for its national defense in 1985.

pitals were located in their neighborhoods, and health insurance enabled them to purchase better health care than ever before. But while the middle class was enjoying a rising standard of medical care, the poor and elderly were still priced out of the health system. Very little changed for them until the 1960s.

When President Lyndon Johnson was elected in 1964, he thrust the prestige of his office behind passage of a health care program for the elderly. In his initial State of the Union speech Johnson announced that he would follow through on President John F. Kennedy's promise to enact Medicare. It was given the highest priority among the Great Society programs. "We are going to fight for medical care for the aged as long as we have breath in our bodies," he proclaimed. Johnson succeeded, but at a price. To win passage, he ceded control of Medicare to the hospital industry. He agreed to "cost plus" reimbursement: The federal government would pay whatever hospitals wanted to charge to treat the elderly. Under this system hospitals would set their own fees and the federal government would reimburse their costs and tack on a profit. Insurance companies were given the task of paying and auditing the hospitals, and the hospitals would pick their auditors.

Joseph Califano, Jr., one of Johnson's top advisers, recalls sitting in the president's small hideaway office in the Old Executive Office Building with Larry O'Brien and Wilbur Cohen, who were lobbying members of Congress on behalf of the bill. Cohen told Johnson, "It'll cost a half billion dollars to make the changes in reimbursement standards to get the bill out of the Senate Finance Committee." Johnson waved a hand dismissively. "Five hundred million. Is that all?" he exclaimed. "Do it. Move that damn bill out now, before we lose it."[2]

Cohen was wrong. Five hundred million proved to be a drastic understatement. Medicare would cost far, far more. By 1967, Medicare had already cost the government $4.5 billion. By 1988 the federal government was spending a total of $90 billion a year on Medicare, with $58 billion going toward hospital care and the remainder to doctors. But even if the true cost had been known, Johnson probably would not have resisted, he was so intent on Medicare's passage. Medicare was passed through Congress with a second program tacked on—Medicaid, which set up a joint federal-state program to pay for the medical care of the poor under the age of sixty-five.

Hospitals that had been born under the Hill-Burton program and nurtured into adolescence by private health insurance reached their maturity under Medicare. While health insurance gave rise to the hospital industry, Medicare would create corporate empires. It would be to the supermeds what tobacco price supports were to North Carolina farmers—a never-ending source of sustenance. David Williamson, vice president of Hospital Corporation of America, said, "Prior to the start of Medicare and Medicaid programs in the mid-1960s, we were like a 'tin cup' industry. Many hospitals actually were sort of 'hand to mouth' operations, trying to find enough revenues to be able to meet expenses. I remember in the period eight to ten years before Medicare, we were receiving about $16 a day for patients sent to us by the local welfare department, which usually ran out of funds in January and our fiscal year started in July. It was really an underfinanced industry as far as operations were concerned. But credit must be given to Medicare and Medicaid for permitting a floor to be established for operational funding of hospitals."[3]

After Medicare was enacted, bureaucrats at the Department of Health, Education, and Welfare took over, and for-profit hospitals wrung further concessions. As the bureaucrats wrote the regulations that would determine Medicare's day-to-day operations, the definition of cost underwent a geometric expansion. The new regulations enabled for-profit hospitals to charge the federal government for a wide variety of expenses. They could fold in interest on loans for constructing new facilities or expanding existing ones. They could charge off the depreciation on their buildings and equipment. And they could ensure that a return on equity would be paid to their investors. Many of these costs were only tangentially related to the care of the elderly. Medicare would end up paying not just for coronary care units but also for nurseries for the newborn. Then, after all these expenses were calculated, hospitals were given a 2 percent bonus for treating Medicare patients. Califano said, "In fact, the two percent was a bribe to get the hospital industry to cooperate with Medicare. With this final windfall, the American Hospital Association promptly passed a resolution calling on all members to support Medicare."

Even more amazing, Medicare reserved a special bonus for for-profit hospitals. They were provided a return on equity that was set at one and a half times the interest on government securities. In effect, these hospitals were promised that their shareholders' investments would be protected. Under this regulation Medicare reimbursements became corporate bonuses from the federal government to corporate shareholders. By 1985 the federal government was paying $200 million a year to for-profit hospitals in return on stockholders' capital. The payments represented 38 percent of the hospitals' annual profits on patient care, according to the Department of Health and Human Services. Its inspector general, Richard Kusserow, said that supermeds were reaping "windfall profits" from the federal government's largess.[4]

Moreover, these payments were essential to the for-profits' growth. They needed funds to expand, and Medicare was a ready underwriter. Through the federal government's return on equity payments, the hospital chains were able to tap into the corporate bond market for long-term financing. In this respect, Williamson said Medicare was "a second Hill-Burton program." As he explained, "Investor-owned hospitals demonstrated that investors could be protected and could expect to receive a reasonable return on their investment. The investor-owned hospitals showed that they could make a reasonable return on investment and they could accumulate capital by going to the financial markets and not be dependent on government or philanthropy." In fact, the federal government was helping to demonstrate that a "reasonable return" was possible.

The supermed era was beginning. The for-profit hospitals owned by local doctors rapidly came to resemble the mom-and-pop grocery stores of the past. Just as supermarket chains bought out those stores, so hospital corporations began to absorb independent hospitals. The hospital corporations expanded into nationwide chains with the federal government's assurance that Medicare would help to pay their acquisition costs, secure their credit lines, and guarantee new investors a return. Corporate empires were being built with taxpayer dollars. In the mid-1980s, for example, taxpayers were being charged $2.9 billion a year by the for-profits, about 7 percent of the entire Medicare budget, in depreciation write-offs, interest payments on loans, and hospital leases. As the supermeds bought and sold, merged and acquired, taxpayers were financing the consolidation of the health care industry. Medicare was an invitation for the supermeds to loot the federal treasury legally; unsurprisingly, they accepted.

The bills can be exorbitant. In a major supermed acquisition, Hospital Corporation of America spent $650 million to buy fifty-four hospitals plus eighteen nursing homes and medical office buildings from Health Affiliates International in the early 1980s. Afterward Medicare spent so much in additional costs that the U.S. General Accounting Office launched an investigation. To finance its purchase HCA borrowed heavily. As a result Medicare was forced to spend an extra $62.5 million, a 300 percent increase in interest payments. In addition, depreciation costs rose rapidly on the newly acquired hospitals. HCA did nothing to improve the properties immediately after the acquisition. The facilities weren't upgraded; the properties remained substantially the same under HCA ownership. But through a totally legal accounting sleight of hand, HCA could claim that they were worth more and collect an additional $8.4 million a year, nearly a 90 percent increase in depreciation. Capital costs rose $70.9 million at the acquired hospitals during the first year although HCA lowered corporate overhead by $15.7 million. In the final bill taxpayers were charged an extra $55.2 million for those expenses alone. To put that figure into perspective, if the federal government had spent those $55.2 million differently—reimbursing consumers for their health care costs, for example—some fifty-five thousand Americans would have received free medical care that year.

The federal government did not question the legality of HCA's action, but it questioned if its action was appropriate and if HCA was taking advantage of a loophole in the law to raise prices to its corporate advantage and the detriment of the Medicare program. After the acquisition, HCA inflated the prices of existing services at its new hospitals. Calculating the Medicare billings at just two hospitals, the federal government found taxpayers spent $600,000 more so that HCA could render the same medical treatment to the elderly after the buy-out. For all fifty-four hospitals the additional charges could be as high as $16.2 million a year.[5]

When supermeds buy individual hospitals, the charges can also be staggering, according to the U.S. General Accounting Office. In Newnan, Georgia, a small town southwest of Atlanta, the public hospital was failing when Humana, Inc., began an aggressive pursuit. The hospital had only 144 beds; still, in a city of only 11,000, it could keep less than half filled. Moreover, many patients who came to Newnan Hospital didn't pay their bills. Hospital trustees watched losses approach $1 million a year. In the year before the hospital was sold, the situation worsened. Confronting the grim balance sheets, the trustees wrote off 6 percent of their unpaid accounts, nearly $500,000, as bad debts that would never be collected. Another $1.7 million in outstanding bills, representing 21 percent of their total revenues, also appeared uncollectible. Humana kept Newnan, now rechristened Humana-Newnan, open, but the taxpayers paid a steep price. The trustees valued the hospital's assets at $7.4 million at the time of the sale. Over the next nine months Humana, Inc., recalculated the assets at $12.3 million. As a result of the reappraisal alone Humana was permitted to increase its Medicare charges for capital costs by 43 percent, or an extra $68.34 per patient. Humana raised other Medicare charges, too. Administrative costs exploded. As a publicly owned hospital, Newnan spent $226.03 per patient for administrative costs. Humana, however, raised administrative costs to $744.77 per patient, a 229 percent increase. On top of those charges taxpayers were required to bolster Humana's profits. These return-on-equity payments amounted to $355.15 per patient.

The U.S. General Accounting Office found that the supermeds didn't have to buy out hospitals to take advantage of the federal government's benevolence. They are entitled to subsidies when they merely rent facilities. Hospital Corporation of America, for instance, decided to lease rather than buy East Pointe Hospital, an eighty-eight-bed nonprofit facility in Lehigh Acres, Florida. When HCA spotted the tiny hospital, only 68 percent of the beds were occupied regularly but the lack of patients was scarcely surprising. East Pointe Hospital was located on the edge of the Caloosahatchee National Wildlife Refuge, twenty miles inland from the nearest town, Fort Myers, which was hardly a major population center. Lehigh Acres had a history of unpaid bills and mounting bad debts. Yet HCA agreed to pay over $1 million to lease the facility for thirty months. Without Medicare subsidies the lease would have been a reckless decision. After HCA signed the lease, Medicare was charged $36,000 a month, nearly half the total payment, for rent. HCA was receiving $409 a month per bed, occupied or not, from Medicare. And half the time only fifty-nine beds were filled. HCA was making money even when East Pointe Hospital had no patients. Under HCA's new management, moreover, Medicare subsidies weren't limited to the lease payments. Medicare paid an extra $184.12 per patient, a 138 percent increase, to cover capital costs. Moreover, Medicare was billed an additional $112.28 per patient, a 28 percent increase, to cover administrative costs. And finally, Medicare began paying a profit margin of $151 per patient. Despite its unlikely location, with the help of Medicare's support East Pointe Hospital proved to be a lucrative investment. The Department of Health and Human Services discovered in 1986 that East Pointe was the most profitable hospital in the state of Florida. On Medicare revenues of $6.6 million it earned $2.5 million, a profit margin of over 37 percent. Its return on equity was nearly 41 percent. HCA had chosen well; only the taxpayers lost.

The U.S. General Accounting Office reported that Humana-Newnan and East Pointe Hospital were typical examples of the high cost of for-profit growth. After studying forty such acquisitions, the GAO concluded hospital acquisitions produced "significant increases" in hospitals' capital costs, administrative expenses, and profit subsidies under the Medicare program. Capital costs, including interest, depreciation, and lease payments, jumped an average of $87.32, or 109 percent, per discharge, while administrative costs rose an average of $132.69, or 86 percent, per discharge. New return-on-equity payments added $101 per discharge.[6]

Hospitals dearly loved the cost-plus system of Medicare reimbursement. There was no incentive to hold down expenses; restraints were totally lacking. Instead, hospitals were encouraged to spend as much as possible as quickly as possible. To make money and keep Medicare funds flowing, they needed only to keep supplying services, running more tests, and adding procedures. As a result, costs exploded. Between 1966 and 1982 Medicare hospital payments grew 20 percent a year, according to the U.S. House Subcommittee on Health. Hospitals were deriving 50 percent of their revenues from Medicare by the mid-1980s. Hospital charges reflected the irresistible urge to provide endless service. In a typical example, Doris Young of Hudson, Florida, complained to Congress about her bill from Bayonet Point Regional Medical Center, a Hospital Corporation of America facility. In 1983 her husband, Norman, was admitted to the hospital one day at 5:45 P.M. and died at 8:45 P.M. the next day after emergency surgery for a stomach aneurysm. The bill contained an itemized charge for twenty-six pints of blood. "I cannot fathom administering that many pints of blood in about seven or eight hours," she wrote Congressman Michael Bilirakis. Still, the transfusions were just one charge that stood out on a total bill of $12,553.70. Mrs. Young said, "I feel the hospital staff did everything possible for him, and I was told there was no chance of him pulling through, but I can't quite imagine how his care could possibly have amounted to $12,553.70 for twenty-seven hours. Incidentally, this does not cover the surgeons' fees, for which I have not yet been billed."

Hospitals were Medicare's major beneficiaries. While hospitals were enriched, the elderly were spending as much as ever for health care. Before Medicare's passage the elderly were paying 20 percent of their total income for health care. Twenty years later the same percentage of their income was still being spent on medical expenses. The promise of Medicare, while unexpectedly blossoming for the supermeds, was unfulfilled for the elderly.

The hospitals were draining Medicare, and the impact of the costs didn't escape notice. As far back as 1975 Medicare trustees were warning that the Hospital Insurance Trust Fund, which pays for beneficiaries' hospital care, would be exhausted by 1990. Congress, however, chose to ignore the crisis just over the horizon. Irwin Wolkstein, a former Social Security official, suggests, "Politicians' slowness to act to correct the trust fund imbalance since the early 1970s probably reflects their political commitment to the elderly and need to postpone, as long as possible, any bad news for this constituency."[7] It took another seven years before Congress confronted the financing crisis.

While Congress dallied, the state of New Jersey was passing legislation that would start a revolution. In 1978 the legislature realized New Jersey hospitals were in serious trouble. Costs were skyrocketing throughout the state; yet inner-city hospitals were unable to pay their bills. The legislature decided to jettison cost-plus reimbursement and institute a new prospective payment plan for New Jersey hospitals. After the system was adopted, hospitals could no longer calculate their bills after delivering services and expect the state to reimburse their costs fully. Instead, under prospective payment, they would know in advance precisely what the state was willing to pay. To calculate the payments, New Jersey used a standard of measurement worked out by Yale University professor Robert Fetter. Fetter had broken down admissions at Yale-New Haven Hospital into 468 separate categories of illnesses known as diagnosis-related groups or DRGs. In New Jersey the DRGs were used to establish reimbursement schedules. Once a patient was diagnosed, the hospital could consult the DRG schedule to find the flat rate for that admission. The DRG rates were based on the standard cost of medical treatment. By averaging the costs, New Jersey introduced enterprise into hospital management. If a hospital treated a patient for less than the DRG schedule allowed, it could keep the savings, but if it spent more, the hospital would have to absorb the extra cost. With prospective payment New Jersey hospitals were put on a fixed budget that paid more for doing less.

New Jersey was still testing DRG schedules in its hospitals when a liberal Democrat pounced on prospective payment in 1983. Congressman Andrew Jacobs, Democrat of Indiana, tacked the sweeping measure onto a desperately needed Social Security financing reform bill. Jacobs said, "Health care was being financed like defense procurement, cost-plus and no sense that it mattered what the final bill came to. Something had to be done to encourage free-market thinking." Prospective payment sped through the House and Senate with virtually no debate in committee or on the floor. Few members were aware that they were voting for a total overhaul of Medicare. Although studies had yet to prove that New Jersey's experiment actually saved money, it now became the basis for Medicare's prospective payment system. The federal government adopted the same DRG categories and flat rates. Hospitals could expect to be paid $2,790 for a heart attack victim, for example, whether the patient was released quickly or stayed far longer than the national average of 7.6 days. Nationally, hospitals were now given the same incentive to reduce services that they already had in New Jersey.

The for-profit hospital industry had lobbied for prospective payment from the start. As Humana founder David A. Jones predicted, "Our profits on that business [Medicare patients] will be double or triple our present level." Under the new system there were winners and losers, and the supermeds were clearly among the winners. The DRG system left unchanged the industry's most cherished policies—the interest and depreciation write-offs, the profit subsidies—and skewed the new payment formula to the for-profits. The supermeds, for example, were favored by flat rates that calculated labor costs on a national, rather than regional, basis. Supermeds tend to have lower wage costs because they avoid union strongholds and concentrate in the South and West. After the national wage rates were phased in, supermed hospitals reaped an estimated $1 billion extra from Medicare. More important, while the prospective payment system appeared to clamp down on a profligate hospital industry, hospitals were in fact being encouraged to profit from Medicare patients. The supermeds believed they had the expertise to minimize costs and maximize profits under prospective payments. Jones prophesied that prospective payment would produce "the most exciting year in our short history." He was right.[8]

More investors began discovering the enormous profit potential in the hospital industry in the late 1970s and early 1980s. By the early 1980s the prices of hospital chains were up. Their profits were growing 10 to 15 percent a year while their per-share earnings were expanding 30 to 50 percent a year. In 1982 Standard & Poor's index of hospital management stocks zoomed 68 percent, making the otherwise healthy 14.8 percent rise in the Standard & Poor's index of 500 industrials appear anemic by comparison. Supermeds were the darlings of Wall Street. To take two examples, *Forbes* found that Humana returned a 34.2 percent profit to its investors in 1983. A share of Humana stock bought for $4.00 in 1974 was worth $403.20 by 1984.[9] American Medical International investors also profited handsomely, with a 22.4 percent return in 1983 while per-share earnings averaged a 28.6 percent growth rate in the preceding five years. In 1983 supermeds earned $6.5 billion or 5.1 percent on revenues. Even better times lay ahead, however. When Medicare switched to prospective payment, profits soared to an all-time high of 6.2 percent, $8.3 billion after expenses. Compared to the 2 percent and 4 percent annual profits earned in the 1970s, the increase was astounding. Humana reported a 10.4 percent profit, while Hospital Corporation of America earned 8.2 percent. Under the federal government's prodding to hold down costs, hospital profits surpassed that of many industries. In contrast, the airline, automobile, and retailing industries reported profits ranging from 2.2 to 5.8 percent.

The Reagan Administration wasn't surprised to see the hospital industry booming as never before under the new reimbursement system. Henry Desmaris, a Medicare official, told the House Select Committee on Aging, "The system ensures greater predictability of revenue for the hospital. All evidence would indicate that hospitals are doing very well under [the prospective payment system]." In describing the benefits flowing to hospitals under PPs, Desmaris sounded remarkably like David Williamson when he explained the advantages of passage of Medicare—more certainty, more federal largess.

Prospective payment was a bonanza to the hospital industry. In Florida, where 60 percent of all hospital patients are over sixty-five years old, the impact was immediately obvious. According to the Florida Hospital Cost Containment Board, hospitals reported profit margins that averaged 11.8 percent, three times higher than ever before. For-profit hospitals benefited especially. Their after-tax profits rose nearly 80 percent or $198.8 million, while average profit margins approached 16 percent. Hospitals that were losing money turned a comfortable profit. Nineteen of the twenty-eight hospitals in Dade County, for example, made more money under prospective payment than under cost-plus reimbursement. In a dramatic turnabout, Westchester General Hospital, which lost 2.6 cents on every dollar in 1983, rebounded to show an after-tax profit of 12.3 cents on every dollar in 1984. Five percent of Florida hospitals reported average profits of $5.4 million.

Nationally, hospitals also thrived. The inspector general of the Department of Health and Human Services found that 82 percent of the nation's hospitals were profiting under prospective payment. By stimulating cost efficiency, prospective payment was producing $5 billion a year in new profits for the hospital industry. The inspector general also discovered that for-profit hospitals wrested nearly a 25 percent profit margin from Medicare, measured as a return on equity, under the new, supposedly tightfisted fixed rates. Throughout the industry, margins averaged 15 percent. Although the number of admissions and length of stays declined, revenues went up. The supermeds sharply escalated the average cost per hospitalization to $5,420, a 17 percent increase, and the average cost per day to $915, a 19 percent jump.[10]

Hospitals quickly realized that they could increase revenues if patients were assigned DRGs that paid well. By 1985 almost 8 percent of their patients were assigned new, more costly classifications. Medicare officials labeled this "upcoding." More bluntly, it was beating the system, squeezing untold millions, from taxpayers for unneeded and perhaps undelivered care. Patients with lung disease were being admitted to hospitals diagnosed erroneously—but far more profitably—as suffering from heart failure or cancer of the bladder. Some hospitals were making these "mistakes" in one out of every four Medicare patients. Such errors were unlikely to happen by sheer chance, but the result was extremely lucrative. These misdiagnoses alone added $23 million a year to Medicare's costs. Meanwhile, patients who showed no symptoms of lung disease were assigned to the "chronic obstructive pulmonary disease" DRG, a frequently ascribed diagnostic category. But the inspector general of Health and Human Services found that up to 60 percent of these patients exhibited no lung disease and that another 5 percent shouldn't even have been admitted. In the pursuit of money, hospitals were willfully disregarding medical evidence. Through this upcoding they increased revenues by $41 million a year. Moreover, 40 percent of patients who were assigned the lung cancer DRG were incorrectly categorized and 7.5 percent were admitted unnecessarily. Officials reported that ten midwestern hospitals collected an extra $6.3 million because of their mistakes. The inspector general concluded, "These coding errors suggest deliberate choices on the part of the hospital personnel to manipulate the DRG system."[11] By 1988 the miscoding was worse. The inspector general reported that 20 percent Medicare claims were inaccurate and that the errors were costing more than $300 million a year.

Soon hospitals spied an even larger loophole. While the DRG's determined reimbursement on hospital admissions, outpatient care continued to be paid under cost plus. The discovery precipitated a medical shell game. By estimating their payments through both systems, hospitals could calculate if a patient would generate the most money in or out of the facility. Supermeds like American Medical International were particularly adept at shifting patients. AMI reported that admissions were down 7.4 percent, but outpatient visits soared 14.9 percent in 1985. In the next two years its outpatient revenues grew 70 percent. Humana sought to expand, too, and earmarked 60 percent of its $350 million capital budget in 1986 for outpatient facilities and services. According to the U.S. Prospective Payment Commission, while hospital admissions dropped 2.5 percent in 1986, outpatient visits jumped 8.1 percent, a record increase that surpassed the previous record of 4.5 percent set in 1985. Outpatients contributed 17 percent of all hospital revenues by 1986. The growth was greatest in ambulatory surgery. Over one in three operations were being performed in outpatient clinics in 1985 compared to less than one in five in 1980. The number of centers grew from 87 in 1983 to 838 in 1987.

The new shell game could be enormously profitable, as cataract surgery demonstrates. Cataract surgery is one of the most frequently performed operations on the elderly, and Medicare pays most of the bills. A decade ago cataract surgery was a major operation that required a three-day hospital stay and follow-up visits to fit and adjust the patient's heavy spectacles. But surgical advances have refined the operation to a delicate but simple procedure that can be performed in three hours in an outpatient clinic. This shift might have been expected to reduce costs. Instead they were magnified. The U.S. House Subcommittee on Health and Long-Term Care found that hospitals could more than double their Medicare reimbursement by switching the procedure from an operating room to an ambulatory clinic. A hospital typically collects $5,700 under cost-plus payment for outpatient treatment, in contrast to only $2,400 under the DRG schedule for a hospital procedure. Not surprisingly, the subcommittee found that almost all cataract surgery was being performed in outpatient clinics. While the hospitals won, the taxpayers and Medicare lost. Through that maneuver hospitals pocket an extra $1.2 billion a year, a practice that still continues.[12]

With Medicare's passage in 1964 the federal government created for-profit medicine; with its 1983 reform it abetted the expansion of corporate control of health care throughout the United States.

The thirty-four hundred community hospitals that deliver most of the health care in the United States are in trouble. Increasingly, they will find survival difficult if not impossible. These hospitals, the product of the Hill-Burton building boom, are now thirty and forty years old. They desperately need to be renovated or replaced. Seth Shaw, a Wall Street analyst, thinks that raising the money to pay for these improvements will be a formidable task. An estimated $150 billion are needed for construction costs alone. Many community hospitals lack the funds for extensive modernization and, unlike the supermeds, their ability to raise funds is limited. They can't issue stock, and tax-exempt bonds, a major source of funds in the past, are becoming harder to market. Even profitable community hospitals will be hard-pressed to find the necessary sources of financing. Their trustees will be pressured to accept whatever money is offered.[13] Hence the selling of Harvard.

On August 1, 1983, psychiatrists at McLean Hospital, a teaching facility of Harvard Medical School, awoke to discover their institute had been sold to Hospital Corporation of America. The news was startling and totally unexpected. There had been no rumors or whispered gossip in the hallways before the public announcement was made. The doctors and research staff had been totally unaware that the hospital trustees were even considering a sale. Many heard the news on their car radios as they were driving to work. "It made me think that we were being sold like chattel," one scientist said.

In fact, it was triage. McLean Hospital was being sacrificed to save Massachusetts General Hospital, another Harvard Medical School teaching facility. McLean, a 172-year-old facility located on well-clipped grounds that recall an elite college campus, was relatively rich. McLean's patients could afford their treatment or they wouldn't be at the private psychiatric facility. Its uncollected debts ran about 2.6 percent of revenues, far below that of most hospitals. Massachusetts General, however, was not rich. It had more prestige than money, and it was growing old without particular grace. More than $200 million were needed to renovate and expand the hospital for its second century. Trustees could tell from a cursory review of its budget that such an enormous sum would be difficult to raise. The trustees who oversaw both hospitals scanned the balance sheets and decided the solution would be to sell McLean Hospital and use the proceeds to revitalize Massachusetts General.

When Hospital Corporation of America, already the owner of twenty-five psychiatric hospitals, came calling, trustees were ready to invite the supermed into the boardroom for sherry. (Describing the confrontation, a staff doctor said, "Harvard meets Godzilla.") HCA was willing to spend handsomely for the Harvard affiliation. Under the draft proposal's generous terms HCA would purchase McLean for somewhere between $40 million and $60 million, spend $35 million on its renovation, and donate $6.25 million to Harvard Medical School to endow five professorships. McLean would be given a new board that would control policy but not, significantly, the budget. The board would be dominated by Harvard and Massachusetts General appointees and headed by the dean of Harvard Medical School. The offer was impressive, but then HCA was buying Harvard. A company started by the Kentucky Fried Chicken king knew the value of a good brand name.

Most of the Harvard Medical School faculty was outraged by the sale. A feeling of betrayal, of violation ran through the entire Harvard community. As a faculty committee reported to Harvard officials, the doctors weren't opposed to the HCA sale per se; they believed that the sale of any Harvard facility to any supermed was unethical. "These ethics hold that the operation of hospitals, and particularly teaching hospitals, should not be influenced by the motivation for profit," the committee said. The opposition that mounted throughout that summer and fall was so relentless that the trustees were forced to abandon their plans.

Harvard trustees were thwarted, but only temporarily. In 1986 McLean Hospital and American Medical International announced the formation of a joint venture, McLean Health Services. Through the new company AMI would help underwrite McLean Hospital's research and teaching program and finance the construction of major new buildings at the Belmont, Massachusetts, campus.[14]

If Harvard Medical School must go to the supermeds, the prognosis for many less prestigious hospitals is grim. The capital crunch is expected to be so severe that Kenneth Abramowitz, a health care analyst at Sanford C. Bernstein & Co., predicts that community hospitals will all but vanish from the United States. "Virtually all free-standing hospitals will soon have to sell out to for-profit hospitals, merge, or affiliate with a nonprofit system to avoid bankruptcy," he states.[15] While these changes will be traumatic for community hospitals, the supermeds will be entering a period of exciting opportunities. As community hospitals flounder, the chains can expect new acquisitions at bargain prices. When this era concludes, the chains will be positioned to imprint their corporate brand names on health care. By the mid-1980s supermeds were poised to monopolize hospital care in many areas. HCA, for instance, owned the only medical facility in sixty-five to seventy communities in the United States. If this trend continues, the supermeds will achieve unprecedented power to dictate the quality and availability of care.

These consequences should have been obvious in 1983 when Medicare reimbursement was redesigned. Ironically, in seeking to clamp down on medical costs, the federal government may be losing the ability to influence health care in the United States. Congress was so intent on controlling expenses that it disregarded the real impact of its reform. Health care was snatched away from the policy specialists and given to the budget experts. This was an abrupt departure. Up until 1983 the federal government had worried about the needs of consumers. Who was getting care, and who was being denied it? Should more money be spent on community mental health or on rural clinics? Were there enough doctors in the right places to provide adequate health care? Now, however, the federal government was driven by the need to reduce spending. The new worry was: How much did it cost, and who was going to pay for it? As Senator David Durenberger, Republican of Minnesota, an expert on health care, explained, "Health policy improvement in America is being pushed to the back of the bus by the rowdies from budget policy."

The federal government promised the changes would reduce costs. Yet, under prospective payment, the elderly found their costs were increasing. The federal government announced the largest increases in the Medicare deductibles, paid by beneficiaries, in years. In 1986 the elderly were billed $492, a 23 percent increase, for the first day of a hospital stay. In 1987 they were charged $520, another 5.7 percent increase. As hospitals released patients sooner, expenses were spread over fewer days, thus increasing both the cost of the first day and the charge to the elderly. The federal government, however, paid little attention to the rising cost to the elderly as long as its expenses were lowered.

The message to hospitals was clear, too. The federal government was deregulating hospitals; laissez-faire had arrived. As long as the government spent less, the hospitals would be unfettered. Abramowitz said that prospective payment offered a "very ingenious solution to a politically intractable problem." Under DRGs, he said, "Instead of paying hospitals according to how much money hospitals spent, hospitals will be paid according to how much money the government has. Since the government promised 30 million [elderly] people too much, the only way to get out of that promise is to pay 7,000 hospitals too little. Someone has to get stuck holding the bag and the government has decided that it will not." Reports circulated that hospitals were discharging critically ill patients if the profit margin, provided by the DRGs, was exhausted. A few congressional committees held hearings on these alarming disclosures, but while testimony filled pages in official reports, nothing was done. No legislation was passed; policies were unchanged. The elderly's traditional champions in and out of Congress complained surprisingly little about hospitals' new "quicker and sicker" discharge policy. As John K. Iglehart, editor of *Health Affairs*, commented, "Quality assurance under DRG's didn't prove a problem for policymakers as long as people weren't dying in the streets."

Congress was in tune with the times when it passed control over health care to the supermeds. Power flowed to the corporations because, suddenly and quite unexpectedly, the supermeds were the only place for it to go. Government no longer wanted it. The supermeds fit the conservative firmament of the Reagan Administration. The intellectual and political fashions of the mid-1980's—a lack of confidence in government, a belief in the blessings of competition, and faith that private enterprise could do better than the federal bureaucracy—were a hospitable Petri dish for the growth of the supermeds. Executives like David A. Jones were featured on the cover of *Parade*. The Reagan Administration pledged to reduce the size of the federal government; of all its efforts to privatize government, health care may have been the outstanding success. And the supermeds were there waiting.

CHAPTER FOUR

•

Good-bye to Dr. Marcus Welby

FEBRUARY 1986 was not kind to Chicago. In winter's final frenzy the city turned slate gray. Chunks of ice littered the Oak Street beaches, and the Chicago River was a metallic slash through downtown. A stinging mist settled over the luxury hotels and department stores along Michigan Avenue. The snow no longer fell; it hovered in an elusive morning light. At nine degrees below zero, with the temperature still dropping, the cold was relentless, numbing both body and spirit.

Inside the Chicago Marriott, where over one thousand doctors were attending a conference on the future of medicine, the atmosphere was equally bleak. These doctors, far more than celebrity superstars like William DeVries, represented the real medical establishment in the United States. They were the elected leaders of medical societies in small towns such as Boalsburg, Pennsylvania, and Lakeland, Florida. They were mostly male, overwhelmingly white and middle-aged, with telltale bifocals and thinning gray hair. In their sport jackets and loafers they looked as if they spent their Saturday nights at country clubs in Amana, Iowa, or Tyler, Texas, dancing with the wife of the bank president, swapping city hall gossip with local councilmen. During the next three days, however, they learned that they were in the midst of losing their power, prestige, and affluence, and if they wanted to keep even a semblance of their privileges, they would be forced to alter their professional and personal lives drastically.

Such a gathering would have been unimaginable even five years earlier. In fact, when the AMA first discussed holding a conference on the revolution in the health care industry, they wondered if their members would even be interested in the subject. They had never held a conference where the sessions concentrated on the outlook for the practice of medicine instead of the advances in medical science. But conference organizers worried needlessly. It turned out to be the most popular conference in their history. Although doctors wouldn't acquire new medical knowledge or sharpen their ability to treat patients, with luck they might gain enough business skills from the marketing experts and health care consultants for their practices to survive.

The conference was a symbol of the great changes that are shaking up medicine, and organized medicine's belated recognition of this transformation. For the past twenty years AMA leaders had been warning doctors that their biggest threat came from the federal government and its support of "socialized medicine" through the funding of health care programs for the poor and elderly. As the AMA fought the federal government, however, they failed to perceive that the emerging health care conglomerates posed a far larger danger to the medical profession. It wasn't until this meeting that the AMA acknowledged the new menace with sessions on "Meeting the Health Care Needs of the Twenty-first-Century Corporation," "Influencing the Changing Environment of Medicine: Enhancing Physicians' Ability to Compete," "Physicians and Wellness: Dollars and Sense," and "Marketing."

Many doctors attending this conference were already smarting from competition from supermeds that had moved into their communities. The others got their first glimpse of the pressures being brought to bear on the medical profession from the keynote speaker, Roger B. Smith, the chairman of the board of General Motors. Smith was an unlikely adversary. He was not only the grandson of a Chicago doctor but also the head of one of the country's most conservatively run corporations. But, as he told his audience, General Motors was no longer being traditional in its approach to the health care of its employees. General Motors was encouraging its employees to join health maintenance organizations because it couldn't afford for them to visit doctors in private practice and still compete with foreign manufacturers.

"Today we're building companies for the twenty-first century—companies that are fully competitive with foreign producers in the two vital areas of quality and cost," he began. "We must reform any procedures that don't contribute to this objective. That means that twenty-first-century companies must have twenty-first-century health care systems—systems that are just as competitive in quality and cost as any other part of the business. We need those systems to help keep jobs in the United States and ensure our very survival—and the survival of a competitive industrial base to keep America strong."

The doctors who settled back comfortably at the beginning of his speech were on the edge of their folding chairs by the time Smith delivered his last, harsh rebuke: "Inefficient practices on the part of health care providers also contribute to excessive costs. . . . Unless we can get health care costs under better control in this country, there is a danger the entire health care system will collapse under its own weight."

A question-and-answer period followed, but the doctors seemed too stunned by his speech to approach the strategically placed microphones. As Smith waited patiently at the podium, a single flustered young man bore down on a microphone, identified himself as a medical student, and said, "I'm worried that the changes in medicine may make it more difficult for me to establish a practice. If corporations like General Motors are going to a more mechanized system, I wonder if I will be able to establish a doctor-patient relationship, if it won't make it more difficult for me to practice medicine. I worry about my future."

But Smith countered, "I think that with health maintenance-type organizations we get better care, better coverage, and, frankly, I like the plan. I've joined one myself. I commend you for getting through school—just don't try to make all your costs back on your first patient."

The AMA could not have chosen a better keynote speaker to dramatize the trends in health care. If Smith and General Motors were attacking doctors, then they would have to search far for understanding friends, and they weren't to be found here. In session after session the experts warned unsympathetically that doctors were losing control of their profession to the health care conglomerates. Tom Hoban, executive vice president of the Hennepin County (Minnesota) Medical Society, said, "We've had five years of illusion. The health care industry doesn't realize yet the power it has, and physicians don't realize how much they've lost. We have less than two years left. By then doctors will either be directly involved in trying to mold the [supermed] companies or we will be working for them. We're in the middle of an alligator-infested pool." Equally pessimistic, Jeff Goldsmith, president of Health Futures, Inc., said, "It's easy to conclude that the end of the world is at hand." And Michael J. Goran, a management consultant at Ernest & Whitney, warned, "For the young physician the old solo practice life will no longer be possible."

Before the conference ended, the doctors knew that the world would be a far less pleasant place than they once imagined. As John McGrath, president of the American Psychiatric Association, concluded, "I think our future is behind us."

He was right. The private practitioners who make up the bulk of the American Medical Association membership are becoming an anachronism. Dr. Kermit Newcomer, president of the American Group Practice Association, said, "The middle-aged, midcareer physician today is like the blacksmith who earned a living shoeing horses in the 1920s. There will always be an important niche for some individual practitioners—for some physicians will not want to move into a corporate environment. After all, there are still a few blacksmiths around today, but not as many as in the 1920s and 1930s." The changes are occurring rapidly. In the 1960s doctors were at the pinnacle of their power; in the 1980s they are little more than an army of pushcart vendors in an age of medical supermarkets. How did it happen? What went wrong?

In the decades immediately following World War II, the U.S. economy boomed and the medical profession benefited mightily from the general prosperity. Doctors saw more patients as health insurance became more widespread in the 1950s. Millions of middle-class Americans, previously unable to pay for such luxuries as annual checkups, were brought into the health care system. And with the advent of Medicare in the 1960s, the number of people who could afford to see doctors expanded dramatically. Some eighteen million elderly, the heaviest consumers of medical services, were freed to seek health care, knowing their bills would be paid.

In addition to the new patients in their waiting rooms, doctors acquired a previously unknown financial security. For the first time in the twentieth century they could be assured their bills would be paid. During financially hard times their bills were paid slowly if at all. In the midst of the Depression, for instance, 66.6 percent of their bills went unpaid for longer than six months. The net income of California doctors fell from approximately $6,700 in 1929 to $3,600 in 1933. The first health insurance plan for payment of medical fees, Blue Shield, was set up by physicians to guard against a repeat of that financial disaster.

Together the private insurance industry and the federal government set up a system that would sustain the economic privilege of doctors for the next thirty years. Private health care insurance paid a little over $20 billion a year to physicians in 1984, while Medicare spent $31.1 billion in 1987. Through Medicare a substantial portion of the federal government's wealth began to be transferred to doctors. To pay their bills the program uses premiums from elderly beneficiaries and taxes paid by working Americans. Unlike Robin Hood, who robbed the rich to pay the poor, the federal government did the reverse. Middle-income Americans were taxed to enrich the nation's doctors. While doctors attacked socialized medicine publicly, they eagerly welcomed it in private. The federal government was bankrolling over 20 percent of all money spent on doctor bills in the United States, and physicians were receiving more than 23 percent of their total income from Medicare. By 1985 it became their leading source of income. In the years following the passage of Medicare, with the government guaranteeing payment for a large share of their bills, doctors began raising their fees an average of 11.3 percent a year. Two decades after Medicare's passage, doctors were increasing their fees so rapidly that their bills were the fourth-largest domestic expense and the fastest-growing segment of the entire federal budget. Congress, desperately seeking to bring costs under control, froze physicians' fees in 1984. The attempt failed. By circumventing the freeze, doctors increased their Medicare payments by 11 percent, an extra $16 million, the next year.

These were the glory days. As the number of potential patients expanded, the number of private practitioners actually declined. For a variety of reasons doctors were drawn to clinical research, medical school teaching, and federal government employment during these years. Between 1940 and 1957 the number of doctors caring for patients dropped from 108 to 91 per 100,000 people. The remaining doctors had only to open their offices, sit back, and watch their practices flourish. Doctors who were seeing 50 patients a week in the 1930s were treating at least 100 a week in the 1950s. Doctors had the best of all possible worlds.

Although the federal government was underwriting physicians' financial success with Medicare, at the same time it was pursuing policies that would later prove their undoing. The federal government observed the growth in health care benefits and worried that there might be too few doctors to take care of the demand. Predictably, the government ordered a study. The resulting 1959 report projected a doctor shortage in fifteen years, and the government responded as it usually does: It created a program. To head off the doctor gap, the government spent freely to establish new medical schools, increasing their number from 88 in 1964 to 126 in 1980. In the process the government created a doctor glut.

The program was an absolute success, producing a bumper crop of doctors. In 20 years medical school graduates more than doubled, from 7,409 to 16,347 new doctors a year. The doctors in active practice increased dramatically. In 1950 there were 209,000 physicians. A decade later, their numbers had increased only slightly, to 247,300. By 1982, however, there were 465,000 doctors. Between 1970 and 1983, general practitioners almost doubled, from 187,637 to 305,755. The flood of medical school graduates increased the number of private practitioners by 41.9 percent during the 1970s, then by another 12.8 percent between 1980 and 1983. Before the year 2000 the number of doctors is expected to increase yet another 21 percent, to 700,000 physicians.[1]

The federal government, however, hasn't been promiscuous in

its subsidies. Numerous policies promote medical specialization. Medicare subsidies to teaching hospitals for residency programs help medical school graduates continue their training. Medicare paid nearly $2 billion in 1986 to support 76,815 residents. Moreover, doctors are encouraged to specialize by Medicare's reimbursement policies. Specialists are paid far more for their time and services. Medicare will pay four to five times more an hour for inpatient surgery than for office visits, for example. Specialists who see the highest percentage of Medicare patients tend to report the highest incomes. Radiologists, who derive approximately 28 percent of their income from Medicare, for example, have some of the highest incomes, with 50 percent averaging over $150,000 a year in 1985. With their advanced training doctors began flooding the best-paying specialties. And the situation of the 1950s and 1960s started to reverse itself.[2]

The federal government was creating an economic fiasco for doctors already in practice and for the new medical school graduates. Suddenly the number of doctors was growing faster than the population. Doctors began watching their thriving practices shrivel. In 1960 there were 14 doctors per 10,000 Americans. By 1982 there were 20.5 per 10,000 Americans, and their ratio continues to climb. Projections call for 23.8 doctors per 10,000 Americans by 1990 and 26.4 doctors per 10,000 Americans when the twenty-first century begins. Doctors already complain that there is a surplus and too much competition. An Arthur Andersen & Company survey found that 71 percent of the doctors believed specialists would be in significant oversupply and 61 percent felt physicians in family practice would be in slight oversupply by 1990. The excess could reach 185,000 doctors.

The competition, however, could easily be worse. In addition to the doctors who are pouring out of American medical schools, the numbers of foreign-medical-school graduates are also increasing. According to the American Medical Association, foreign-trained physicians have doubled from 58,543 in 1971 to 112,005 in 1983. Some 13,000 foreign-medical-school graduates were in advanced training programs in the United States in 1985. In some inner-city hospitals they account for more than 50 percent of the residents. At Methodist Hospital in Brooklyn, New York, 95 percent of the residents and 38 percent of the full-time medical staff were educated abroad.

Added to this pressure is yet another. Americans are paying fewer visits to their doctors. Americans who visited their doctors almost three times a year in 1976 came in only two and a half times annually in 1981. Doctors saw 12 percent fewer patients a week between 1982 and 1984. And because fewer patients are hospitalized, doctors make 20 percent fewer hospital rounds, further reducing their income. The trend is expected to continue.[3]

The consequences are clear. Doctors will be earning less in the decades ahead. Dr. David Hilfiker, an inner-city physician who laments that medicine has abandoned the poor, says that his $22,000 a year salary plus housing allowance is "hardly sacrificial."[4] He is in a distinct minority, however; most doctors would consider that abject poverty. The average physician had a net income of $113,200 in 1985, but in some specialties it was far higher. Surgeons averaged $155,400, while the average income for anesthesiologists was $140,200, and just below them were obstetrician/gynecologists, with average incomes of $122,700. The average physician enjoys an income five times greater than that of the typical American worker, but in relative terms physicians began falling on financial hard times in the mid-1980s. The American Medical Association found that physicians' incomes began to stagnate in 1983. The typical doctor saw his income grow by only 2 percent, not enough to keep up with inflation. In the decade between 1975 and 1985, after adjusting for inflation, some specialists—internists, pediatricians, psychiatrists, and others—actually watched their incomes drop. Only surgeons, radiologists, and anesthesiologists experienced real increases in earnings. Doctors just starting out had an even tougher time. Their incomes began to decline in 1970. Throughout the 1970s and into the 1980s they were unable to keep up with inflation. Young doctors, often straddled with over $60,000 in student loans, are seeing the return on their investment in a medical education plummet. In the 1950s a young person could expect those four years to bring lifetime returns of 15 to 18 percent a year, one of life's safest and best investments. That era is gone.

Henry-Evans & Pierce Co., a leading health industry consulting firm, predicts that the average doctor can expect a 25 percent drop in income by 1990. Dr. John W. Pollard of the Carle Clinic in Champaign, Illinois, warned a Group Management Association meeting: "To deny that physician income is going to go down in the future is like the captain of the *Titanic* insisting that his ship isn't going to sink."[5] Dr. Donald Kelly of Healthgroup International put it even more boldly: "For the past forty years everyone in medicine has had a license to steal." This is no longer true. A medical license is just a permit to compete in a world of steadily diminishing resources. Physicians are so alarmed that even home test kits, sold over the counter to diagnose pregnancy, high blood pressure, and the like, are considered a financial threat. Dr. Hugh R. K. Barber warned readers of *The Female Patient* that the multimillion-dollar industry could have a "devastating impact" on doctors. "Do-it-yourself testing may be the most formidable challenge the medical profession faces at the end of this century and the beginning of the next," he added in cataclysmic tones.

At medical conventions and in professional journals doctors sound as if it's December 7, 1941, and they are swaying, helplessly alone, on the prow of ships in Pearl Harbor. They talk about being under siege and of lost wars and battles. When they write articles for the *American Medical News* titled "A View from the Twenty-first Century: How Medicine Met Its Demise," they sound hopeless and confused. They also sound outraged and bitter in articles such as the one headlined "Medical Schools Preach Long-Gone Fantasy." Its author, Dr. Joseph D. Wassersug, wrote, "Nowadays, if we teach medical students 'idealism,' we are teaching fantasy, deception, and fraud, and are not preparing them for the harsh realities of current medical practice. . . . For much less than what it costs to become a physician, one can obtain a McDonald's franchise. Here, too, great good is done. The hungry are served, the young are entertained, and the housewife's lot is made easier. In spite of what medical schools may teach, you don't have to be a physician to be of service."[6] Doctors feel as if they have been victimized. All they have prepared for and known is slipping away. Although doctors are troubled by their declining practices and incomes, money is only a symbol of the real source of their distress.

They are losing their earning power because of a fundamental restructuring and realignment of power in American medicine.

Throughout the first half of the twentieth century, doctors were at the center of a health care system that was organized for their convenience. During the Hill-Burton hospital boom administrators eagerly courted the physicians in their communities. While doctors need hospitals, the hospitals needed the physicians far more. Only doctors could admit patients to hospitals, and without their allegiance hospitals couldn't keep their beds occupied and eventually would go broke. Doctors were essential to their economic well-being, and little was spared to keep them happy. Hospitals invested in the latest technology, built new wings, granted liberal admitting privileges—anything the doctors desired that would keep their patients coming. In effect, physicians were Fuller Brush salesmen for the hospitals. Hospitals still need patients, but since the arrival of DRGs they have been demanding that patients produce profits as well as fill beds. This new selectivity is altering the relationship between doctors and hospitals.

Community hospital administrators still believe that doctors may be their most important market. If they can sell physicians on their facility, they can swell the stream of patients passing through the hospital. "Doctors are our only future in the hospital industry. They are the driving force behind return on investment. They are the key to the hospital front door," said George Gray, Jr., of Baptist Health Services in Gadsden, Alabama. As the health care conglomerates expand, community hospitals, unable to match their aggressive marketing, may need physicians more than ever. Richard G. Gray of Memorial Care Systems in Houston advises his fellow administrators to think of doctors as "a direct sales force of the hospital."

A trade newsletter advises hospital administrators, "Too many doctors treat marketing as a dirty word. Don't let them get away with it. Be direct. Ask doctors how they plan to send their kids to college. Share marketing data. Offer names of [other] doctors who can use their services." If they need further encouraging, readers are reminded, "Just one busy surgeon means $1.5 million per year for the average hospital. One busy internist $750,000. One busy ob/gyn $600,000. A busy GP? $500,000."[7]

Supermeds need doctors, too. As Hospital Corporation of America says, "The most important factor relating to the occupancy rate of a hospital is the number of doctors using the hospital." HCA considers the number of referring doctors a more important factor than the number of competing hospitals or the demographic or economic makeup of a community. But while supermeds acknowledge that doctors are necessary, they also consider them a threat. In their facilities the physicians can be too independent, undermining corporate structure, injecting an element of uncertainty that weakens corporate control and the sureness of profits. Because physicans determine 91 percent of all hospital costs, according to the U.S. Office of Technology Assessment, supermeds need to manage physicians in order to control profits.[8]

Supermeds don't just need doctors; they need the right kind of doctors. They need doctors who practice supermed medicine. Toward this end health care conglomerates are seeking to instill an entrepreneurial ethic in their doctors. In large measure they are succeeding. The supermeds are helping to change the values of a medical profession that shows diminishing resistance. For decades doctors found that idealism was profitable. They could live very well while they talked about serving humanity. They could ignore the business of medicine and still watch their incomes climb. This luxury no longer exists. Increasingly doctors are forced to concede that they are also running a business. The supermeds arrived at precisely the right time to capitalize on doctors' anxiety about competition and the changing practice of medicine. They are able to attract physicians who might have spurned corporate ties in the past.

Supermeds try to attract doctors by offering numerous inducements to calm their financial worries. When Humana sought pediatricians for a group practice in Springhill, Louisiana, it guaranteed each physician a $5,500-a-month income for the first six months and projected a minimum first-year income of $150,000. In addition, it promised "absolutely no business or office overhead expenses" for the first year. The company would pay for a nurse, secretarial help, office equipment furniture, "and more." Other enticing fringe benefits included free health/dental/life/malpractice insurance, a car, moving expenses, and a paid membership in the local country club.[9]

The supermeds encourage doctors to use their hospitals by building adjacent medical offices. HCA owns eighty-five medical office buildings with approximately 1.6 million square feet of office space for physicians. Humana operates forty-nine medical office buildings near its hospitals and is constructing twenty-six more. Humana rents its offices at far below the going market rate. In fact, it loses money on almost all of them, but it expects to recoup its losses from the patients who are referred to its hospitals. Doctors aren't required to admit their patients to Humana hospitals in exchange for the favorable leases, but if they don't, they may soon be looking for new office space or renegotiating at a higher rate. Staff doctors, however, may be kicked out if they don't funnel patients to Humana hospitals. At Humana's St. Petersburg (Florida) General Hospital, staff doctors are expected to meet an annual admissions quota. In 1985, according to a hospital memorandum, they were told to admit "at least" twenty patients. The hospital reviews its doctors' performance annually, and in deciding whether a doctor will be reappointed, St. Petersburg General considers "his use of the hospital's facilities for his patients." Doctors who don't use the hospital's facilities or meet their quota are threatened with the withdrawal of their admitting privileges. In a small city where over half of the hospitals are owned by Humana, such requirements can jeopardize a doctor's livelihood. A St. Petersburg radiologist, warned that his privileges were about to be rescinded, protested, "Humana has introduced a new dimension into the practice of medicine which I do not think is entirely healthy, namely a profit-driven facility. . . . It is my notion that this provision is not only unfair but is detrimental to the public welfare since the physician's prerogative to practice in the hospital, and at times even to make a living in the community, should not rest with this economic barrier."

Doctors have been losing control of medicine to the supermeds largely because of doctors' growing numbers. In the medical world the laws of politics don't apply. Unlike other professionals, doctors don't gain power if their numbers increase. The exact opposite applies. Within the health care industry their power lies in their patients. The more patients doctors have, the more powerful they are. If they can admit fewer patients, they are less able to dictate the conditions of those referrals. In their dealings with health care conglomerates they become weaker, not stronger. The supermeds are attempting to exploit that vulnerability through marketing strategies that are intended to appeal directly to patients. National Medical Enterprises, for example, conducts extensive community surveys to determine the needs and demands of its potential customers. As John C. Bedrosian, senior executive vice president of NME, put it, "Now the doctor no longer has an exclusive on patient admitting, for he increasingly shares it with PPOs [preferred provider organizations], HMOs [health maintenance organizations], insurance companies, labor unions, and large employers. Moreover, he shares it with the patient himself, who is now presented with economic incentives to exercise other choices." As a result of its marketing program, Bedrosian said National Medical Enterprises has been able to establish "extremely aggressive, market-oriented advertising campaigns at all our facilities."

Moreover, doctors can no longer claim power solely through technical proficiency. While their skills certainly determine their worth to patients, proficiency is losing its previous value in the medical marketplace. Greg Korneluk, a Lewiston, New York, medical consultant, stresses to his doctor clients, "A successful practice is the result of consistent, successful physician-patient encounters in which the patients leave feeling that their visits were both pleasing and memorable events which will make a positive impact on their personal well-being." As medicine becomes a business, doctors can't trust their survival to knowledge alone. Supermed medicine demands business sense and the ability to cope with corporate managers. The medical world is turning upside down. With a captive market, the supermeds will need doctors less and less financially. Physicians, however, will need their goodwill to maintain a practice. The hospitals will be wholesaling medical services, produced by doctors, to giant purchasers represented by private industry and government. Doctors are becoming just another source of revenue for hospitals, no more and no less than outpatient clinics or ambulatory surgical centers. As a result, supermeds can increase their pressure on physicians. Bedrosian said, "We have instituted physician referral programs to help new residents select a family doctor. This activity, while pleasing to our medical staff members, makes it easier to solicit their cooperation in carrying out our cost-containment programs."

No wonder that doctors are upset. They are squeezed between formidable, increasingly fierce competition from their colleagues inside medicine and escalating outside competition from the supermeds. Louis Stern, marketing professor at Northwestern University, said, "The first reaction of most doctors [to the competition] is, 'If I lie here, it will go away. Just throw a blanket over me and keep me warm.' The second reaction is defensive retreat. It's a Maginot Line psychology." According to Stern, many doctors are going through the same stages of mourning as their dying patients, passing through denial and anger to acceptance. But if they mourn too long, they are likely to find they've lost their practices. Only if they uncurl from their fetal positions can they cope with the changes in medicine. And at that point they may discard their scorn for business techniques and start practicing an entirely new style of medicine.

The television screen flickers and then Dr. Ralph Wittenberg, president of the Washington, D.C., Psychiatric Society, appears. Dr. Wittenberg is describing the classic symptoms of depression —persistent feelings of sadness, sleeping difficulties, fatigue, inability to concentrate, crying, suicidal thoughts. It appears to be a typical public-service announcement, the kind that television stations run regularly, but it is not. It is an advertisement for the four hundred or so psychiatrists who practice in the District of Columbia and the surrounding suburbs. After recounting the ten signs of depression, Dr. Wittenberg adds the zinger, "If you have four or more of these symptoms, you should consult a psychiatrist." In effect, he is telling viewers who may have never considered seeking psychiatric help before to think about it. He concludes with a plug for local psychiatrists. The local psychiatric society, he says, can help viewers find a psychiatrist. At the bottom of the screen flashes the telephone number for the local referral service.

Because of traditionally generous mental health benefits for federal workers, Washington, D.C., has one of the heaviest concentrations of psychiatrists in the United States. The federal government has been curtailing benefits, however, and psychiatrists are feeling the pinch. Local psychiatrists can use an infusion of new patients. When the ads were first proposed, they were controversial enough to split the psychiatric community. Many doctors were adamantly opposed, but a majority of society members agreed to test the response to the ads. They're not the only doctors resorting to television come-ons. The Television Bureau of Advertising reports that spot ads for health care professionals totaled $62 million in 1984, an increase of 51 percent over 1983.

Dr. Robert Schnipper, a Jacksonville, Florida, eye surgeon, for instance, advertises his services between the eleven o'clock news and the late-night movie. "What's evil about it?" he asks. "I'm just trying to hold on to my market share. I can see the wave of the future—isn't that what a good businessman is supposed to do?"

Traditionally, doctors have held themselves apart, repudiating the normal advertising and marketing that other professionals rely on for clients. Even after lawyers, also suffering from an oversupply of practitioners, began advertising, most doctors disdained such crass commercialism. But doctors who once believed that medicine was above marketing have succumbed to economic realities. Doctors who thought that medicine couldn't be sold like floor wax are trying to learn Johnson Wax Company's techniques. Several medical magazines are now being published to educate doctors about the business of medicine. At *Medical Economics* an annual writing contest offers prizes for true-to-life stories that help their readers cope with the New Medicine. Titles of winning stories have the lurid flash and appeal of a true confessions magazine: "How I Beat the Doctor Surplus," "Our Walk-In Clinic Beat Hospitals to the Punch," and "I'm Tired of Being a Fall Guy for Hotshot Specialists." And in *Private Practice* a pediatrician describes how he builds his practice with a simple rule: "Give Your Patients More Than They Bargain For." Dr. M. Lawrence Podolsky lists the lures that can build a doctor's following—gum, candy, rings, toys, plastic dinosaurs, puzzles, dry cereals, balloons, pennies, beads, pencils, baby bibs, marbles, love buttons, drinking cups, badges, "My Doctor Loves Me" stickers, erasers shaped like alien creatures, space raiders, soft cuddly balls with eyes called "weepuls," clickers, magnets, toy soldiers, and dolls. Consumer activists might question the nutritional wisdom of candy or the safety of some of these toys.

But Podolsky advises his fellow doctors, "With the intensified scramble for patients, the doctor who gives a little extra is more likely to succeed against the competition, assuming all other factors are equal. Furthermore, there are no practice-builders or advertising schemes that cost less or accomplish more than a gift or handout. . . . Lagniappes have become almost essential to health and business practices."[10]

To survive the competition, doctors are adopting strategies unthinkable even five years ago. Some doctors, like the Albuquerque gynecologist who sends a hot-air balloon emblazoned with a stork wafting across the city, are using flamboyant techniques, but most are more circumspect, limiting themselves to flyers for neighborhood residents and newsletters on medical topics. The Keene Clinic in Keene, New Hampshire, sends out newsletters on hypertension during National Blood Pressure Month. An initial mailing brought in two hundred people who wanted their blood pressure tested. A subsequent mailing offering free screening for diabetes during National Diabetes Month was equally successful. Doctors who have never written a headline can turn to companies that provide sample newsletters and advice on design, illustration, printing, and bulk-mail rates.

A new breed of consultants have sprung up, selling physicians a variety of marketing help at $300 an hour or $2,000 a session. Some redesign waiting rooms, banishing sliding glass windows and installing flower-bedecked receptionist desks so patients will feel more welcome. Others gather "focus groups" of six to ten patients in hotel rooms where they discuss their feelings about their doctor and his practice. The sessions are recorded and the results, with interpretations added, offered to the doctor. A few even explain the use of "corporate espionage," spy techniques that can ferret out the practices and marketing strategies of rival medical groups.

The emphasis on marketing medicine is so rampant that the American Medical Association draws this picture of the day in the life of a typical doctor not too far in the future:

Five patients are already thumbing through magazines in the waiting room when the doctor arrives. Rushing past them, he enters his office to find a pile of computer printouts on his desk. Glancing through them, the doctor discovers a report on his profits from hospitalized Medicare patients, marketing advice about competing with a nearby health maintenance organization, a medical flow chart on a difficult patient, billing forms, and a financial review of his practice. The doctor worries about cost overruns on one of his Medicare patients and decides to call the hospital later to find out why Mabel Jones exceeded the Medicare allowance for her heart ailment. He calls his secretary and asks her to find out the promotional cost of a mailing to the thirty-five-year-olds in the neighborhood who seem to be enrolling in the HMO.

Only then does the doctor signal that he is ready to see his first patient, whose waiting time had been considerably lengthened and anxiety heightened. The doctor, however, is serene, knowing that action is being taken to replace his lost patients.

There is nothing wrong about attractive waiting rooms. They can make the lengthy waits more pleasant while doctors peruse their computer printouts. Patients can learn useful information from health care newsletters. Ads that avert a single suicide are worthwhile. These advertising and marketing campaigns have quite a different purpose, however. If they benefit consumers, that's a plus. Their real intention is to benefit doctors. In fact, doctors are cautioned by some marketing gurus not to adopt practices that would be of advantage to their patients. William Trombetta, a Philadelphia consultant, warned doctors that they shouldn't lower their prices to compete. "If you're a competitor of mine and you drop your prices by 20 percent tomorrow, I have no choice but to drop mine 20 percent, so where are we now?" he said. "Anybody can match price." It's far more useful, he tells his clients, to open up new offices in locations that can bring in new patients. Patients, however, might well prefer reduced fees to a newly designed waiting room in a luxury medical condominium.

Most patients have limited skills to evaluate a physician. They don't have the medical background to distinguish among doctors' medical abilities or credentials. For the most part they choose their doctors haphazardly and take a leap of faith that the doctor can be trusted. If their doctors are spending their time choosing paint for their reception areas rather than perfecting their clinical skills, that trust may be misplaced. In this era of new medicine the stress is on style rather than substance. In fact, doctors are often advised that only style matters. According to this new breed of medical consultants, doctors have more to gain from reading *Architectural Digest* than the *New England Journal of Medicine*. Bouquets of flowers in the reception area are prized above continuing medical education. Selecting the right lamp for the waiting room ranks higher than keeping abreast of the medical literature. Nathan Kaufman, vice president of marketing for National Medical Enterprises and a frequent lecturer at medical society meetings, tells doctors that quality of care isn't a factor at all. Instead, he says physicians will get ahead in their practices if they have attractive waiting rooms, hire a pleasant office staff, and are charming to their patients. "If a doctor does those things right, the actual quality of clinical ability doesn't matter. That's the unfortunate thing," he says. "You need class and taste to sell health care." Another consultant admonishes, "Convenience may be more important than quality—believe it or not."

In the fever-pitch competition many doctors are willing to defer to these recommendations. But not all physicians are happy about the marketing of medicine. In *American Medical News* Dr. Jack Hyman rebukes his fellow physicians: "Once medicine is marketed like soap or hamburgers, once the sales pitch wins out over the quiet personal performance of a confident physician, our profession, as we know it, is gone. . . . If the practice of medicine should, God forbid, ever become simply another profit-making business, instead of that sacred convenant between physician and patient, we will have forfeited our claim to the transcendental position the profession of medicine has always occupied."[11]

Not all doctors have succumbed to the profit principle. Dr. Luis Perez, president of the Florida Medical Association, is an internist and cardiologist who has practiced medicine for twenty-five years without ever taking out a single ad in his local Sanford, Florida, newspaper. He refuses to advertise and holds scathing opinions of those who do. "To me medicine is a science," he said. "I don't believe in prostituting it in any way. We cannot go down into the gutter and go on television like these lawyers are doing."[12]

Dr. Richard J. Feinstein, a Miami doctor, likewise paints a devastating portrait of the future of medicine, decrying doctors who advertise their wares like common merchants. He predicts that in the twenty-first century private practitioners will work out of storefront offices where videocassette recorders continuously run tapes touting their expertise and attractiveness over colleagues who are using the same technology to market their practices. He forecasts, "As competition to the fee-for-service solo medical practitioners began to develop, many physicians became selfish and greedy. . . . As the fabric of the profession began to unravel, more and more physicians abandoned their professionalism like rats abandoning a sinking ship."[13]

Advertising has come to represent the medical world's internal debate on the new health care. Throughout the 1980s it has been a symptom of the changes in health care. While consumers might benefit from advertising that accents price and credentials and injects rationality into the selection of doctors, most commercials and ads contain little information to inform patients' choices about prospective doctors. According to a highly regarded medical sociologist, doctors, too, have nothing to gain from the vigorous self-promotion. In his description of the American medical profession's rise to power, Paul Starr commented, "[T]he profession's success in establishing its sovereignty in medical care depended on the banishment of profit-making businesses from medical education and hospitals as well as from medical practice itself." In their scramble to keep their market share, a concept almost unknown a decade ago, doctors are helping to undermine their own power. By adopting the mentality of the supermeds and competing on the same basis, they are relinquishing their last vestiges of moral authority. The medical profession is trying to adopt the techniques of the supermeds and still stay aloof from them. It is an untenable position and, unfortunately for physicians, they are losing on both counts. They don't have the power or the money to compete with the supermeds. And by figuratively shedding their clinical white coats for Madison Avenue suits, they are throwing away patient trust.

In the end, doctors can survive only by hanging on for dear life to the patients they have or by stealing them from other physicians. Young doctors are particularly bitter about the division of medicine into hostile camps. A Virginia internist, the son of a doctor, said, "If I had to do it over again, I would never, ever go into medicine. I worked a hundred hours a week during my residency and for what? I barely survive and there's always another doctor around waiting to steal the patients I do have. I've had patients go to the emergency room of a hospital and say I'm their doctor. Yet I'm never called. The doctors in the emergency room don't care. They're just interns and residents, happy to steal my patients and assign them to the doctors who are on the teaching staff so they can get good ratings from them. They take away my patients to curry favor with their supervisors. The interns and residents who steer the most patients into the medical school faculty have the most influence with the professors. Sometimes they do it because they want a good recommendation from the doctors on that service to further their careers and sometimes they do it because they get extra money for doing so. Either way, I'm never notified. Sometimes I can't pay my telephone bill; I'm mortgaged to the hilt but I'm better off than a lot of the guys. I know doctors who can't even afford to buy a house. I know doctors at these HMOs who are being paid less than the receptionists."

In areas where competition is brisk, there's a whiff of desperation in the air. In 1984, Jacksonville, Florida, was one of the most competitive medical markets in a highly competitive state. There was an ample supply of doctors and enough extra hospital beds to close down two entire hospitals. Jacksonville physicians and hospital administrators thought they knew all they cared to know about competition. Then the Mayo Clinic, one of the world's most prestigious health care facilities, announced that it would be opening its first clinic outside of Rochester, Minnesota, in Jacksonville.

The Mayo Clinic was brooding about its market share, too. While the clinic still had more than its share of patients, the directors realized that the Midwest market was not growing. People who were potential patients were moving to the Sun Belt. The directors reasoned that Jacksonville, which could attract patients from the entire Southeast, would be a logical site for expansion. With its heavy concentration of Medicare beneficiaries, Florida was a natural market. Even affluent Latin Americans, already accustomed to shopping trips to Miami, might schedule an appointment with Mayo doctors while in the United States. Then, too, competition was already so stiff in Jacksonville that doctors there looked like easy targets. W. Eugene Mayberry, chairman of the board of governors, said that Jacksonville was picked because "There are not a lot of integrated group practices." In short, many Jacksonville doctors were still practicing medicine 1950s style. And while they might be fighting each other, they would be no match for the Mayo Clinic.

Jacksonville is a conservative southern city, dominated economically by traditional banking and insurance industries. So little changes there that residents have reelected the same congressman, Representative Charles Bennett, since 1948, and no one remembers the last time he faced serious opposition. The city has been relatively unscathed by the influx of drugs, a surging refugee population, and unbridled growth that rocks the rest of the state. All of this undoubtedly contributed to its appeal for the Mayo Clinic.

The Mayo Clinic proposed to introduce 1980s-style medicine to Jacksonville. It set aside $20 million to $30 million for initial costs for its new satellite. The directors announced that the clinic would be staffed with thirty Mayo-trained physicians. The clinic would expand rapidly to employ one hundred doctors and five hundred medical support personnel. Superspecialists from Rochester would be visiting. Mayo also promised the community that it would be spending $100 million a year on medical education and research. The new clinic would consist of six stories of postmodern ziggurat architecture to be built at an estimated cost of $10 million. It would be built on 140 acres of land donated by James E. Davis, a frequent patient at the Mayo Clinic and founder of the Winn-Dixie grocery store chain. Many doctors in Jacksonville believed the civic leader had betrayed the community.

The Mayo Clinic could easily locate in Florida only if state medical licensing laws were changed. Under the existing laws doctors who wanted to practice in Florida needed to have passed a licensing exam within the past ten years. Otherwise they would be forced to take the Florida examination, one of the toughest in the United States. The Florida medical exam was intentionally difficult to protect doctors already practicing in the state. But the Davis family not only gave the Mayo Clinic their land but also through their political clout set about changing the laws to accommodate their doctors. They had plenty of influence. For years the Winn-Dixie political action committee had been one of the major campaign contributors to state politicians. Almost all of Florida's leading politicians had received donations from the Sunbelt Good Government Committee. Now the Davis family wanted a little understanding from the state legislature. They found a sympathetic listener in Steve Pajcic, a member of the state House of Representatives from Jacksonville.

Pajcic and Dempsey Barron, onetime president of the state Senate and still its single most powerful member, introduced legislation that gave the Mayo doctors precisely what they needed. Under its terms doctors would be granted Florida licenses automatically if they were associated with a nonprofit corporation that employed more than six hundred physicians and that spent at least $75 million in 1984 for medical research.

Florida doctors were outraged by the bill that let over one hundred new Mayo doctors escape the grueling medical exam. The Florida Medical Association, the biggest contributor to political campaigns in the state, strongly opposed it. Dr. Jack Sapolsky, president of the Duval County (Jacksonville) Medical Society and the leading opponent, argued, "Florida has always licensed individual physicians. A physician should be licensed on his or her own merit. Every physician in Florida today has gone through that process. Our position is the licensing laws are tight to keep out bad doctors, not good doctors. The Mayo Clinic has good doctors. They don't need this legislation exemption. They just frankly don't want to be bothered with taking this examination." Sapolsky said that Florida doctors were worried about the precedent that might be established by the law. If the exemption were granted, he said, Mayo doctors might not be the only ones who would be able to slip into the state. Supermeds like Humana, which has a nonprofit subsidiary foundation, might also be able to move their doctors in.

The doctors, however, were outmatched by the grocery store owners. The Winn-Dixie exemption was approved by the Florida legislature, and Jacksonville became a wide-open city. It was an historic event. For the first time Florida doctors no longer controlled their profession. Politics now governed who would and who would not be able to practice medicine in the state. The doctors did have one brief victory: After the Winn-Dixie bill passed, the legislature enacted another law, raising the medical licensing fee for out-of-state doctors from $100 to $1,000. But the Florida Supreme Court later declared that the law was unconstitutional.

Jacksonville doctors were in a thinly disguised state of panic. Less than a year after the Mayo Clinic announcement, they were abandoning their solo practices as fast as they could shed their stethoscopes. They were organizing group practices and new financial arrangements with hospitals that were equally scared by the competition. Dr. Raymond Roberts, medical director of Riverside Hospital, said, "There are a few doctors still left in private practice in Jacksonville but in a matter of months they won't have any patients left." Jacksonville billboards, once trumpeting the comforts of Holiday Inns to travelers, were being reserved by doctors: "Need a physician? Call 393-2203."

Hospital staffs pushed their administrators to market services aggressively, hoping to establish a specialized niche and medical brand identification before the Mayo Clinic could open. St. Vincent's Medical Center proclaimed itself the local heart-lung institute. Baptist Hospital advertised itself as the regional cancer center. University Hospital told prospective patients that it was the only hospital with facilities to treat severe trauma. Some, like Memorial Medical Center, genteelly cloaked their advertising in educational garb, but others, like St. Vincent's, budgeted $350,000 for television programs that combined education and hype. Its "Health Matters" show was equal parts documentary and Phil Donahue schmaltz. After a brisk explanation of health issues, viewers were invited to call in questions to St. Vincent's doctors. Memorial Medical Center sought a niche as Jacksonville's women's center through offers of *in vitro* fertilization, breast cancer screening, and plastic surgery programs. But the results didn't come quickly enough for Memorial physicians. Six of its emergency room physicians set up two emergency clinics in direct competition with the hospital. They aggressively plastered their names and telephone numbers on billboards, handbills, even placards at bus stops. While some physicians might find such advertising distasteful, it succeeded. Before long the clinic was handling as many patients in fourteen hours as Memorial Medical Center was in twenty-four hours. In fact, said Richard A. Nixon, vice president of Clinicorp of Florida, Inc., the clinic's holding company, "Everyone has followed our lead on advertising, except for the bus stop benches—and those may be tacky but they work."

This frenzy occurred before the first Mayo Clinic doctor ever took his luggage off the airport carousel. It illustrated physicians' massive professional insecurity and the lengths to which they were willing to go to safeguard their fiefdoms. And as it turned out, they were right to be worried. After evangelist Billy Graham presided over the official opening of the Mayo Clinic late in 1986, clinic doctors were booked immediately for routine appointments through the middle of 1987.[14]

Elsewhere doctors spotted the trend toward corporate care early on. They realized that if they didn't want to be forced into alliances with the supermeds, they would have to form alliances of their own choosing. Their colleagues reacted to such self-protection with the kind of hostility usually reserved for supermeds.

Outside Rochester, New York, the highway billboards might say, "Welcome to the doctor wars."

In the countryside dairy cows contentedly nibble the grass beside 26 acres of farmland now sprouting glass-and-brick medical buildings. The three buildings, constructed at a cost of $30 million, offer 120,000 square feet of office space. The developers envision 6 more buildings that will contain an additional 250,000 square feet of space. The medical campus is similar to the ones being developed by National Medical Enterprises, but in this case the developers are local Rochester physicians.

The developers are a curious blend of medical practitioners who seem to have little in common—two separate groups of ophthalmologists and psychiatrists. Medically, they don't. But the doctors who head the two groups took a hard look at medical practice in the 1980s and drew similar conclusions.

The thirteen ophthalmologists who formed Rochester Ophthalmic Associates (ROA) in 1984 realized that the federal government was encouraging outpatient care and through technical quirks in the Medicare law would pay even higher rates for some procedures, previously limited to hospitals, if they were performed in ambulatory clinics. Led by medical director James Aquavella, they set out to develop safe, high-quality care in a new facility with the very latest technology. They now run the largest freestanding ophthalmic ambulatory surgical center in the United States.

The nine psychiatrists who make up Westfall Psychiatric Associates (WPA) also looked at the trends in health care and concluded that if they didn't change their medical styles, they could easily lose their practices. Potential patients were switching in droves from Blue Cross to health maintenance organizations that offered far fewer mental health benefits. With WPA the psychiatrists hoped to move into the expanding HMO market through prepaid services. They also saw lucrative opportunities in a New York State law that required HMOs to pay for alcohol and drug abuse treatment. They were the third group in the state to be approved for such payment.

Westfall Psychiatric Associates moved into the second building to be constructed in the former pasture. The third medical center leased space to specialists in internal medicine, oncology, neurology, immunology, obstetrics, otolaryngology, and orthopedics. Pharmacies and laboratories moved in, too.

Westfall's entrepreneurial genius was to design a treatment package that fit into the HMO psychology. HMOs hold costs down primarily by keeping patients out of hospitals. WPA specialized in the treatment of acutely ill patients who might otherwise need to be hospitalized. Dr. Joseph Messina, WPA managing partner, said, "In psychiatry this represents an unusual opportunity to demonstrate a truly cost-saving mechanism for treating patients. The average cost of acute care in an office environment amounts to $400 to $600 per week. In a hospital it's about $3,000."

WPA captured the interest of the HMO that pays for 30 days of in-patient psychiatric care, only a fourth of the 120 days covered by Blue Cross. Richard Greene, president of the Rochester Health

Network, said, "Conceptually, Westfall Associates is moving in the direction that we want to move. Whenever we can agree on a capitated or prepaid price, that's good. In psychiatry it's been extremely difficult because it's very hard for practitioners to estimate what would be reasonable in the future."

Psychiatry is traditionally conservative. Many psychiatrists still rely exclusively on talk therapy and eschew the drugs that are the by-products of research into the chemical basis of mental illness. The entrepreneurial psychiatrist is unlikely to endear himself to his traditional colleagues. And WPA associates didn't. A Rochester psychiatrist said scathingly, "Nobody's going in there to listen to music. It's a fight for turf. They're out to make a buck." Another, however, conceded more honestly, "There is some envy, some jealousy, and some belief that it will fall flat on its face. I also have some concern about the impact on individual practitioners. I don't want to see a large chunk of my practice disappear."

The former chairman of Blue Cross/Blue Shield, David Stewart, attacked the entire undertaking, charging that it would raise the cost of medical care in Rochester. "The community is paying for the facilities that have been built and it is equally clear that those who create the private diagnostic and treatment centers expect the public to pay as well," he said. "Physicians construct these buildings outside of the health care planning mechanism and then, after construction, they try to get back into the health care system for payment."

But the medical experts in Rochester who are more attuned to the future than the past see things differently. Ruth Eckelmann, executive director of Preferred Care, one of the city's fastest-growing HMOs, said, "This is not a conspiracy against one group of folks. The solo private practice psychiatrist is beginning to see what everyone else is seeing—another step in the evolution of what's happening in medicine across the country."[15]

Some physicians are joining unions in response to corporate control of medicine. Their sudden growth spurt is a symptom of the drastic changes engulfing the medical profession. By 1987 the Union of American Physicians and Dentists claimed over 43,000 of the nation's 502,000 doctors. Organizers predict geometric growth in the future. With the issues of declining incomes and eroding authority, union organizers believe they have the grievances to organize effectively.

Union president Dr. Stanley Marcus said, "What will induce doctors to join a union is unemployment, which is right over the horizon. I anticipate that given the ratio of doctors-to-population here, there will be a base line of 10,000 to 15,000 unemployed doctors in this country within the next ten years. That pool of unemployed doctors will be joining unions."

Meanwhile, physicians are joining in the hope that union membership can stanch their losses. Florida, for example, is one of the least unionized states in the country. Yet in 1985 Florida doctors conquered their innate resistance to unionization and formed the seventeenth local of the Union of American Physicians and Dentists. It was not happenstance. Florida is not only a ruthlessly competitive health care market but also in the midst of rapid colonization by the supermeds. Lured by the heavy concentration of Medicare patients, health care chains have bought out nearly half the hospitals in the state, own a hefty share of the nursing homes, and are expanding their prepaid health care plans as fast as they can print enrollment forms.

Florida doctors didn't need to be educated about the impact of corporate medicine. They could see its effect on their individual practices daily. When organizers advertised the initial meeting, stressing the union's ability to negotiate fees and services with HMOs, hospitals, and insurance companies, hundreds of doctors showed up. Within weeks the newly formed union had 250 members in Florida's five largest cities. Union organizer Arthur L. Hall, a family practitioner from Orlando, said, "Physicians don't have any choice. Overhead costs are increasing, our liabilities are increasing, and at the same time we're having to compete with corporate medicine that is siphoning off the paying patients."

Within medicine a spirited turf battle is emerging between the unions and the American Medical Association for the allegiance of doctors. The AMA adamantly opposes the union movement because it believes, correctly, that it is a threat to its own ability to speak for physicians. The AMA argues that it is already organized to do for doctors what the union promises to do. But the unions appeal to many doctors precisely because they feel that the AMA is not coping with the realities of the new medicine. AMA membership is down sharply among doctors under the age of forty because they see the association as stodgy, hidebound, and opposed to change. To fight the union's appeal, the AMA warns physicians that membership could violate the federal antitrust laws forbidding restraint of trade, although organizers say no legal problems have arisen. The AMA argues, too, in perhaps its most compelling rebuke, that physicians can't be doctors and union members at the same time. Ultimately, the AMA says, doctors in collective bargaining will be forced to choose between their duty to treat the sick and to strike. Union organizers dismiss this argument. They say that doctors don't have to pocket their stethoscopes to have power. All they need do is put away their pens, refusing to sign hospital charts and release forms to force concessions from administrators.

To a certain extent, though, the American Medical Association may be correct. The Hippocratic Oath may not be fully compatible with unionization, but a lot has changed in medicine since the third century before Christ. Hippocrates himself didn't practice in a society of prepaid medical plans and health care conglomerates. Certainly Hippocrates never heard about productivity quotas.[16]

It was productivity quotas that incensed physicians at the Group Health Association, Washington, D.C.'s, largest prepaid health plan, with 145,000 members, and led them to authorize a strike when their contract expired in 1986. The confrontation between GHA and the 160-member Capital Alliance of Physicians, a local union unaffiliated with the Union of American Physicians and Dentists, was a classic power struggle, foreshadowing many more still to come. The issue was not money, as it frequently is in labor disputes. The doctors who averaged $91,000 a year for a thirty-five-hour week weren't seeking salary increases. The issue was control over their working conditions. They believed the contract being offered by GHA would negate that control, forcing them to practice medicine under terms dictated by their employers. In particular they opposed a clause being sought by GHA that would require them to spend between twenty and thirty-five hours of their workweek exclusively on office visits. They would no longer be able to count the time devoted to hospital rounds and other duties in their weekly total, and they would also be required to work more evening shifts. To enforce these changes GHA was proposing an incentive system to increase the doctors' productivity. GHA would place 5 percent of their salaries in an escrow account. If the doctors were able to meet newly implemented patient quotas, they would get the money back—with a 5 percent bonus.

The outraged doctors quickly labeled the proposed contract "assembly line medicine." Union president Dr. Nieves Zaldivar, a pediatrician, said, "The basic issue here is that we physicians insist on continuing to have enough time with each patient to assure quality medical care."

GHA saw the situation differently. It was struggling to cope with strenuous competition and mounting costs. GHA, the oldest health maintenance organization in the Washington, D.C., area, was founded in 1937 to offer low-cost medical care to members who couldn't afford private physicians. It was a bold departure then, and almost fifty years passed before the rest of medicine caught up. Historically, GHA was not only proconsumer but also prolabor. In the three years since GHA and the Capital Alliance of Physicians sat down to bargain, however, the number of prepaid medical plans in the Washington area had proliferated. In 1986 its administrators believed it could no longer afford their liberal policies. They were convinced GHA might not survive unless they implemented new work rules. Months before negotiations were to begin, its executive director, Robert Rosenberg, invited union leaders to dinner at a French restaurant near GHA headquarters and forewarned them that negotiations would be far more difficult on the upcoming contract. To impress them with his earnestness, he announced that for the first time a corporate labor lawyer had been hired to bargain for GHA.

As Rosenberg, a pediatrician like the union president, said later, "You have to understand we are living in a very serious competitive environment and our major issue is to provide access to medical service at a reasonable price. This is not revolutionary. It is consistent with the way many physicians [now] are being reimbursed." Rosenberg described the new contract clauses as "modest changes" that would provide a badly needed boost to GHA's competitiveness.

The union rejected this argument. Doctors voted overwhelmingly to go out on strike. The doctors announced they would help with emergencies, hospitalized patients, and childbirth but would refuse to handle all other patient care. Zaldivar said the doctors deeply resented the patient quotas, which they claimed would inevitably lower the standard of care. The doctors were insulted by "the affronts to their professional ethics and standards" that were embodied in the GHA proposals. Two days after the contract expired, doctors started picketing GHA facilities. It was a strange sight. Doctors wore placards emblazoned with, "We Say 'No' to Assembly Line Medical Care" and moved briskly to keep warm in the early-morning freeze. A majority of the doctors heeded the strike call and stayed home. A substantial number of the Registered Nurses and Physical Therapists Association, another local union that had struck GHA in the past, refused to cross the picket lines.

The strike lasted for twenty-five days, costing GHA more than $1 million and forcing five thousand patients to reschedule appointments. In the meantime, the Federal Mediation and Conciliation Service tried to fashion a compromise. The resulting contract gave both GHA and the doctors a little of what they wanted. The doctors would keep their thirty-five-hour weeks but agreed to spend a few more hours a week on office visits. GHA could introduce the bitterly opposed incentive pay, rewarding doctors for treating more patients, but only after a joint labor-management committee and an arbitrator, rather than GHA alone, agreed on standards. The bonuses, however, would not exceed 3 percent, and doctors would receive a 5 percent raise over the next three years.

Both sides professed happiness with the new contract. Rosenberg said, "I think it is a fair contract which allows GHA to improve its accessibility to members." He said GHA would be better able "to generate a positive bottom line." Labor lawyer Abraham Zwerdling felt that doctors would be able to maintain their professionalism under the contract. Zwerdling said, "GHA doctors are sincere, dedicated professionals who came to practice quality medicine and didn't want to hustle patients." Of the doctors, federal mediator Emmett DeDeyn said, "They want a decent life-style appropriate to a physician, but their predominant concern was not financial status. It was patient care. . . . It was unusual to find people who were not just interested in their own self-interest and gain."

The unionization movement has begun slowly. Doctors in general haven't wanted to identify themselves, as one doctor put it, as "tradesmen." Yet economics can be far more powerful than philosophy, and doctors are beleaguered in and out of medicine as never before. They are losing out to discount doctors in organized prepaid health plans. They are being outbid by young graduates, products of the doctor boom, willing to work out of necessity for longer hours at lower pay. They are being overtaken in the competition for patients by the supermeds, who are wholesaling their products to employers. They are ceding authority to insurance companies and the federal government, which demand previews of hospital admissions and other procedures. It hasn't been easy for physicians, with their inherent philosophical biases, sliced into sometimes competing specialties, to recognize a common interest. Although patients may criticize doctors for their clannishness, the reality is different. As a doctor joked at the AMA conference, to a roomful of laughter, "The only thing that two doctors can agree on is the quality of a third's practice. It's always worse."[17]

Doctors may cherish their freedom, but as the century draws to a close that freedom is becoming an historical illusion. It belongs to a world where doctors made house calls. Doctors are becoming employees either in fact or in effect. A growing number of young doctors are seeking employment instead of setting up private practices. They need the guaranteed income to pay off their medical school loans and live comfortably at the same time. According to the American Medical Association, over 25.7 percent of physicians were employed outright by prepaid health plans or corporations in 1985, while another 20 percent, many drawing salaries, are paid directly by hospitals.

Doctors may very well need unions, but this question remains: Do their patients? Unions exist to further the economic interests of their members. They will try to frame those interests so they also appear to be in the public interest whether they are or not. The public is more likely to be sympathetic to a strike if they can be persuaded that their care is threatened than if they believe that doctors don't want to work longer shifts in the emergency room. But consumers may have less to fear from a doctors' strike than they might think. When Los Angeles surgeons announced during a strike that they would postpone all elective operations and perform emergency surgery only, the number of deaths in Los Angeles County fell for the next five weeks. During the work slowdown deaths declined by one third. When the surgeons went back to work and resumed their normal schedule, the death rate returned to normal.[18]

CHAPTER FIVE

•

Getting Less but Paying More

MEMORIAL HOSPITAL'S ADMINISTRATOR was reluctantly wrestling with a typical predicament of modern medicine. One of his staff, Dr. Jack Press, who had been at Memorial since his medical school graduation twenty years earlier, was practicing medicine as if it were still 1958 and he were kindly Dr. Marcus Welby. He had yet to grasp that while it was all right to be kind to patients, hospitals had to produce a profit in 1987. Press frequently hospitalized his elderly patients for periods that exceeded Medicare's prospective payment guidelines. Press didn't seem to understand or care that the longer a patient stayed, the less money the hospital made. At the administrator's request Memorial Hospital's chief of staff tried to explain the new medical economics to Press. After that failed to produce results, the administrator instructed the business office to compile a meticulous account of Press' patients—their diagnosis, their length of stay, and Memorial's profit or loss per admission. The administrator shuddered when the computer printout arrived. The hospital was averaging a $4,500 loss on each Medicare patient. If Memorial kept accepting Press' patients, it would eventually be bankrupt. After reviewing the computer graph, the administrator concluded unhappily that Memorial could no longer afford Press. The administrator was supposed to ensure that Memorial was run soundly, and as long as Press remained and resisted change, he would threaten its financial solvency. Press would have to be removed from the staff, his privileges and his right to admit patients revoked. The decision was economically correct, but the administrator wondered if Press challenged Memorial's action, as he very well might, whether it would be upheld in court.

Dr. Jack Press and the Memorial Hospital administrator's hypothetical problems were posed to health care experts at a Washington, D.C., conference on medical practice in the 1980s. Although the situation was conjectural, doctors and hospital administrators recognized the problem instantly. If they weren't confronting a similar dilemma, they knew a colleague who was. The chief of the medical staff at Rochester, New York's Highland Hospital said, "I think all of us will have to face this in the next year in order to survive. I think the action is justified." A New Jersey doctor agreed, pointing out that a state court had upheld the right of a hospital to dismiss a doctor on economic grounds. Another noted that Summit Health Ltd., a Los Angeles-based for-profit chain, was assembling extensive profiles on its doctors, statistically documenting their spending habits right down to the count and cost of their surgical sponges.

The doctors and administrators believed that the future of the health care industry lay in cost acounting. But to achieve this they required a strategy to handle the recalcitrant doctors, the real Dr. Jack Presses who refused to care as much about the cost of surgical sponges as their surgical skills. They needed to devise a procedure to withdraw the privileges of their money-losing physicians and avoid a lawsuit.

As they debated, a doctor from Milwaukee, Wisconsin, stood up. "What about the interests of the patients?" he asked. "Certain DRGs we know are money-losing DRGs and we may try to avoid them if this kind of action is going to be initiated by a hospital against a doctor. Then he may try to avoid certain losing DRGs and those patients will be dumped somewhere else and we may not want to care for them. If a hospital is going to be like a Big Brother watching us, if you have organizations keeping profiles on us—what we spend for a given treatment, if those are going to be taken into consideration in keeping our appointment on a medical staff—then I think care will suffer in the long run."

In fact, care is already suffering, and the likelihood is that quality will deteriorate further as a result of prospective payment. The diagnosis-related groups are reversing three decades in health care. During those years health insurance insulated hospitals and doctors, separating medicine and money so that costs were removed from the marketplace. With prospective payment the federal government reconfigured cash and care, calculating the worth of care independent of the cost of rendering it. The old system produced spiraling health care inflation; the new system is apt to create a steady decline in quality of health care for most Americans. John Morse, who runs Humana's Care Plus, said, "Only the very rich are going to be able to afford the kind of health care system that existed in this country from the inception of Medicare in 1964 through the early 1980s, when the government decided to end the cost spiral. We're in a dilemma. We can't afford what we've got and we don't want to give it up."

The elderly are not the only ones who will be affected, although they are the first. Prospective payment is being steadily adopted by private insurers for patients who are under age sixty-five. Blue Cross and Blue Shield, which process Medicare claims in many states, were the first to grasp that if prospective payment was extended to all patients, insurers could cut costs. Blue Cross was operating on Medicare's cost-plus reimbursement system. It paid hospitals for the costs of their services plus a profit, and it was watching those costs increase by 15 to 20 percent a year. To be sure, Blue Cross passed its costs on to consumers through rate increases, but its officials began to worry that premiums might become so expensive that the average American could no longer afford them. Blue Cross realized that prospective payment might be able to contain costs and forestall further premium increases. By 1987 Blue Cross was applying the Medicare system of fixed payments based on illness to policyholders in New Jersey, Kansas, Oklahoma, Arizona, and Nebraska. Pilot programs are being tested in Florida and Michigan. Superficially, consumers have seen few changes. They still pay their insurance premiums, their deductibles, and their copayments. Behind the scenes, however, everything has changed. The insurance companies are telling hospitals that they will pay so much and no more to treat policyholders. In doing so, they are enlarging the number of patients who can produce profits for hospitals if their costs are less than the fixed rate. Neal L. Maslan, vice president of American Medical International, said, "From a purely cost perspective, it's the only way to go. The question is whether you want it to apply to your family."

While the supermeds and DRGs are natural allies, nonprofit hospitals are being transformed, too. The combination of fixed rates and supermed competition is pressuring nonprofit hospitals to review their operations and behave more like for-profits. A "profits first" atmosphere is being fostered in these institutions. The upheaval has been so great that Dr. Merlin K. DuVal, president of the American Healthcare Institute, which represents nonprofits, said in 1987, "The nonprofit hospital will likely disappear from the scene as we now know it."

Under the prospective payment arrangement doctors like Jack Press can jeopardize profits. Doctors have the authority to order services and procedures that may cost the hospital more to provide than they can expect to get paid. Hospitals naturally find that objectionable, but doctors oppose restraints on their power and their wallets. Physicians earn over 50 percent of their income from the delivery of services to hospital patients, according to the Department of Health and Human Services. Even while the supermeds have been increasing their profits through DRGs, the federal government has provided an impressive weapon against physicians, the Professional Review Organizations. PROs are private for-profit companies staffed by doctors, nurses, and other health care professionals and that contract with the federal government to review hospital cases. They oversee hospitals' performances under the fixed-rate system. The PROs, one for each state, search through Medicare claims for dubious care or unnecessary hospital admissions. They have the authority to deny payment to a hospital if they find the care was unjustified. If they deny a sufficient number of claims, the federal government will renew their contracts. If they aren't so meticulous in their denials, their contract may not be continued. In short, the PROs stay in business if they help to ration care. The PROs are thriving with an average profit of 8.3 percent. In 1987 HHS charged that some PROs were making "excessive profits" of 20 percent or more. The PROs and for-profit hospitals are natural collaborators because they have a common financial incentive to restrain care.

PROs have broad powers, and doctors say those powers are used capriciously. Dr. Edward McKenzie, a general surgeon in a small North Carolina town, told a Senate hearing about a urology patient who was hospitalized for a bladder tumor. It was cauterized and three days later the patient was discharged; then she began to bleed and was readmitted. McKenzie said, "The first [payment] was denied because the guidelines indicated admission was not necessary. The second [payment] was denied because the patient was discharged too soon from the first admission."[1]

Despite these complaints the PROs are determined to change the way that medicine is practiced. Their announced goals are to cut hospital admissions by nearly 300,000, shift almost 600,000 patients from hospitals to outpatient clinics, and eliminate another 425,000 admissions to targeted hospitals by specific doctors. In its arbitrarily defined quotas, Health Care Review, Inc., the Maine PRO, for instance, wrote the Department of Health and Human Services, "Health Care Review, Inc., projects that approximately 394 Medicare admissions will occur during the contract interval for total knee replacements. Health Care Review, Inc., will reduce the admissions by 86 cases resulting in 308 admissions. . . . Health Care Review, Inc., projects that approximately 684 Medicare admissions will occur during the contract interval for total hip replacements. HCR, Inc., will reduce the admissions by 203 cases resulting in 481 cases." The PRO then went on to translate these statewide target figures into quotas for individual hospitals. Their orders were explicit and extraordinarily precise. Different hospitals were told to cut their number of procedures by 1.8 or 6.6 or 11.4 cases.[2]

When the New Jersey PRO issued guidelines on hospital admissions for abdominal hernias, the surgical staff of Morristown Memorial Hospital protested that they violated standard medical practice. According to *Principles of Surgery,* "All hernias of the abdominal wall should be subjected to prompt surgical correction." But the New Jersey PRO said that surgery should be restricted to patients who were under the age of seventy-five, in pain, and who could not be treated by alternate procedures. Dr. Warren D. Widmann, a surgeon for eighteen years and an assistant professor of surgery at Rutgers Medical School, protested in a letter to the PRO, "The elderly are being singled out for a form of treatment that carries recognized risk, and I gather that if they choose to proceed with surgery, there would be no reimbursement for the hospital or surgical fees engendered. This represents, as best I can see it, discrimination against the elderly."

The PROs put extraordinary pressure on hospitals, but hospitals are learning to use that pressure to modify their doctors' behavior and boost profits. Dr. Clarence Avery, a San Leandro, California, surgeon and former president of the California Medical Association, said, "This is the first step in the rationing of health care in this country—and it's being directed primarily toward the elderly."[3] The American Medical Association started a study of prospective payment shortly after the program began. The results were immediately obvious. Some 42 percent of the doctors complained of pressure from hospital administrators to compromise medical care. Their grievances are compelling:

- "As a practicing urologist in a small community hospital, I find the patients, physicians, and hospital personnel in great disarray, confusion, and displeasure. . . . The patients are treated callously and harassed by an attempt to expedite procedures. . . . I, as a physician, have found it very difficult to practice quality medical care in this environment of harassment, urgency, and cutting short corners."
- "There is no question that during the medical staff meetings, the administration is no longer concerned about the welfare of the patient. The only concern that we ever discuss in staff meetings, much to my objection, is the economics of the patient."
- "We have the hospital administration telling us to treat one medical problem at a time: clearly contrary to our training to treat the total health problems of the patient in the most efficient manner. We are under unsubtle pressure to cut days and utilization of services: clearly a compromise of our right to exercise our best medical judgment."
- "Our administrator has initiated a system of yellow and red

stickers to be placed on the charts as the magic allotted figure [of days allocated for that DRG] nears consumption. It is very disconcerting to see these stickers on charts of patients who are critically ill and recently post-op."

- "[The fixed-rate system] has affected relations among administrators and physicians, since physicians are being told they cannot maintain patients in the hospital at a stay longer than what the hospital is able to afford even if the patient should still be in the hospital, but the hospital cannot afford this [and still make a profit]. It is creating stress between administrators and physicians and between physicians and utilization review physicians."[4]

Dr. John Dawson, a Seattle surgeon and AMA board member, told the U.S. House Select Committee on Aging, "While physicians have been trained to be advocates for and protectors of their patients' health, physicians are increasingly being pushed into the uncomfortable and objectionable role of being the advocate and protector of the federal budget. Physicians who err on the side of patient advocacy are, at a minimum, subject to challenge; at worst, they are subject to severe sanctions." Moreover, many physicians don't seem to be resisting. They may complain to the American Medical Association, but they aren't objecting loudly enough to the hospital administration. Doctors who have endured rigorous training, who confront death and disease daily, seem to quail before hospital administrators. Dawson conceded that doctors had not protested vehemently, but he explained, "Physicians and hospitals have had a love-hate relationship not too dissimilar from some marriages for years." When doctors are urged to put their hospital above their patients, Dawson said, many do because they don't want their hospital to fail. If it closes, they may have trouble locating a new staff appointment at a convenient facility. In short, they go along because it is convenient and because they worry about retaliation. As one doctor told the AMA, "I think the handwriting is on the wall, however, that hospitals will keep 'physician profiles' and from these may eventually determine that it is not profitable to keep certain physicians on the medical staff."

The fear is legitimate. Dr. Karl K. Kellawan of Bakersfield, California, told the U.S. Senate Special Committee on Aging, "I have a profile in one of the hospitals [where] I practice. Right now I am a good guy because I make money for them. But next week I may be a bad guy because they lose money. They can coerce you in many ways. You want to admit patients to the hospital; they say, well, no, there are no beds available. They can intimidate you by endeavoring to get you kicked off the staff when you do not do your charts on time. I am not a surgeon, but, for example, I do certain endoscopic procedures, [and] they can make it difficult for you scheduling patients. We do not have time to do it; we can do it next week for you. So there are a lot of techniques that are being developed to so-call punish you."[5] Some specialists are particularly vulnerable to these profit-and-loss evaluations because of their practices. Dr. Joseph C. Barbaccia, a specialist in geriatric care at the University of California at San Francisco Medical School, testified, "From the hospital's perspective, the most desirable patient the doctor can admit is one whose diagnosis is paid for most generously, consumes the 'right' number of services during the hospital stay, stays for as few days as possible, and when ready to leave will do so as quickly as possible. Obviously, the patients of some specialists, e.g., of cardiovascular surgeons who require coronary bypass procedures, are very welcome, while those of other specialists are not, e.g., the chronic pulmonary patient who has no family, is in repeated pulmonary failure and unlikely to recover but requires a prolonged hospital stay."[6]

Doctors are reluctant to complicate their lives unduly, and in Thomasville, North Carolina, doctors responded as Dawson predicted. Dr. Thomas H. Byrnes, a physician on the staff of Community General Hospital, told the U.S. Senate Special Committee on Aging that he understood and sympathized with the hospital administrators. "The hospital cannot afford to encourage admissions in cases where arbitrary retrospective review may lead to denial of payment and the additional risk of potential sanctions or other penalties on the hospital," he said. "This system promotes the unavoidable effort on the part of the hospital to discourage any but the most obviously indicated admissions. This inevitably causes the Medicare beneficiary to suffer unnecessary pain or risk of bad results. . . . Even the most competent and qualified physician cannot avoid being unduly influenced by the pressure."

In the first two years under prospective payment, there were one thousand fewer Medicare patients in the hospital; the average length of stay dropped from 7.5 days to 6.3 days. The hospital responded by closing one wing and eliminating thirty-five jobs. Yet, according to Medical Review of North Carolina, the state PRO, too many Medicare patients were being admitted. The PRO required that doctors call its utilization panel and receive prior approval before hospitalizing Medicare patients. Otherwise the federal government would refuse to pay the bills. Moreover, the PRO sent a speaker to a meeting of the hospital's doctors. Perry T. Jones, the hospital president, recalled, "A review organization spoke to our medical staff and said, among other things, that if you have a certain number of admissions denied, you will end up on what amounts to a blacklist. That had an effect on my physicians' behavior. . . . [N]o physician wants to be on any kind of a blacklist where he looks bad compared to his peers or in the eyes of the general public." The doctors began to change. They tried to admit patients only if reimbursement was assured. Dr. James Hunter, an internist and chairman of Community General Hospital's utilization review committee, testified that unfortunately local doctors no longer can rely only on their medical texts and expertise to decide if a patient should be hospitalized. Instead they also consult a DRG handbook published by a North Carolina hospital for physicians.

Since the doctors changed their habits, both the hospital and their patients have been affected. Hospital finances have improved dramatically. Its Medicare reimbursement rate has gone up 10 percent, from 63 to 73 percent of its charges. Jones said, "This certainly is a positive step and one for which we are very appreciative."[7] Patients, however, have not fared nearly as well. Hunter said, "We are really powerless to admit patients that common sense and compassion dictate belong in the hospital." As an example, he cited an eighty-two-year-old woman in excruciating but intermittent pain from breast cancer that had spread to her spine. He said, "Both her family and she desire admission to our local hospital, but this cannot be done unless orders are written for intramuscular injection of pain relievers at least three times daily, medication she may not need that often." The cancer patient was denied admission because the hospital couldn't be absolutely certain her bills would be paid.

Financial risk and economic reward have intruded into the doctor-patient relationship in a previously unimaginable manner, according to Dr. Marianne J. Legato, a professor at Columbia University College of Physicians and Surgeons. At a New York Academy of Medicine conference on physician-patient relations she explained the cynical calculations that influence hospital admissions. According to Legato, a doctor now must question not only whether a patient needs to be hospitalized but also whether the decision can be justified to Medicare or the insurance company. If payment is refused, the doctor must speculate if the patient can pay or if the hospital will be liable. And the doctor must wonder if he has the time to challenge a denial. In the end, Legato said, the doctor must decide if the patient can be treated at home with far less trouble and financial risk. "And," she said, "if there is a financial catastrophe, the patient is seventy-two years old—that's really enough time to have lived anyway."

If physicians are troubled by that calculus, hospitals can exercise an extraordinary array of powers to influence their behavior. Dr. Sigmund Greenberg, professor at Temple University Medical School and an internist in Abington, Pennsylvania, testified at a Senate hearing to threats. "Things have reached the point that if enough of the physician's patients cause a deficit in reimbursement to the hospital, he may be threatened with dismissal from the staff, the loss of privileges, or else invited to join the staff of another hospital that can, quote, 'afford him,' unquote," Greenberg said. "Paid hospital staff, persons whose livelihoods depend on the goodwill of the hospital administration, call doctors . . . to pressure them into . . . alter[ing] records of discharge diagnoses in order to obtain as much money as possible. We are asked to rearrange the discharge sheet listing the illness treated in such a way to get the most financially out of the patient's admission. The aim is for the hospital to profit from the DRGs."

One of Greenberg's patients was admitted to a nearby hospital for treatment of diabetes, where it was discovered that he had incurable cancer of the pancreas, cancer that had spread to his liver and skeletal system. The cancer was causing the diabetes. Shortly afterward, still in the hospital, the patient died of cardiac arrest. Three weeks later, a physician on the hospital utilization review panel asked Greenberg to revise the patient's records. The physician told Greenberg, "If you put down that the patient has cancer, metastatic, of the liver and the bone, we will get [an extra] $1,600." Greenberg said, "At first, I fought. But after a while, you get tired of fighting. You only have so many hours a day. And then you say, 'Yes,' because really, you are not saying anything that is not truthful. You are just rearranging in a numerical way the diagnosis." The legal niceties and ethics are shoved aside, and the next time the doctor, who has acquiesced once, may not protest at all.

Greenberg claimed that many patients are discharged to die. "Doctors are coerced into sending patients [like his cancer patient] out of the hospital long before it is medically, morally, or ethically reasonable. They are forced by the cold-blooded use of the so-called utilization review committee. Without regard to the emotional impact on the patient or the family and without recourse to any appeal process, these people willingly force the discharge of this kind of patient," he said. "The hospital feels it is more important to be in the black and in a positive financial state than to try to cure the patient or to make life easier for the family."

At Greenberg's hospital doctors are sent regular computer printouts on the amount and source of revenue that they're generating. The bimonthly reports give the diagnosis, the total amount of Medicare reimbursement, the hospital charge and cost, and the profit or loss to the final penny. In 1985 the reports showed that the hospital was losing money on Greenberg's patients. Between January and March Greenberg admitted 368 patients whose care cost the hospital $24,083.59 more than it was reimbursed by Medicare. Earlier the hospital administration had notified its medical staff, "Everyone should be familiar with the 'ground rules,' have an opportunity to ask questions, and then I believe peer acceptance will be followed by peer pressure to make the system work smoothly."

Greenberg charged that the hospital mobilized his fellow physicians and enlisted their help in its campaign against him. He said it began at an April staff meeting when he and two other physicians were identified as sources of lost revenues. The two physicians were reported to have hospitalized heart attack patients unduly long but "after some discussion and exchanges of letters," the doctors were now discharging more quickly, according to a hospital memorandum. "The changes in statistics were viewed by those present as representing satisfactory improvement although somewhat slow," according to meeting minutes. But Greenberg presented a slightly different problem. The hospital was losing money because, after reviewing his patients' medical histories, Medicare was denying payment for their admissions. Greenberg was responsible for over 40 percent of all hospital denials and, as the minutes pointed out, this could cause yet another problem. "If the denial rate goes above 1 percent, Blue Cross will withdraw our advance utilization review privilege, which is very undesirable," the medical staff was informed. "The problem with [Dr. Greenberg] has continued into 1985. There has been a sharp increase in the number of denials by Blue Cross and we are above the 1 percent rate presently endangering our advance review privilege." Unless Greenberg changed, the revenue loss would continue and the rest of the staff would suffer a major inconvenience. Like the North Carolina doctors, they would need the PRO's prior approval to hospitalize patients. In June 1985 two members of the utilization review committee and Greenberg met for two hours to discuss his practice patterns. In July the chairman of the department of medicine complained that Greenberg's chart notes were inadequate on a recent admission. "It is evident that the patient was really here for a long time and it may have been possible to shorten that stay," he wrote. "The issue is communication. It would have been most useful if you had written a direct response to the [utilization review] committee's inquiry, which was placed in the chart on several occasions in the form of the orange sticker. At no point did I see it clearly expressed that 'this patient needs to be in the hospital because . . .' "

In September 1985 Greenberg testified before the Special Committee on Aging: "There is more to this than another cumbersome bureaucratic burden. There is a basic corruption of the system here. . . . The aim is for the hospital to profit from the DRGs. . . . I should not be penalized because I choose to care for complicated, very sick patients or because I care for patients of limited means." In the present hospital environment, Greenberg said, "I have great difficulty maintaining the quality of care I am trained to administer because of the constant badgering of the utilization review committee."[8]

If hospital and peer pressure fail, hospitals can try financial inducements. Paracelsus Healthcare, a for-profit chain based in Pasadena, California, instituted its Physicians' Sharing Cost Savings Program at its fourteen hospitals in 1985. Under its incentive plan doctors were given a cash rebate whenever they helped the hospitals break even or make a profit on Medicare patients. The doctors were paid on a graduated, complex formula that increased as the amount spent by the hospital on the Medicare patient declined. Paracelsus added up its charges and Medicare payments once a month and then wrote a check to individual physicians. If the Medicare reimbursements for Dr. Smith's patients were $5,000 above the hospital charges, for instance, Dr. Smith would receive $3,275 that month as his rebate on the hospital's savings. Paracelsus' president, Ron Messenger, dismissed criticism of the immediately controversial plan, arguing in an interview on the AMA's cable television network, "The payment to the physician for each individual patient is so small that physicians would not want to jeopardize themselves from a malpractice or legal point of view by giving lesser quality care. The physician receives reimbursement for the whole population of patients he treats within a period of one month."

Paracelsus officials said that the plan was a prudent business decision, set up with the advice of attorneys who assured the corporation it was legal, and that participation in cost savings was voluntary. Doctors weren't being forced to accept the rebates, but as Bruce Harris, the chain's director of reimbursement, said, "We've had no complaints when the checks were issued." However, the American Medical Association, which called for a federal investigation, wasn't convinced that the plan was either legal or wise. Dr. Mitchell Carlin, president of the Los Angeles Medical Association, said, "There is a temptation for physicians to be led by monetary interests to admit patients more frequently, to admit patients who may not have to be admitted to an acute care hospital or could be treated as an outpatient, or to ping-pong patients by admitting them again and again."[9]

After investigating the Paracelsus plan, the U.S. General Accounting Office (GAO) also concluded that physicians were likely to be tempted by such enticing financial rewards to their patients' detriment. Physicians could shuffle their practices, the GAO said, so that many low-cost patients were admitted to Paracelsus hospitals in a month. To accomplish this they had simply to postpone admitting seriously ill patients or send them to another hospital. They could also order fewer services or discharge the patients before they were sufficiently recovered. The GAO concluded, "We believe that certain features of the plan make the incentives too strong for physicians to underprovide services or admit patients to the hospital who might not need hospitalization." Congress passed a law in 1986 that would forbid such incentive plans after April 1, 1989. A spokesman for Congressman Fortney Stark, Democrat of California, who sponsored the law, said, "It puts too much of a financial conflict on the physician who's got two kids entering college."[10]

Surveys conducted beginning in 1985 by the American Medical Association and the American Society of Internal Medicine reveal that hospital pressure is constant and widespread.* Doctors in all medical specialties throughout the United States reported it. At least 80 percent of physicians said that hospitals are pushing them to change their style of practice. Nearly that many said they have been asked to discharge patients faster. Ten percent were asked to reduce the number of elderly patients they hospitalized, while 21 percent were asked to increase the total number of patients they admitted. Over 17 percent were specifically told not to admit patients with certain money-losing diagnoses or encouraged to send them to other hospitals. Another 17 percent complained that hospitals were trying to identify and deny or restrict privileges to doctors who lost the facility money. Over 50 percent said they had been asked to limit the use of expensive diagnostic tests or reduce

*In 1978 the American Society of Internal Medicine released an updated survey that confirmed its initial findings.

the number of procedures that are done on inpatients. Eighteen percent said that hospital care previously considered medically necessary was being denied.

Such intense pressure can continue only so long before patients begin to be hurt. Consumers are at risk in numerous ways. If patients need to be hospitalized, they may not be admitted. If they don't need hospital care, they may be admitted unnecessarily. An alarming number of doctors agree that patients are being harmed. In 1985 over 66 percent told their medical societies that the quality of care in their hospitals was declining. Some 40 percent conceded that they are discharging patients faster. Almost 35 percent of the doctors said that in the month preceding the survey they readmitted a patient who had been released recently, a telling indication that the discharge had come too soon. Nearly 10 percent said they readmitted five or more patients. Astonishingly, in view of their legal and moral obligations, virtually every doctor who admitted that a patient was discharged early also conceded that the patient suffered as a result. Half said that their patients became sicker or died. Significantly, 27 percent of doctors on the staff of for-profit hospitals say they have less freedom to make these clinical decisions than their colleagues in other hospitals.[11]

Doctors aren't the only ones who believe that care is declining. Patients also feel that callous treatment and life-threatening conditions exist in the nation's hospitals. Louis Harris and Associates reported in 1986 that a broad cross section of Americans are affected. An estimated 2.6 million Americans a year are discharged prematurely, according to the polling organization. A majority said they experienced continuing or worsening medical problems as a result, and nearly eight hundred thousand said they were readmitted to a hospital. People most likely to say they left too soon had household incomes under $15,000 or were on Medicaid. Humphrey Taylor, president of Louis Harris and Associates, said, "The data suggest very strongly that premature release is a major and quite rapidly increasing problem." Yet if 12 percent of respondents said they were discharged too early, 9 percent felt they had stayed too long. Taylor suggested that hospitals may try to keep some privately insured patients because of financial incentives to prolong treatment.[12]

While hospitals search for the economically attractive ill and pressure the staff to produce them, patients and their families who are unaware of these financial manipulations can be plunged into chaos. As they recuperate, the hospital administrator may send a notice like the form letter sent on October 3, 1984, to a patient of Dr. Sigmund Greenberg:

> The Utilization Review Committee has reviewed your medical record and has determined that continued hospitalization in an acute care hospital is no longer medically necessary and/or appropriate. You no longer require twenty-four-hour continuous attention of trained medical and paramedical personnel and further hospitalized care is no longer needed.
>
> Your attending physician, Dr. S. Greenberg, has been contacted. The Hospital Administration and the Business Office have been notified of this decision. The Medicare program will cover your hospital stay for an additional one day from the date of this letter to allow you or your representative to make arrangements for transfer. Therefore, after October 4, additional expenses incurred during this admission will not be reimbursed under the Medicare Program of the Social Security Act.
>
> This means that after October 4 you will be personally responsible for the payment of any charges incurred during your stay.

For a seriously ill patient to be confronted with an immediate order to leave within twenty-four hours or to start paying hundreds of dollars a day for care is frightening. Most patients aren't able to pay the bill for their continued care. They may be too sick or unsophisticated to challenge the hospital administration. They may not be able to trust their doctor to intercede. Many will react to such a notice like the sixty-eight-year-old man who was admitted for treatment of vomiting and shortness of breath. He suffered, too, from severe emphysema and heart failure. In the hospital he was diagnosed with a hiatal hernia, and his lung problems worsened. Nevertheless, even though his vomiting and breathing difficulties continued, the patient was told to leave after eight days. According to Senate investigators, the man panicked and insisted on leaving because he was unable to pay for extra days in the hospital. He left, but he never arrived home. He died in his own driveway.

Senator John Heinz, Republican of Pennsylvania, convened a series of hearings that revealed the devastating impact of hospitals' drive to maximize profits. During the hearings Heinz coined the phrase "quicker and sicker" to describe the hospital practice of discharging patients before they were ready. Heinz accused hospitals of judging patients by their profit potential and doctors by their revenue-generating ability.

Betty F. Kratt of Bakersfield, California, described the problems that began when her eighty-five-year-old mother required hospitalization. Her mother was ill with multiple ailments including kidney failure, high blood pressure, and a heart condition. She was also blind and hard of hearing. On January 9, 1985, Kratt took her mother, suffering from a heart attack and kidney failure, to the hospital. Kratt said, "She was so weak and unable to feed herself. She was on oxygen twenty-four hours a day, and her heart was so bad that her skin color had turned blue. During her hospital stay my mother required around-the-clock oxygen, she had a catheter, IV tubes, and a feeding tube." By almost any standard her mother was seriously ill. Kratt testifed to the Senate committee about what happened next. "Then, on January 29, I received a call from the hospital stating that my mother would have to go to a nursing home because she no longer needed their acute level of care," she said. "On January 31 they sent for an ambulance and transferred her to a nursing home. . . . I did everything I could to prevent them from moving her, but they told me that Medicare would not let her stay any longer and they were losing money on her. To make matters worse, the hospital informed the nursing home that she was able to feed and bathe herself and also had bathroom privileges. This was absolutely not true. She could not move at all. My mother passed away on February 1, just fourteen hours after entering the nursing home."

Kratt has nightmares about her mother's death and dreams about her own solitary death. "I still wake up at night trying to sort out all the events and what can be done to stop this from happening to our older people," she said. "I am sixty-five years old myself and my husband is sixty-six years old and we are heading down this same road and I do not want any part of it. I have been very angry over all this. I feel like all of this is what has killed my mother. It is just like murder to me."[13]

Dr. Karl K. Kellawan, her mother's physician, was not consulted about the transfer. He, too, was dismayed by the hospital's action. Calling the discharge "inhumane," Kellawan asserted that his patient was released in an unstable condition. "[T]o state that this patient was stable and in a condition to be transferred to a nursing home was a lie," he said. Kellawan added that in his opinion the hospital could be sued successfully for malpractice with an award ranging up to $250,000. No suit was filed.

Hospitals have discovered that some patients who aren't generating revenues can become money-makers if they're discharged and readmitted. Hospitals ping-pong patients from ward to home and back again. Harrison Seeley, seventy-two years old, began his odyssey through Milwaukee hospitals when his doctor spotted a small tumor on his bladder. The tumor, malignant but localized, was removed successfully. After a week Seeley was sent home, although he now had a new problem. He was suffering from back pain so excruciating that he could barely walk. The hospital, however, had admitted Seeley for bladder surgery, and his allotted time for postoperative recovery was up.

A week later a new physician, an orthopedic specialist, sent Seeley to a different hospital, where he was put in traction. After six days the doctor walked into his room, stood at the foot of his bed, and informed Seeley that once again his Medicare stay was nearly over and he would be released the next day. Seeley's seventy-year-old wife, Dorothy, who was also in poor health, protested, "I can't handle him. How can I take care of him when he's in such pain?" The doctor brushed aside her worries. "Dorothy," he said, "I have to put on a different hat now. The hospital administrator is on my back, and Harrison has to leave. I know he's not ready to go home and you know he is not ready to go home but he has to go home." Seeley was discharged in such pain that an ambulance was needed for his trip home. When Dorothy Seeley recalled the episode later to the U.S. House Select Committee on Aging, she was still outraged: "Can you imagine, I drove him to the hospital so that he could have his back pain treated. Yet when the hospital let him go, he was in such bad shape, they had to call an ambulance."

The couple struggled through the weekend. Seeley was rendered helpless by his pain, unable to turn over in bed unaided, barely able to get to the bathroom. The Seeleys cried for two days. On Monday Dorothy called the doctor; on Tuesday Seeley returned by ambulance to the hospital that had discharged him only three days earlier. He had a CAT scan; then the ambulance took him home. On Thursday the doctor called the Seeleys. He had bad news: The CAT scan showed Seeley had cancer of the spine. The doctor ordered Seeley to the hospital a third time, for radiation therapy. Again he went by ambulance.

Dorothy said, "We asked ourselves: Why in the world didn't the doctors at the first hospital look at his spine when he went for bladder surgery? Why wasn't the diagnosis made before he was sent home in such pain from the second hospital? Why was everyone so much more anxious to get him out of the hospital than they were to find out why his back hurt so much? The people we trusted to take care of Harrison seemed to put Medicare payment first. To them the cancer hiding in his spine was secondary. This should not have happened to us."[14]

The Seeleys and Kratt offer eloquent testimony that hospitals can't always generate maximum profits unless quality of care is sacrificed. Because of that William Hoffman, director of the Social Security department at the United Auto Workers Union, believes that for-profit hospitals threaten the nation's health. He told a hearing of the Institute of Medicine, a federally funded independent research organization, "The competition [for-profit institutions] are advocating is between profits and quality of care—with the consumer caught in the middle." The supermeds are breeding a generation of corporate medical buccaneers who are willing to place profits ahead of quality. As Wall Street analyst David Lothson points out, "If Medicare is not paying its way, if insurers are demanding greater and greater cost concessions, a decline in the standard and quality of hospital care may be inevitable. . . . The concept of downgrading the product delivered is a standard response in virtually every other industry; we believe it is an inevitable response in the hospital industry given the demands of the providers."[15]

There are frightening indications that patients with the same conditions or hospitalized for the same procedures may be more likely to die in supermed facilities. The possibility that supermeds may be hazardous to their patients' health emerges from millions of statistics that the federal government has been collecting since prospective payment began. Before the establishment of diagnostic-related groupings, hospitals could not be judged easily on their performance, and comparisons among them were difficult. But by classifying treatments and procedures into categories, DRGs set up a mechanism that could be used to measure performance. Information on hospitals and Medicare beneficiaries has been filed in government computers since 1983. At the punch of a button the computers can spew out individual hospital profiles that enable comparisons to be made on charges, levels of reimbursements, lengths of stay, and mortality rates. The same information can be used to draw comparisons between for-profit and nonprofit facilities. Statistics have been released despite the adamant objection of the hospital industry, and it is obvious that wide disparities exist. Patients die more frequently and are charged higher rates at some facilities than at others in the same community.

When mortality rates were compiled on the twenty most frequent DRGs at South Florida hospitals during a nine-month period, the results, as reported by the South Florida Medical Review, were startling. Patients weren't just more likely to die of some causes at many supermed hospitals; in many instances their chances of dying were geometrically higher. While several Florida supermed hospitals compiled death rates in the double digits for some DRGs, many other hospitals in the same community reported no deaths at all.

Five Humana hospitals accounted for the highest death rates for six out of twenty DRGs. For example, patients were thirty-three times more likely to die of cerebrovascular disorders at Humana Hospital-Bennett than at Mercy Hospital, a church-operated facility. Almost one out of three patients who were admitted to Humana Hospital-Bennett with this diagnosis died; Mercy Hospital reported no deaths out of sixty-seven admissions. They were twenty times more likely to die of chronic pulmonary obstruction at Humana Hospital-Bennett than at twenty-three other South Florida hospitals, which reported no deaths. Patients who were admitted for major bowel procedures were almost fifteen times more likely to die at Humana Hospital-Biscayne than if the procedure were at nonprofit South Miami Hospital. Patients died of digestive disorders at Humana Hospital-South Broward almost five times more often than at twenty other nonprofit hospitals. At Humana Hospital-Cypress patients who were admitted for prostate surgery were about four and a half times more likely to die than at twenty other hospitals.

But Humana wasn't the only supermed whose South Florida hospitals had notably high death rates. At Doctors Hospital of Lake Worth, a Hospital Corporation of America facility, patients died of pneumonia almost twenty-one times as often as at Mercy Hospital. At AMI's Southeastern Medical Center, patients died of kidney infections eleven and a half times more frequently than at four other hospitals. At Republic Health Corporation's John F. Kennedy Memorial Hospital, patients died of cardiac arrhythmias seven times as often as at seventeen other hospitals. At National Medical Enterprises' Delray Community Hospital, patients who were admitted with back problems were twice as likely to die as at thirty-one nonprofit South Florida hospitals.[16]

Similar differences showed up between mortality rates at some supermed facilities and other hospitals in data that were released in 1987 by California Medical Review, Inc., the state professional review organization. California Medical Review released the death rate for patients in common diagnostic-related groups at individual hospitals and the statewide averages. While patients with heart failure had an average mortality rate of 9.2 percent, the mortality rate at Summit's Santa Ana Hospital Medical Center was 21.5 percent. Patients with pneumonia had average death rates of 12.3 percent, but at National Medical Enterprises' Granada Hills Community Hospital the mortality rate was 22 percent. Stroke victims had a 15.6 percent death rate statewide, but at AMI's Medical Center of North Hollywood their mortality rate was 26.2 percent. At NME's Placentia-Linda Community Hospital the death rate for stroke victims was also 26.2 percent, while at Twin Cities Community Hospital, another NME facility, it was 23.7 percent. Heart attack patients had an average death rate of 20.4 percent in California, but at NME's Doctors Hospital of Montclair it was 32.8 percent and at its Ojai Valley Community Hospital it was 30.9

percent. The mortality figure was also above average, 33.3 percent, at AMI's San Dimas Community Hospital. Patients who underwent heart bypass surgery had an average statewide mortality rate of 7.2 percent, but at HCA's Brotman Medical Center their death rate was 13.5 percent.[17]

In 1988 the Public Citizen Health Research Group, a Ralph Nader organization, compared the death rate for severe acute heart disease at hospitals operated by nonprofit Kaiser and AMI. Sixty-five percent of the Kaiser hospitals fell into the lowest-mortality category for that DRG as established by the Department of Health and Human Services; only 7 percent of AMI hospitals did. No Kaiser hospitals were in the highest-mortality category; 20 percent of AMI facilities were.

There may not be a single explanation of these varying mortality rates, but the reasons may very well lie in different medical styles that are practiced at the hospitals. Evidence already exists that supermed hospitals are inferior in significant respects to their nonprofit competitors. According to the Institute of Medicine, supermeds hire fewer personnel, and as a result their patients receive three hours a day less of staff time than patients at nonprofit facilities. Supermeds hand out staff credentials more freely, screening doctors who apply for admitting privileges less rigorously and, as a result, their doctors tend to be less qualified. Supermeds have fewer staff doctors who have passed the competency tests that are administered by the medical specialty boards. Many of their surgeons, in particular, lack board certification. At supermed hospitals about 67 percent of surgeons were board-certified compared to nearly 80 percent at private nonprofit hospitals and 76.5 percent at nonfederal government facilities. Many of these differences were attributed to the for-profits' need to bring in revenue and produce profits. By expanding the medical staff, they increase the number of potential patients.

Even physicians who practice at for-profit hospitals question their ability to deliver proper care. According to the Institute of Medicine, among these doctors 24 percent say that patients receive better care in nonprofit hospitals, while 28 percent say that a hospital can't be operated properly as a for-profit corporation. Among all doctors a mere 7 percent say they would prefer to practice at a for-profit hospital, perhaps because only 9 percent believe they have the same amount of clinical freedom in those facilities.[18]

Certainly, Dr. Norman Silversmith, a West Palm Beach, Florida, psychiatrist, believed that the administrators of National Medical Enterprises' Lake Hospital interfered with his attempts to treat patients properly. Silversmith became disturbed by the conditions at the Lake Worth, Florida, facility and wrote a lengthy memo in August 1982 detailing threats to patient safety and well-being. He says he received no reply and the administration took no action to correct conditions at the small psychiatric hospital. Troubled by the lack of response, Silversmith, then head of geriatric services, talked to a local newspaper reporter and contacted the Florida Department of Health and Rehabilitative Services, which began an investigation in October. The state found ample evidence to justify Silversmith's concern. Its report documented numerous deficiencies at Lake Hospital that included inadequate safeguards in storing and preparing medications, patient rooms that failed to meet state standards of eighty square feet per bed, and insufficient bathroom facilities, forcing patients at times to wait in long lines.

A month after the state intervened, Silversmith, who had been associated with the National Medical Enterprise facility for six years, was fired. He says hospital officials charged he was not "sufficiently supportive" of the administration. Hospital administrator Alan T. Penn subsequently sent Silversmith a memo, dated February 19, 1983, that stated the reasons for his dismissal. According to Penn, Silversmith was fired because of "failure to inform management of existing problems, circumvention of the existing management team, and attempts to discredit the hospital by contacting not only the Department of Health and Rehabilitation Services but also a local newspaper reporter." Penn seemed to suggest that Silversmith was removed from the staff because his efforts to correct dangerous conditions created a public-relations problem. Under Florida law, however, staff privileges can be revoked only for specific causes that include malpractice, negligence, and physical or mental impairment.

Silversmith decided to fight back. He filed suit charging that the Lake Hospital board violated his constitutional rights to due process by terminating his staff privileges in a closed meeting. A Palm Beach County jury heard the case in 1986, ruling, after a five-and-half-week trial, that Silversmith was denied due process. Moreover, the jury found that Lake Hospital's corporate officers and administrators were acting maliciously when they conspired to fire him and, not satisfied with his dismissal, intentionally disrupted his business relationships with physicians still on staff. The jury awarded Silversmith $4.35 million in compensatory and punitive damages. The case is currently on appeal. "As my case shows, a physician does not get a fair hearing before a corporate board of directors," Silversmith said. "I never got a hearing from the medical staff, a hearing from my peers." Although Silversmith possessed the time, money, and perserverance to undertake a lawsuit, many physicians do not. Silversmith says he hopes that his case will provide a precedent for doctors who are likewise dismissed unfairly. Just as likely, however, it could serve as a warning about the dangers of defying corporate power.[19]

Supermed hospitals are distinguished not only by the quality of care they offer but also by their costs. Although supermeds profess to be cost-efficient, that efficiency may go no farther than the business office. In fact, while the for-profit hospital industry claims that competition will reduce costs, Stephen L. White, associate professor of health policy and management at the University of South Florida, presents fascinating evidence that such battles actually raise costs. In a paper prepared for the Florida Hospital Cost Containment Board, White found that hospitals engage in "conspicuous consumerism," competing for prestige and physician allegiance through the purchase of the latest high-tech gadgets. At the same time hospitals tried to attract patients through expensive media campaigns and amenities such as romantic steak and champagne dinners for new parents. But the market competition didn't produce price wars. White said, "Paradoxically, then, competitive pressures in the hospital industry in the past contributed to, rather than moderated, escalating costs." Moreover, White said that for-profit hospitals were unlikely to cut prices in the future because of high debt and capital costs: "These studies suggest that investor-owned hospitals will not be in a position to compete more vigorously in terms of prices and, thereby, cast doubt on the claims that such competition will help contain hospital costs. In fact, it may be that these institutions will force more active nonprice competition and thus contribute to ever higher hospital costs." In his report on competition and costs, White concluded, "[T]he greater the competition, the greater the cost of hospital care."

On average, supermed hospitals charge substantially more than their nonprofit competitors. For example, according to the Institute of Medicine, the federal government paid 8 percent more to treat Medicare patients at for-profit facilities, while private patients paid 24 percent more for their care. Overall, because of inflated prices, the Institute of Medicine found, for-profits add $470 million a year to the nation's health care bill.

Supermeds earn money in very precise ways. For-profits might break even treating patients who need little more than bed rest, but their facilities would be unlikely to earn profits. Some wouldn't break even. Hospitals frequently price room and board at or below their costs; they are not particularly profitable activities. Supermeds make money by bombarding patients with diagnostic tests, special services, and medical supplies. Supermed doctors regularly request more services for their patients than doctors who practice at nonprofit facilities. In particular, they order laboratory tests and drugs, two of the most profitable services, with far greater frequency. Clinical lab services were used 10 percent more frequently per admission at for-profits, while pharmaceutical services were requested 50 percent more often. Through higher markups and charges, supermeds make far more from these services than their nonprofit competitors.[20]

At the same time supermeds, to raise profits, price their ancillary services higher than nonprofits. Supermeds manage to produce almost 40 percent more revenues per day from such ancillary services as drugs, clinical laboratories, respiratory therapy, blood banks, anesthesia, physical therapy, renal dialysis, and radiation therapy. These services account for 60 percent of their revenues. Researchers examined hospitals in various parts of the country, measuring costs and prices on both a per-admission and a per-day basis. They concluded that in both instances for-profits charged more. In an extensive study, undertaken in 1984 for the Hospital Alliance of Tennessee, consulting firm Booz-Allen and Hamilton analyzed the performance of profit and nonprofit facilities, representing almost 95 percent of the hospitals in Tennessee. The sixty-five for-profits and seventy-three nonprofits were matched by location and number of beds, then compared for costs and charges. With only two exceptions, patients paid more on average to be hospitalized in for-profit facilities. Patients were charged an average of 58 percent more per admission and 30 percent more per day at the for-profit facilities. When charges were examined on the basis of diagnoses, the for-profits also were consistently higher. For gall bladder surgery, patients paid up to 38 percent more. Patients with back problems received bills that ran 27 percent higher at the for-profits. Heart attack victims were charged 48 percent more. Women were charged up to 85 percent more to be treated for menstrual disorders and up to 58 percent more to give birth at for-profit hospitals. Patients paid more to be treated at the for-profit hospitals because of their aggressive markups in four major ancillary services: medical supplies, pharmaceutical drugs, inhalation therapy, and laboratory tests. Patients living in the same community and being treated for the same diagnosis paid up to 44 percent more at for-profit hospitals than at the nonprofit hospitals.[21]

The Florida Hospital Cost Containment Board, which reviews hospital budgets, has amassed information, including costs and charges, on state hospitals' fiscal practices.[22] By examining the relationship between $1.00 of charges and $1.00 of costs, the board found that supermed hospitals reported higher markups for their services than government, nonprofit, or state facilities. In 1985, supermeds charged $1.59 overall above cost compared to $1.40 for state, $1.35 for government, and $1.32 for nonprofit hospitals. There was a 26 percent difference between supermed and nonprofit prices. The supermeds charged the highest price of all hospitals on all their services. All facilities marked up their ancillary services substantially, but at supermeds the overall markup was $2.16 compared to $1.73 at nonprofits, a 20 percent difference. On some ancillary services the price difference was even higher. In almost every instance, once again, supermeds charged the highest prices while nonprofits charged the lowest. At the supermeds markups were higher for electrocardiograms by 25 percent, for anesthesiology by 27 percent, for blood banks by 35 percent, and for physical therapy by 30 percent. The supermeds had the highest charges for other services such as ambulances and surgical clinics, too. The supermeds billed $1.06, only slightly above the break-even point, but the government hospitals charged $0.89, below cost, and 16 percent below the supermeds. All types of hospitals lost money on basic medical services such as coronary and intensive-care units, but the supermeds came closest to making a profit, charging $0.97 for every $1.00 of costs. Nonprofits charged 5 percent less, only 92 percent of costs, the least of all hospitals.

When the Florida Hospital Cost Containment Board compiled charges by diagnostic categories, supermeds were still expensive. While their charges were not always the highest, they were usually close to it. They were rarely the lowest. In South Florida two AMI facilities, Southeastern and Parkway, charged the most for thirteen out of twenty diagnoses. The price difference averaged $6,662 but ranged up to $15,115 for major bowel procedures. Only two supermed hospitals, both owned by Hospital Corporation of America, had the lowest charges in the twenty categories. Doctors Hospital of Lake Worth charged the least for kidney infections, while Palm Beach Martin County Medical Center had the lowest charges for prostatectomies.

The Florida board found the same relationship between high charges at supermeds and low charges at other facilities throughout the state. When hospital charges were combined into high and low average charges, exceedingly wide variations existed. At the low-priced hospitals, for example, mothers were charged $459 for normal childbirth. At supermed hospitals they paid at least 50 percent more and sometimes 250 and 300 percent more. At North Florida Regional Medical Center, a Hospital Corporation of America facility, new mothers paid $4,525, nearly ten times higher. Geometric differences also existed for other procedures and services. Stroke patients who were charged an average of $1,720 in Florida hospitals paid $11,051 at Republic Health Corporation's DeePoo Memorial Doctors Hospital, $12,415 at Humana Hospital-Daytona Beach, and $16,521 at AMI's Palmetto General Hospital. Patients who were admitted for cataract lens procedures paid an average of $668 in Florida hospitals but $7,105 at AMI's Southeastern Medical Center and $3,673 at Humana Hospital-Brandon. Patients with back problems could be treated for an average of $710 in Florida hospitals, yet were charged $4,580 at HCA's Plantation General Hospital and $4,246 at National Medical Enterprises' Palms of Pasadena Hospital.[23]

In short, supermed medicine can pose serious problems for their patients—less care for more money.

CHAPTER SIX

•

The No-Care Zone

MISFORTUNE struck twice in 1984 when Gloria Jackson entered a for-profit hospital to give birth to her second child. She and her doctor anticipated a routine delivery, but in the middle of labor there were complications. After childbirth Jackson required immediate surgery on her urinary system. The surgery went smoothly, but as she lay recuperating with the catheter from the operation still in place, a member of the hospital's administrative staff visited her room. Jackson was informed that her Medicaid coverage had lapsed and no longer covered her hospitalization. She was told she could start paying for her care or she could leave—at once. Without savings or private health insurance she was forced to leave.

Afterward Jackson, sick, frightened, and frustrated, with a newborn infant in need of care, sought financial assistance. Through a welfare rights organization Jackson was steered to a social service agency that was willing to cover the costs of her remaining care. Jackson was able then to leave her two children with her mother and return to the hospital. Once assured that the bills would be paid and profits wouldn't suffer, the hospital welcomed her back, removed the tube, and continued her postoperative care. "The hospital clearly demonstrated that it cared more about my financial problems than it did about my health," she told the Mississippi Human Services Coalition.

As supermeds expand, Americans who lack health insurance are finding that their ability to find medical care is contracting. More Americans are experiencing more difficulty in getting medical treatment they want at a price they can afford than at any time since World War II. The paradox is clear. In the midst of a surplus of doctors and hospital beds, many Americans are being refused medical care.

Hospitals have traditionally served their patients and society, delivering consumer services to people who could pay and public services to people who could not. But the supermeds haven't become billion-dollar companies by doling out charitable care. In the world of the supermeds money and care are intimately—and simply—related. People who can't pay may not get treated. Through their "profits first" policies supermeds are restructuring medicine into distinct product lines to be bought and sold like all other consumer merchandise. As a result medical care is becoming less of a right and more of a negotiable commodity.

Among supermed executives this attitude is widespread. Hospital Corporation of America officials Helen King Cummings and James P. King explain, "A health care industry based on market economics and provider efficiency is emerging. In such an industry, the financial survival of providers will be determined by their ability to deliver services to those patients whose care is explicitly financed."[1] John C. Bedrosian of National Medical Enterprises explains, "We are finally witnessing the great demystification of health care which now joins the twentieth century as a business driven by market influences. . . . Gone will be the perception of health care as a free birthright."[2] Humana, Inc., official Ira Corman echoes, "We have the world's greatest health care system . . . if you have the money." American Medical International lobbyist Rebecca Kupper argues, "If Safeway doesn't give away food, why should we give away medical care?"

This corporate philosophy governs the operation of local hospitals. For-profit hospitals in Florida, for instance, limit their charitable expenses to approximately $13 million a year, thus helping to lift after-tax profits above 6 percent. Government-owned and nonprofit hospitals spend, respectively, over four and five times that amount on indigent care, as reported to the state Hospital Cost

Containment Board. According to Niels P. Vernegaard, the associate director of Miami's Humana Hospital-Biscayne, which enjoys a before-tax profit of 7.5 percent, this is an accurate reflection of the hospitals' obligations to the poor. Vernegaard said, "In South Florida there are certain hospitals that receive millions of tax dollars to treat the poor in our communities. Therefore, when a patient that can't pay is seen at our hospital, we will try and transfer the patient to one of those hospitals. Not because we are terrible people, but because the government has decided to centralize their resources at particular hospitals. We do not, however, transfer anyone who is not medically stable." Vernegaard does not feel that by accepting a variety of tax subsidies the supermeds have incurred an obligation to treat the indigent.

The United States has yet to adopt Bedrosian's belief about medical treatment, but his attitude is increasingly common among health care professionals. According to a 1984 Arthur Andersen & Co. survey, 98 percent of medical leaders believed that all Americans were entitled to a "minimum level" of health care. Only 12 percent agreed, however, that all patients had a right to the "same level" of care, while 45 percent strongly disagreed that all patients should receive equal care. Almost 90 percent of the experts predicted that people without money or insurance would receive significantly worse care by 1995. In the future medical treatment will be the prerogative of those who can afford to pay.

Middle-class Americans may accept this notion reluctantly. They have come to expect that when they are ill, they will receive the best and latest medicine has to offer. It is not just furbelows that are involved here. A hospital's location and amenities can indicate the quality of care that is being delivered. In the nonprofit outpatient clinic at Chicago's Cook County Hospital, for example, three physicians must see 275 patients a day. Doctors who are so besieged can keep exhaustion at bay for only so long before their judgment must suffer. When medicine is distributed on the basis of money, health care will separate into price categories that provide far better care to the rich and middle-income than the poor and uninsured. The distinctions between the haves and the have-nots that began to blur in the 1950s will sharpen again.

In supermed hospitals, where patients are considered profit or loss centers, health insurance is the price of admittance. An Institute of Medicine study found in 1986 that insurance covered a "significantly higher proportion" of patients at investor-owned hospitals than at nonprofit or public hospitals. The supermeds are insisting on insurance at a time when working Americans are finding that their policies cost more and cover less than they did a decade ago. Since 1980 companies have been trimming insurance benefits, according to the Employee Benefit Research Institute. Over 70 percent of employees were required to pay a larger share of their hospital bills, while 74 percent paid higher deductibles before they could collect on their policies. Employees were encouraged to avoid hospitals and check into "surgicenters" or ambulatory care facilities that had begun to be covered under group insurance policies. If that was impossible, they were told to get a second doctor's opinion or seek preadmission clearance by a consulting panel before their insurance would guarantee payment. As a result, even with insurance, patients have seen their out-of-pocket health care costs rise 13 percent a year throughout the decade.

Moreover, because of the rising cost, the number of people who can afford health insurance is dropping. Blue Cross/Blue Shield policyholders in Pennsylvania, for instance, watched their premiums escalate 95 percent in the early 1980s until some, like the farmers in rural Sullivan County, simply let their policies lapse. Chester L. Reed, executive director of the Pennsylvania Farmers' Union, said he has observed a steady decline in Blue Cross/Blue Shield subscribers. "We receive letters from subscribers every month telling us they have decided to drop their health insurance completely because they just cannot afford the premiums," he said. As Sullivan County resident Leon Molyneaux explained, "Sullivan County has the lowest net income per family of any county in the state and 17 percent unemployment. I'm a farmer and I do lumbering. I only made $6,400 net last year and there is no way that I could afford to keep up my Blue Cross/Blue Shield, [not with] premiums over $2,000 or more a year."

Middle-class Americans comprise a steadily growing number of the uninsured who are apt to be denied care from the supermeds—even in an emergency. The U.S. House Select Committee on Aging reported in 1986 that working adults and their dependents comprise the overwhelming majority of the uninsured. One out of five people who lack health insurance earns over $10,000 a year; one out of ten makes over $20,000. By traditional definitions they aren't poor; yet they are too financially strapped to buy insurance. They may be self-employed or employed only part-time or they may work in new high-tech or service-related companies where health coverage is not a traditional fringe benefit.

Twelve years ago Helen Freimund of Racine, Wisconsin, worked in a automobile plant where union members took health insurance for granted. When the plant closed, Freimund, then fifty years old, looked for full-time employment but couldn't find it. Finally she was forced to accept a part-time position at a company that doesn't provide health insurance. Freimund bought her own policy and is struggling to pay the premiums. She said, "A health insurance rate which steals 30 percent of my annual earnings from minimum wage employment . . . is clearly the straw that is breaking the camel's back. My insurance premiums will send me to work every day until the moment I can qualify for Medicare coverage. Many people will listen to my story and recommend that I drop my health insurance or go on welfare to cover these needs. These are not choices that I feel Americans should be forced to make."

While for-profit medicine magnifies the importance of health insurance, the American Medical Association reports that up to 37 percent of all Americans under sixty-five were uninsured or underinsured in 1985. Some 9 percent had no health insurance, another 9.4 percent were uninsured sometime during the year, and the remaining 18.6 percent were underinsured and vulnerable to financial devastation by unexpected medical bills. Other experts feel that the number of Americans who are unprepared for a medical emergency could be far higher. More than two hundred million Americans, 85 percent of the total population, lacked adequate protection against catastrophic illness according to the U.S. House Select Committee on Aging. Many Americans would be thrust into financial turmoil by even small medical bills. About 4.3 million middle-income Americans would face severe financial hardship if their medical costs exceeded $2,200. Another 6.4 million would be ruined if their bills amounted to 5 percent of their incomes. Medical treatment has become so expensive that the U.S. House

Subcommittee on Health and Long-Term Care estimated that one million Americans were pushed below the poverty line in 1987 by catastrophic health care costs.

Joyce and Fred Gordon of Fort Washington, Maryland, are typical of the American families who learn suddenly that their coverage stops when they need protection the most. Both Gordons hold managerial positions at major corporations—Joyce with American Telephone & Telegraph Company and Fred with Safeway Stores, Inc. They never really thought about health insurance. Both have group policies through their employers and they assumed that their family was protected. It was the least of their worries until their telephone rang one Friday night.

Karen Gordon was seventeen years old, bright, energetic, the kind of daughter who makes her parents proud. She sang in the Grace United Methodist Church youth choir and was active in extracurricular activities at Friendly High School. She marched beside the school band in her color guard uniform when it played at football games. At about 9:00 P.M. on November 15, 1985, Karen was returning from a church fellowship meeting with her sister Indya and three other teenagers. Less than a block from her house, as their Cadillac rounded the final curve, an oncoming car's headlights flashed across their windshield. The Cadillac swerved to avoid a head-on collision and hit a utility pole. Karen suffered severe brain damage. She was flown by helicopter to Prince Georges County General Hospital. By the time her parents arrived Karen was in a coma. She needed a respirator for a month to breathe and stayed in intensive care until New Year's Day. In January she was transferred to a rehabilitation center.

After six months Mrs. Gordon was informed that her daughter was languishing in a semicomatose condition and was likely to remain there indefinitely. She was also told that their health insurance would no longer pay for Karen's therapy. She said, "We decided to bring Karen home as opposed to placing her in a nursing home and continue her care as much as we could after we were told by the staff at Mount Vernon that due to Karen's slow progress our insurance companies would no longer cover her hospital costs." On their salaries the Gordons couldn't possibly pay the $8,000 a week that was necessary to continue her care at the rehabilitation center. They took her home to the small suburban brick house near Washington, D.C., and the bedroom where she once played with dolls. Her family has hopes that, surrounded by familiar things and their constant love, Karen may one day get better. The Gordons are paying $2,000 a month for her medical care at home, but their savings are dwindling rapidly.

Mrs. Gordon remains astounded by this experience with the health care system and the financial arrangements that pay for complicated medical care. Under their insurance policies Karen was provided 150 days of care; their doctor told them that her recovery could take up to two years. Mrs. Gordon said, "My husband and I had always considered ourselves among the fortunate, good jobs with good benefits, good kids, an overall good life, but the emotional and financial stress of this catastrophic illness has created a tense environment. Add to this frustration and helplessness in looking for help. We find that because we are classified as 'middle class,' own a home, and are not on the brink of bankruptcy—we qualify for no assistance. We are among the underinsured—that growing number of people due to the wonderful technology of modern medicine which is saving more and more lives."

While the middle class is finding that catastrophic care may be priced beyond their reach, the poor and elderly are discovering in the 1980s that they are being pushed out of the health care system altogether. Under the leadership of President Ronald Reagan and a compliant Congress, major cuts have been made in their health care programs. According to the American Federation of State, County, and Municipal Employees, between 1982 and 1986 Medicare benefits for the elderly were reduced over 7.4 percent, or $24.9 billion, while Medicaid benefits for the poor were cut by over 8.7 percent, or $10 billion. Since 75 percent of Medicaid funds are spent on nursing home care for the elderly, very little remains to pay the medical expenses of the poor who are under sixty-five years old. Moreover, eligibility requirements have become so restricted that fewer people qualify for benefits. In 1975 the income of the average Medicaid beneficiary was 67 percent of the federal poverty level, but ten years later the Employee Benefit Research Institute found the average income had slipped to only 38 percent.

Almost two thirds of the poor had been disqualified. Half a million elderly and seven hundred thousand children lost their Medicaid coverage. As a result, the National Citizens' Board of Inquiry into Health in America estimates that two hundred thousand Americans have been denied emergency care and eight hundred thousand denied routine care at hospitals because they lack the ability to pay.

Hidden within those statistics is death and brutality to the young and old alike. In North Carolina's Halifax County, expectant mothers delay baby showers until after infants reach their first birthday. Jennifer Henderson, director of the North Carolina Hunger Coalition, told a National Citizens' Board of Inquiry hearing that this was the custom because of the high infant mortality rate—the sixth highest in the nation. Many babies, born into families that can't afford prenatal care, never live that long. The elderly also suffer. In Washington, D.C., social worker Lin Romano of the Community for Creative Nonviolence testified at a board hearing, "Imagine being an insulin diabetic with no refrigerator storage, eating soup kitchen fare. The dual pain of watching your own leg balloon out of your pants, yet, to your mind, having no place to turn for help . . . imagine the anguish of the man who, just three weeks ago, allowed a shelter volunteer to change an old hospital dressing on his foot and when the bandage came off so did his toe."[3]

Without private insurance or government health care benefits, Americans of all ages, people like Linda Lee McCoy, are being squeezed out of the medical system by the supermeds. McCoy was two months pregnant when doctors discovered complications that required immediate surgery. The local tire-service center that employed McCoy's husband didn't provide health care benefits. And while he earned $9,600 a year, they lacked the $500 down payment that Riverton Memorial Hospital, a Hospital Corporation of America facility, demanded before they would accept uninsured patients. Memorial Hospital was Riverton's only medical facility; the nearest county hospital that might have accepted McCoy was fifty-five miles away. The McCoys chose the only course they thought was available. Linda Lee delayed the operation for a month so the McCoys could apply for financial help through a county program.

While she waited, McCoy said, she bled internally and suffered enormous pain.

Judith Waxman, an attorney with the National Health Law Program, cites another instance of HCA's reluctance to offer care that is not explicitly financed. In 1985 in Nashville, Tennessee, an HCA hospital demanded $500 before it would begin radiation therapy for an elderly cancer patient. When the hospital was asked to reduce its fee because the patient lived with a disabled wife on $328 a month, HCA refused. It said that the HCA policy was to require full payment in advance. The family scraped together $500 so the first of some thirty-five sessions could start. Then the hospital demanded another $500 or it would stop treatment. Waxman said that it took legal action for the care to continue.[4]

In small towns and cities the supermeds' power is magnified. When they set admissions standards, they also determine who will and who will not get care. However, patients can encounter the same difficulty in the middle of Manhattan. A cross section of New York City residents told the Lou Harris poll in 1986 that medical care was becoming harder to find. Nine percent of all respondents and 16 percent of those living below the poverty line complained that they couldn't get needed medical care in the previous year. Humphrey Taylor of the Harris organization said it was the first time since Medicaid and Medicare were enacted that New Yorkers encountered such problems.[5] In still another 1986 survey, reported in *Health Affairs*, Arizona residents said that they, too, were denied care. About 7 percent of the poor families said they were turned away by medical staff when they sought treatment at hospitals. "I was in pain," said a patient. "They only gave me pain pills and told me to go home and rest and stay in bed because of my financial situation and because I didn't have insurance." Nearly half, even those suffering from very serious illness or injury, said they were unable to locate treatment after they were turned down.[6]

According to a third 1986 poll, this one of health care administrators, perceptions of insufficient health care are well founded.[7] Health care administrators themselves admit that they tend to shun the poor and uninsured. Ninety-three percent of fifteen thousand administrators in a 1984 Arthur Andersen & Co. survey said these patients were not welcome at their facility. Some 65 percent described medical care for such patients at their facility as "very inaccessible," while 38 percent said it was "somewhat inaccessible." By contrast, virtually every administrator said that patients with insurance would be welcomed warmly and treated readily.

The poor depend heavily on a few public and private teaching facilities that represent only 10 percent of all hospitals but deliver 40 percent of all indigent care. Yet just when these hospitals are needed the most, their ability to care for the poor is declining. As businesses cut health insurance benefits, the poor as well as the middle class are hurt. In the past, hospitals charged the middle class more than their care actually cost and used the excess to help subsidize care for the poor. Privately insured Floridians, for instance, pay a hidden tax of $144 a day when they're hospitalized to create this subsidy. As long as business acquiesced, hospitals could shift costs around and partially recapture the expense of treating the poor and uninsured. But when businesses began trimming benefits, this subsidy diminished. Hospitals can no longer routinely loot the insurance treasure chest to care for the poor. As employers insist on paying only for their employees and for-profits refuse to deliver services that aren't explicitly financed, the poor place a growing burden on community hospitals. Penelope Anderson, director of the District of Columbia General Hospital, said, "Most public hospitals around the country are a threatened and endangered species. We are threatened by our mission: to service all patients regardless of their ability to pay. This translates into a patient population made up of transfers from other hospitals, the homeless, refugees, illegal aliens, and other special populations historically not served by our elaborate health care system. Public hospitals are further jeopardized because we treat sicker patients: patients with multiple diagnoses, who are victims of infectious diseases, accidents, violence, and substance abuse."

These patients severely strain hospital resources; the financial drain becomes too burdensome for numerous facilities. In the 1980s community hospitals began to fail in record numbers. The U.S. Prospective Payment Assessment Commission reported that forty-nine community hospitals closed in 1985 compared to an annual average of thirty-three between 1980 and 1984. According to the American Hospital Association, seventy-one closed in 1986 and ninety-six shut in 1987. A community threatened by the loss of its hospitals is an appealing target for supermeds. National Medical Enterprises advertises its willingness to help hard-pressed hospitals in *County News,* published by the National Association of Counties. In a memo to county supervisors and commissioners about "your county hospital," NME says reassuringly, "Help for you and your hospital is just a phone call away." NME lists the problems confronting county hospitals: "rising costs, reduced government reimbursements, a declining patient census, the need for new buildings and equipment, and little possibility of new revenues in your county." However, NME promises, "We've assisted other county leaders with great success in solving their hospital problems. And we're ready to help you, too." Under these circumstances a vicious cycle can emerge. Hospitals strained by too many patients and too little money sell out to supermeds. As a result, more poor patients are forced onto the remaining public facilities, and their survival becomes more precarious. In Clearlake, California, Virgil Edwards, the administrator of Redbud Community Hospital, wonders daily if his hospital can continue to operate. Almost 85 percent of the patients are on Medicare or Medicaid. As Edwards said, "This certainly doesn't leave us much room for cost-shifting. Just one patient who stays too long . . . can mean the difference between profit and loss for us during the year." If Redbud Community Hospital closed, the fifteen thousand residents of the Napa Valley would have to travel fifty miles to reach the nearest hospital.

The poor, the uninsured, all the economically undesirable patients shunned by the supermeds lose. Dr. Quentin D. Young, president of the Health and Medicine Policy Research Group, said, "Underfunded patients have increasingly turned to public hospitals for care, creating such fiscal stress that these public hospitals are frequently sold to for-profit hospital chains. However, although the county or city is relieved of the burden of the hospital, in the long run taxpayers pay higher charges and the institutions and capital pass from the health care sector to investor control." The poor were being squeezed out of the health care system as cuts in Medicaid benefits and the growth of for-profit hospitals coincided in the early 1980s. The American Hospital Association found that fewer Medicaid patients accounted for 60 percent of the decline in hospital admissions in 1981 and 1982. Public hospitals were unable to expand sufficiently to meet the need during those years. While the number of uninsured poor rose nearly 21 percent, hospitals increased their charity care by less than 4 percent.

As the poor are redirected to public hospitals, they may be deprived of health care altogether. Their hardship is evident, according to the National Health Law Program, in the directions that a Santa Monica, California, hospital gives to indigent patients who are sent to the nearest county facility. The patients, many physically and mentally handicapped, are told to take:

> RTD #20 or #308 on Wilshire Blvd. to Westwood Blvd. Exit on Westwood. Take the #88 South on Westwood to the LAX Terminal Exit at 98th St. & Vicksburg (LAX Terminal-Los Angeles Airport). Take #232 bus from LAX to Pacific Coast Highway and Torrance Blvd. Exit at PCH and Torrance Blvd. Take #3 Torrance bus east on Torrance Blvd. to Harbor General Hospital. Approximate bus fare for the entire trip $1.00. Approximate travel time 2½ hours.[8]

The uninsured, the sick, and the handicapped are expected to undertake a daunting 2½-hour ride on four different buses to get medical treatment and then repeat the entire trip to get back home. Residents who can't reach a public hospital have lost the ability to find medical treatment. In Los Angeles County's six public hospitals the poor comprised 28 percent of the case load in 1983 but 42 percent of patients by 1985.

Some supermeds have a quick remedy for economically unattractive patients who seek care at their facilities. They get rid of them. As costs become more difficult to shift, many hospitals turn to shifting bodies. In a morbid game of musical chairs patients are rushed from one emergency room to another until they are admitted or die. Although supermeds claim they won't transfer critically ill patients, in Cook County Hospital's emergency room the harried doctors know differently. They see over four thousand patients a year who have been dumped by private hospitals. The number jumped sharply after a nearby hospital was converted from nonprofit to for-profit. Although dumping is illegal under Illinois law, the practice is widespread and growing. According to Dr.

Robert L. Schiff, an attending physician, the number of patients who were dumped soared 500 percent between 1982 and 1986.

Schiff conducted a revealing study, published in 1986, of 437 patients who were admitted to Cook County Hospital from emergency rooms throughout Chicago. Eighty-seven percent were black or Hispanic, 81 percent were unemployed, and 92 percent had no insurance or were on Medicaid. Emergency rooms told Cook County Hospital doctors that 213 patients were being transferred because of lack of insurance; 233 patients were sent to the hospital without prior notice. One out of 4 patients was transferred in a dangerously unstable condition. The transfers may have been fatal. The transferred patients were twice as likely to die as other patients who were admitted directly to Cook County Hospital. Schiff was startled by the high mortality rate. "We had not expected that degree of increased mortality," he said. On some indigent patients the private hospitals spent just enough time—and money—to enable them to survive the ambulance ride to Cook County Hospital. "They treat 'em, stabilize 'em, and dump 'em," Schiff said. Even that wasn't necessarily true. Some poor and uninsured patients were sent away before doctors rendered even minimal services—injecting antibiotics, for example, to fight infections. "The most striking thing was that definitive treatment was not done," he said.[9]

Cook County Hospital's experience is not unique. Over 15 percent of hospitals nationwide adopted explicit policies in the early 1980s restricting admissions to the rich or the well insured. In Dallas indigent patients were dumped on Parkland Memorial Hospital, a public teaching facility, until it became a statewide, then a national scandal. Over two hundred patients a month were transferred by private hospitals that were unwilling to assume financial responsibility for their care. A study of two thousand transfers found that 75 percent of the patients were sent to Parkland Memorial Hospital for financial reasons. Chief operating officer Ray G. Newman recalled a patient who entered a private Dallas hospital to give birth. In the delivery room she mentioned to the doctor that her husband had just lost his job and their health care benefits. The physician then sent her in midlabor to Parkland Memorial Hospital. Emergency room personnel complained that patients were arriving in taxicabs with intravenous needles in their arms and the IV stands dangling out the window because they wouldn't fit in the backseat. The state Board of Health documented five deaths that resulted from the transfers, five people who died simply because they had no insurance and couldn't get care without it. Attracted by Parkland Memorial Hospital's growing notoriety, *Sixty Minutes* aired "The Billfold Biopsy" about the practice of dumping poor people on the besieged hospital. The piece included the following telephone conversation between the employee of a private hospital that wanted to transfer a patient, and a Parkland Memorial Hospital employee.

Private hospital: Listen to me for a minute now, don't give me all that crap. She does not have any insurance. The hospital does not want to take care of her. Okay?

Parkland: Yeah.

Private hospital: This is a private, capitalistic, moneymaking hospital. They're on my back to have her transferred.

Assessing the conversation, Dr. Ron Anderson, Parkland's chief executive officer, told Mike Wallace, "Well, the Hippocratic Oath is sometimes in conflict with corporate policy."

After the deaths and the national publicity Texas adopted regulations to prohibit all economic transfers and to allow medical transfers only after the receiving hospitals agreed. In other states that haven't fallen under *Sixty Minutes*' scrutiny, they continue. After investigating transfers to an Oakland, California, public hospital, for example, Dr. David U. Himmelstein of the Harvard Medical School concluded, "What we found was that the transfers were a form of medical abuse."

Through their annual reports the supermeds project revealing corporate images. Blacks, Hispanics, and other ethnic groups are notably absent from the carefully selected photographs. In these glossy pages hospitals are populated almost exclusively by white, middle-class doctors and their strikingly wholesome and cheerful patients. At HCA's Grant Center Hospital a schoolgirl wearing an accordion-pleated skirt, white anklets, and patent leather Mary Jane shoes clutches a stuffed toy. At National Medical Enterprises' Los Alamitos Medical Center a four-member surgical team prepares to operate on an abdominal tumor with high-technology las-ers. At AMI's Anclote Manor Hospital, "located on eighteen lush and secluded acres on a penisula bordered by the Gulf of Mexico and the Anclote River," a young couple wheel their bicycles onto a weathered gray bridge for a chat. At Humana Hospital-Sunrise a mother cradles a newborn infant on her stomach while an adoring father gazes at both.

Supermeds try to maintain their middle-class preserves by locating hospitals away from the poor. They favor neighborhoods where the poor don't live and aren't well served by public transportation. The strategy is obvious. If indigent patients can't get there, hospitals don't have to take them in. For-profit hospitals also shun services such as obstetrics that attract a high proportion of uninsured patients. According to a 1986 Institute of Medicine study of fifty-four hundred hospitals, supermed facilities offer relatively few services that appeal to low-income groups. Less than one third of supermed hospitals had nurseries for premature infants, for example, while approximately two thirds of the nonprofit and government hospitals did. Supermed hospitals also had significantly fewer family planning services. Such a service would draw low-income women who might return to give birth. Out of ninety-four medium and large supermed hospitals, not one had a family planning clinic, but nearly 23 percent of the nonprofits and 34 percent of the government hospitals did. When supermeds say they don't dump patients, they are almost right. Supermeds try to ensure that they have no poor patients who need to be transferred. When they are forced to dump patients, they are in effect admitting that this strategy has failed.

Some communities have recognized that supermeds may reduce the availability of care to the poor and refuse to issue building permits. Humana thought that Reston, Virginia, where numerous, well-insured federal government employees live, was an ideal location for one of its facilities. It asked the local Health System Agency for permission to build a new $101 million, two-hundred-bed hospital. Before it reached a decision on Humana's application, the agency studied the admissions procedures at fifty Humana hospitals throughout the United States. It discovered that at Humana hospitals Medicaid patients represented only 4.9 percent of admissions compared to the 14 percent national average. The agency also looked at the number of patient transfers from emergency rooms at Humana hospitals and other northern Virginia hospitals, concluding, "[T]he chances of a patient at a Humana hospital emergency room being transferred to another facility were six times as great as for a patient at one of northern Virginia's hospitals." The agency found that poor patients seeking admission to the proposed Humana hospital might be transferred "[i]f they do not have third-party coverage or money for a down payment on their bills and they are not in an immediately life-threatening condition."

Humana's policy is commonplace. In this respect, at least, supermed facilities are interchangeable. Northern Florida, a geographic anomaly closer culturally to the old Confederacy than to Miami's Latin Quarter, is a case in point. In the late 1970s four supermeds—HCA, NME, AMI, and U.S. Health Corporation—owned six of the twenty hospitals in the area and 29 percent of the beds. Just one of those six hospitals provided any indigent care at all between 1979 and 1981, and that care represented only 2 percent of its billings, according to the state Hospital Cost Containment Board. Moreover, that hospital offered minimal care to Medicaid patients. At supermed hospitals Medicaid patients represented only 1.5 percent of admissions, while at other hospitals they accounted for 6 percent. Supermeds had expanded their control of medical care in the area by 1985. Now three hospital chains—AMI, HCA, and Humana—owned eight facilities, but very little changed for the poor and uninsured. AMI's Lake City Medical Center, its Citra hospital, and HCA's Niceville hospital treated no charity or Medicaid patients in 1985. Six of the supermed hospitals reported that indigent and Medicaid patients made up 1 percent or less of all their patients. Humana's Fort Walton Beach hospital offered the most charity care. Almost 8 percent of its patients were uninsured or on Medicaid. In northern Florida and similar areas few if any public hospitals exist. By refusing to treat the ill, if they happen to be poor, the supermeds are helping to determine their medical fate.[10]

The supermeds are unlikely to change without powerful financial inducements or extreme pressure. Such circumstances are rare but not unknown. When Houston's medical boom town collapsed with the Texas oil and gas industry in 1985, local hospital executives suddenly found themselves with fifty-five hundred empty beds. When, on top of that, the Harris County Hospital District proposed razing the existing public hospitals and building two new ones at a cost of $216 million, private hospitals panicked. Led by HCA, supermed hospitals rushed to offer their empty beds to indigents. HCA announced that it welcomed an opportunity to help the community provide medical care to the poor. HCA needed the patients. Its fourteen facilities had a dismal 50 percent occupany rate. It volunteered to waive Medicare deductibles for the elderly and to provide maternity care for an estimated seventeen thousand to twenty thousand poor, pregnant women. Although hospital occupancy rates are declining nationwide, Houston is likely to remain an exception. The chances are far higher that supermeds will reduce rather than expand their services to the poor.

CHAPTER SEVEN

•

The Lovely Gleam of Gray Gold

BEVERLY ENTERPRISES is the largest, wealthiest corporation of its kind in the world, a multibillion-dollar-a-year enterprise whose management inspires gushing praise in *The New York Times*, but is virtually unknown to the general public. Beverly officials aren't troubled by their obscurity; it reflects a deliberate corporate style. The company rarely issues press releases, and its annual reports, unlike the glossy, self-promotional pieces frequently published by other corporations, provide only the sketchiest information about its operations. Yet even if its management sought publicity, Beverly Enterprises might well remain cloaked in anonymity by its very nature, a business that many people find too depressing to contemplate. They are content to let Beverly go about its business of caring for the old and dying quietly, behind firmly closed doors.

Beverly Enterprises is the supermed of the nursing home industry.* It is the leading operator of long-term care facilities in the United States, with 1,025 homes and 115,000 beds in 45 states and the District of Columbia. Its nearest competitor, ARA Living Centers, boasts only a third of its capacity. Altogether Beverly owns 8 percent of the 1.6 million nursing home beds in the country. In addition, Beverly Enterprises is the foremost provider of home health

*According to a company history, founder Roy Christensen named the company after Beverly Hills to give it a "quality, top-of-the-line" image.

services, with over one hundred home health agencies. Beverly is big and getting bigger. Since the late 1970s it has expanded aggressively, buying out mom-and-pop nursing homes and sometimes entire chains, growing at rates varying from 15 to 95 percent a year. In its latest major acquisition, completed on December 30, 1986, Beverly Enterprises bought 69 nursing homes with 7,500 beds in Texas and Arkansas from Stephens, Inc. Beverly intends to add an estimated 15,000 new beds a year to increase its market share in the long-term-care industry to a minimum of 15 percent by 1990. In some communities it has acquired monopoly control of long-term care, owning 50, even 100 percent of the nursing homes.

In less than ten years Beverly Enterprises has fashioned a for-profit nursing home chain with the potential to seize total power over the long-term-care industry. Beverly has consolidated individual homes and small chains into a nationwide chain with headquarters in Pasadena, California. Many of these facilities were being operated for a profit when Beverly bought them, but Beverly added corporate oversight and investor ownership. In the process profits loomed larger, and the new revenues flowing into the corporate treasury are being put to work for shareholders.

Beverly Enterprises typifies for-profit medicine and corporate dominance in health care. It is a senior citizen supermed that possesses the power to determine the kind and quality of long-term care that is available to large numbers of the elderly. It is a formidable power. Beverly offers a sneak preview of the consequences of mixing medicine and money, and it is not a comforting picture.

Despite its lack of public recognition, Beverly is well known to the financial community and consumer organizations. Beverly is perceived so differently by these two groups, viewing the corporation from their widely dissimilar perspectives, that it often appears as if they are talking about two distinct companies. To Wall Street, Beverly, with a history of rising profits, has seemed capable of doing very little wrong. To patient advocates, Beverly, wringing profits from the care of the infirm, cited repeatedly by regulatory agencies for flagrant patient abuse, appears to do little right. Nursing home regulators have documented its neglect of residents. In state after state Beverly has been cited for deficiencies ranging from unsanitary kitchens to neglect that endangered the lives of patients.

While Beverly Enterprises receives billions of dollars from the federal government to provide long-term care to the elderly, the federal government does almost nothing to ensure that the company spends the money wisely. Beverly Enterprises is supposed to comply with numerous government standards, ranging from staffing to housekeeping, from sanitation to nutrition, to qualify for Medicare and Medicaid funds. Enforcement, however, is notoriously lacking. Annual inspections are required by federal law but frequently occur at eighteen- to twenty-four-month intervals. Homes are often notified in advance of impending visits. Under these circumstances nursing home administrators should find compliance with the minimum standards relatively easy. It is a wonder, then, that Beverly Enterprises homes are so often cited for violations.

Mark Turns, a nursing aide who worked at a Beverly Enterprises home in Pennsylvania for fourteen months beginning in 1981, testified before the Pennsylvania Unemployment Compensation Board of Review: "You know, when the state comes to inspect them, I have, you know, I have been standing in rest rooms and stuff when they didn't know that I was there. I didn't try to do it but I have overheard them tell [the management] when they are coming and what they are going to look for."

Turns was fired because he asked to speak to visiting inspectors. They arrived as he was refusing to work on an inadequately staffed shift. "I say the reason I was fired is because I asked to speak to the inspectors. Up until that point I was only suspended for a day," he told the Pennsylvania Unemployment Compensation Board of Review. On the day he was fired, he reported to work at 6:30 A.M. and discovered he was the only aide assigned to a floor with sixty patients, all in need of total nursing care. He punched out and went to the staff lounge. "I did it because I didn't want to be a part of abusing and neglecting these patients anymore," he said. "I didn't want to just quit because jobs are hard to get. And I wanted to try to make it better for these patients. I got, you know, pretty close to some of them and I care about them."

Based on his experience at the facility, Turns might have guessed it was a futile protest. "This isn't something that just happened, you know, an isolated incident," he said. "This is something that has been going on, going on and going on the whole time I worked there. And many of us, especially me, have always voiced my opinion that it is understaffed, you know, it is an operating policy that they are understaffed." Although the state requires two and a half hours a day of nursing care for such patients, Turns charged, "it was never done there the whole time that I was there for the simple reason that four, five, and six people can't do it. You would get your first patient up and you would get them out, you know, in a chair or something and you would be lucky that you could get back to them until a few minutes in the afternoon."

Without adequate staff, Turns said, residents weren't cared for properly. Donald Coller, an elderly patient with circulatory problems, was neglected until an open sore developed in one of his legs, Turns claimed. Then, after a dressing was applied, the staff didn't have time to change it. "Well, one nurse can't pass medications on the whole floor plus supervise the whole floor plus do all the treatments," he said. "So, you know, it wasn't getting done right so she went in there to do it and there were live maggots crawling all over the guy's leg. And I reported that to the state."

But, Turns said, it wasn't only understaffing that caused suffering. "Last winter temperatures of fifty-six, fifty-seven, and fifty-eight degrees [were common] in the whole 900 wing and that's with the [heat] working at maximum capacity. If you turn the thermostat up, that's all you can get," he said. "And that, you know, if they would be honest about, that creates a danger of hypothermia in these elderly patients. And you know nothing was done about it. . . . We dressed people in coats after they got up out of bed and there was nothing done about that. I complained about that. Nothing was ever done about it."

After a year Turns said the home deteriorated further. "The conditions there, they are so horrendous to me, it is just like a warehousing of bodies to me," he said. "It just kept getting worse. . . . In the last three months it got so much worse. It was always bad enough but it got worse."

At the hearing Beverly Enterprises administrators never responded directly to charges about inadequate care, claiming only that state regulations were met. They noted that while the state demanded patients receive 2½ hours of nursing care a day, staffing was left up to the facility. An administrator testified, "I would like to say that while the state does require 2½ hours per patient per day, it is at the facility's discretion how each shift is staffed. . . . And we had had in the past [the] 800 and 900 work units work very well with only five nursing assistants. I would also like to add that although the [nursing] unit secretary does not provide hand [*sic*] on care, she is allowed to be counted in our nursing hours per patient day to meet the state requirements." Without adequate staff, obviously, residents would never receive several hours a day of nursing care. Four untrained nurse's aides could not possibly provide adequate care to two wards of bedridden patients.

After Turns was fired, his wife, another employee at the home, quit. He later met with administrators at the facility and afterward received a polite, noncommittal note, never addressing his specific complaints, from Beverly Enterprises' nursing home ombudsman. In her brief letter she said she hoped that Turns was able to discuss his concerns at the meeting. Beverly Enterprises denied none of Turns' charges.[1]

Wall Street, however, cares little about quality of care. It emphasizes profit-and-loss statements, and Beverly's reports made Wall Street hearts throb faster for years. The financial community's enthusiasm is reflected in the rapturous articles that Beverly Enterprises receives from the business press. *Forbes* published a flattering article in 1981 titled "Gray Gold" that began, "Tales of patient-beatings, druggings and deaths still abound but on Wall Street at least the nursing home business is shedding its Dickensian past."[2] In 1986 *The New York Times* ran a profile of Beverly and its "tireless, fidgety [chairman] who works from 5:30 A.M. to 6:30 P.M." under the headline, "Superstar of Nursing Homes." *Barron's* titled its article, published that same year, "Really Rocking: Nursing Homes Are the Healthiest Thing in Health Care."[3]

Even its adversaries are impressed by Beverly's moneymaking ability. The AFL-CIO Food and Allied Service Trades Department (FAST), which waged a prolonged unionization drive against Beverly, stresses its "spectacular corporate track record." After years of studying Beverly Enterprises, FAST concluded, "Beverly Enterprises is one of the great financial success stories of its time. Among long-term-care companies it is the systems innovator, the financing leader, the pioneer of successful acquisitions, the dominant force in the industry and a Wall Street favorite."[4]

The financial community fell in love with Beverly Enterprises in its adolescence. Jonathan M. Frank, an analyst with *The Value Line Investment Survey*, wrote in 1986, "There's still a place in most investors' portfolios for the nation's leading nursing home chain. . . . We foresee a public desire for a recognizable, trustable name in this fragmented industry. Such a trend could bring advantages similar to those McDonald's had in doing battle with local eateries, like economies of scale in advertising and operations."[5]

Beverly has made itself easy to love. Its financial performance, judged by any measure, was awesome. Between 1980 and 1987 its stock went from $4.60 to $22.50 a share, with three-for-two and two-for-one splits. In the same period its revenues zoomed from $292.8 million to $2.2 billion, and its equally flashy after-tax profits went from $8.4 million to $68 million. Its average annual growth rates never dipped below the double digits. Revenues have grown by an average of 21.5 percent, earnings by 23.5 percent, and dividends by 12.5 percent a year. An investor who bought Beverly stock at its low in 1980 and sold it at its high in 1986 would have made an 800 percent profit.

Beverly is coming of age at precisely the right time. As Chairman Robert Van Tuyle says, "When you look at the demographics this country faces, it's almost scary. There will be so many old people who need care."[6] The bell-shaped curve used by demographers to chart population movements once showed a population concentrated in the middle years with a small proportion of the very young and very old at either end. But over time the curve has listed to the right and now more nearly resembles a tidal wave about to crash down on the population charts. According to the Census Bureau, 28 million Americans were over 65 in 1987, and their numbers are expected to increase by more than 50 percent in the next 12 years. Even more important to Beverly Enterprises' future, the 85-year-olds and up compose the fastest-growing age group in the United States. Their numbers are expected to double to almost 5.1 million by the year 2000; every one is a potential Beverly Enterprises patient. While only 5 percent of people over 65 live in nursing homes, the percentage goes up dramatically as birthdays mount. Nearly a third of the 2.3 million people over 85 are confined to long-term-care facilities.

Moreover, once patients move into a nursing home, they have a slim one-in-five chance of ever leaving voluntarily. For 80 percent of nursing home residents, the only exit is death. They simply have no place else to go. They are old, alone, and afflicted with multiple ailments that destroy self-sufficiency. According to the U.S. House Subcommittee on Health and Long-Term Care, the typical nursing home resident is a 82-year-old single woman or widow whose husband died years ago. She cannot bathe or dress without assistance. She may have trouble seeing or hearing, as a third of nursing home residents do, or she may be incontinent, as 40 percent are. She is likely to have chronic heart trouble or suffer from Alzheimer's disease. The elderly have to die somewhere. By and large, elderly men die in hospitals or at home because they have spouses to care for them. Elderly women are far more likely to die in nursing homes.[7]

Ironically, Wall Street analysts are inspired by this profile of elderly residents too old, too sick, and too isolated to leave a nursing home. Captive patients, forced to buy the product whether they like it or not, are good for business, as Beverly stockholders know. The company enjoyed pretax profit margins on nursing home operations that averaged 14.6 percent in the 1980s, peaking at 16.2 percent in 1986. Joseph D. France, an optimistic health care analyst at Smith Barney, says nursing home residents are "less organized buyers . . . less able to exact concessions." Frequently they were chosen for their financial solvency. "In many cases, particularly nursing home operators catering to the wealthiest sector of the elderly population, they are able to get price increases in excess of inflation," France said. "Presumably for the most expensive of the nursing homes, you have been screened before admission to make sure that you have adequate financial resources. And once you've gotten into a nursing home, it's not often that you're willing to get up and move across town to save $15, $20, $50 a month. . . . People tend to pick out nursing homes in areas where they've lived and where their friends are. And once they've made that difficult decision, they're reluctant to change it."[8]

Profits alone did not cause the bullishness on Beverly Enterprises. It is the promise of still greater future profits as the growing need for nursing home beds collides with the acute shortage of long-term-care facilities. This crisis was created through state regulation of the nursing home industry. In the early 1980s state legislatures passed stringent certificate of need laws that required advance approval before new nursing homes could be built. Many states limited the number of certificates that were issued and imposed a moratorium on the industry's growth. Nevertheless, with its superior ability to issue new stock or sell corporate bonds, Beverly raised the capital to subsidize an ambitious acquisition program. By buying rather than building, Beverly was able to flourish despite the regulations. With competition stifled by state regulators, Beverly Enterprises emerged as the industry leader. By the early 1980s it was operating facilities over 90 percent full, an indication that the demand for beds was not being met by existing nursing homes.

In fact, so many people now need nursing home care and so few beds are available that Beverly can pick and choose among potential patients. As Van Tuyle said, "From a practical standpoint there is no capacity to absorb the patients coming in at the moment, so there's no such thing as competition, as I perceive it. The decision to put Grandma or Mother, as the case may be, into a nursing home is made, usually, by the doctor and the family, and then the place where the patient is admitted is not a matter of free choice for the family. It becomes a matter of, 'Where can I find a bed?' "

Although the over-eighty-five age group grew by 30 percent in the 1980s, the number of nursing homes increased by only 15 percent. In 1986 the federal government eliminated certificate of need laws and allowed, in effect, unfettered competition. With $500 million in assets and projected revenues of $3 billion a year before 1990, Beverly is well poised to take advantage of deregulation. The opportunity is substantial. Van Tuyle estimates that the demand is three times the supply, while the American Health Care Association estimates that one 120-bed nursing home would need to be built every single day for the next decade to accommodate the anticipated patients. Putting the growing need in a slightly different context, Van Tuyle told a 1986 health care conference sponsored in Texas that the nursing home industry would have to raise $4.2 billion to build another 169,000 beds by the 1990s. As he reported to stockholders, "Exciting times are ahead for Beverly."

These estimates are based on current population projections of the number of people over sixty-five and their future health. They may very well underestimate the need. Medical advances that reduce the death rate from cancer or heart disease, for instance, could easily double or triple the demand for nursing home care. Moreover, poor health alone does not determine the demand for nursing home care. Social elements are almost as important as health factors. The elderly can be forced into nursing homes when they lack family support or the financial resources to hire care. It is this combination of needing help yet not being able to find it outside an institution that drives so many elderly women into long-term-care facilities. The social changes of the past decades—more divorces, fewer children, more working women, fragmented and geographically dispersed families—are likely to impel more elderly into nursing homes.

Van Tuyle was sixty-five years old when he became president and chief executive officer of Beverly Enterprises in 1971. He knew almost nothing about nursing homes. Van Tuyle was a chemical engineer by training who spent over three decades at Emery Industries in Cincinnati, Ohio. He drifted around several corporations, gathering the reputation as a "Mr. Fix-It" for ailing companies, before arriving at Beverly Enterprises. He discovered that Beverly was an unruly collection of businesses, acquired over the previous eight years, with little in common. The company possessed little cash and almost no working capital. Van Tuyle quickly stripped the company of its interests in plastics, printing, hospitals, and a deficit-ridden real-estate-development company. To symbolize his new, pragmatic management style, he moved headquarters from the penthouse of a corporate spire to more modest headquarters. Then, left with a company owning only seventy nursing homes, he began to build a new corporate empire that would provide long-term care to the growing number of infirm and disabled elderly.

Beverly has been relentless in the pursuit of profits in long-term care, but it wasn't the first to glean gold in the nursing home business. Other, less successful attempts have been made to capitalize on the graying of America. In the midst of the go-go stock market of the 1960s, numerous companies, many totally lacking experience in the industry, began to enter the long-term-care market. In 1969 Richard Elliott, Jr., appraising the market for *Barron's*, wrote, "A kind of frenzy seems to grip the stock market at the merest mention of those magic words: 'convalescent care,' 'extended care,' 'continued care.' All euphemisms for the services provided by nursing homes, they stand for the hottest investment around today. Companies never before near a hospital zone—from builders like ITT's Sheraton Corporation, National Environment and Ramada Inns, to Sayre and Fisher . . . have been hanging on the industry's door." An investment banker told Elliott, "Nobody can lose money in this business. There's just no way."[9] He was wrong. Companies did lose money; some lost substantially, and their shareholders, anticipating unrealistic returns, watched their stocks hit bottom.

New nursing home corporations titillated potential investors with prospectuses that boldly predicted returns of 20 to 25 percent a year. As a result, nursing home stocks sallied forth as some of the highest fliers in a buoyant stock market. Their price-earnings ratios, a measure of the market's confidence in future earning capacity, soared. In those years such stocks approached forty times the price-earnings ratios of the blue chips—the stocks of the major companies, such as IBM Corporation—that are the very spinal cord of the American economy. Speculative fever pushed the price-earnings multiple of Medic-Home to 179 and of Unicare to 700 in 1969. Not even the hottest market could sustain such hope, and by the early 1970s, prices collapsed. Medicenters of America stock, for example, was carried to almost $60 a share by the high-flying market of the late 1960s before crashing to $4 a few years later.[10]

During this period the nursing home industry was rocked by scandals. As the stocks soared, the chains became increasingly visible, inviting scrutiny by the press and regulatory officials. Newspaper reporters and investigators, representing state agencies and congressional committees, began probing the quality of care in nursing homes. They quickly discovered widespread evidence of neglect and abuse, of residents roped to chairs or left to lie in their own wastes. The unsavory conditions led to one headline after another. Publicity, highlighting the wretched care at many nursing homes, helped dampen investor enthusiasm but alone would not have toppled stock prices.

These exposés, however, were followed by revelations of financial irregularities in the industry. The Four Seasons Nursing Centers, the most widely publicized chain and the first to list its shares on a major exchange, was the catalyst. Speculators drove the price of Four Seasons stock up to $100 a share, but the stock had tumbled to $0.06 a share when the Securities and Exchange Commission suspended trading in 1970. The SEC undertook an extensive investigation into Four Seasons' unexpected bankruptcy, which disclosed shocking evidence of massive fraud in its operations. The scandals had a cumulative impact. The market cooled; investors looked to different industries to deliver the returns once promised by the nursing home chains.

Even without the scandals most companies that lurched into the long-term-care field in the 1960s would not have survived. They simply didn't understand the business. And in modern times it has almost always been a business.

Beverly Enterprises had its origins in the almshouses, charitable institutions that cared for the destitute and infirm elderly from the 1700s into the 1930s. A popular tune of the Depression was "Over the Hill to the Poorhouse." When President Franklin Roosevelt pushed Social Security through Congress in 1935, over a hundred thousand aged Americans were living on poor farms. With the passage of Social Security, the elderly were guaranteed a retirement income for the first time in U.S. history. And with the guarantee of federal dollars a new industry was created; for-profit nursing homes opened. The homes offered health services and long-term care to elderly who had resources through Social Security to pay for it. An estimated twelve hundred nursing homes were operating in 1939, but their numbers escalated rapidly as the population of elderly qualifying for benefits grew. By 1950 the number of nursing homes increased to nine thousand. According to the U.S. Department of Health and Human Services, the elderly were spending $187 million a year for nursing home care, 1.5 percent of all national health expenditures.

With the passage of Medicare and Medicaid, long-term-care benefits dramatically increased. In 1965 there were 460,000 nursing home beds; by 1973 there were 1.1 million, a 139 percent increase. Since 1965 the federal government has been paying a steadily increasing amount for nursing home care, rising from $1.3 billion in 1965 to $16.5 billion in 1985. Through the 1970s and 1980s long-term-care spending has increased at an average annual rate of 15.6 percent. In the late 1980s nursing home care absorbs 8.3 percent of all health care spending, and the state and federal governments pay approximately half the bills.

Spurred by the growth of federal funds, corporations have rushed into the nursing home business. As the government's reimbursement policies created the supermeds, they have also stimulated the growth of for-profit nursing home companies such as Beverly Enterprises through financial incentives. Following passage of Medicare and Medicaid, for-profit companies rapidly expanded their penetration into the nursing home industry. Slightly over 64 percent of nursing home beds were controlled by for-profits in 1969; in the next six years corporate ownership of nursing home beds increased to almost 84 percent. In some years the chains grew by 25 or 30 percent. In 1988 two-thirds of nursing homes are controlled by for-profits, and there are ten major for-profit chains. The growth has come mainly from the acquisition of existing facilities by profit-making chains. Only a tiny handful of investor-owned nursing homes were registered with the Securities and Exchange Commission before Medicare and Medicaid, but with federal funds surging into the economy, this changed rapidly. In 1969 alone nursing home corporations sold stock worth $340 million.

Many of those companies had never been near a hospital zone before and fatally misjudged the federal government's willingness to pay for long-term care. They assumed that Medicare's "take what you want" reimbursement policies for hospitals would be extended to nursing homes. In fact, however, the elderly could qualify for nursing home benefits under Medicare only if they had been hospitalized first. Even then Medicare would reimburse the complete cost of nursing home care for the first twenty days only, and coverage ended altogether after one hundred days. Moreover, Medicare wouldn't pay for any custodial care. To their regret, many companies learned that patients who couldn't pay their own bills would have to depend on Medicaid, which was far less benevolent in its reimbursement policies, because patients were forced to exhaust almost all of their assets before they could qualify. Moreover, while the federal government paid half the costs, the states determined Medicaid eligibility and payment.

Throughout the 1970s and 1980s Beverly Enterprises profited from almost every development in the long-term-care industry. It picked up new nursing homes at firesale prices as numerous companies, exhausted by wrangling with fifty different state agencies about reimbursement rates, gave up and left the business. Beverly noted in an annual report, "There is little if any competition in price, services or quality with respect to Medicare and Medicaid patients."

Under Medicaid substantial profits were possible, but it took a determined company like Beverly to realize them. With its centralized operations, sophisticated computer resources, and single-mindedness, Beverly was able to manipulate the state reimbursement systems successfully to secure maximum income. By 1983 Beverly Enterprises was so skillful at extracting Medicaid money that it was getting three cents out of every Medicaid dollar spent in the United States. Moreover, Beverly reported increasing profits through the 1980s, when almost 60 percent of its patients were on Medicaid. By comparison, only 36.4 percent of its competitors' patients were on Medicaid.

Van Tuyle explained Beverly Enterprises' success: "This is what I call a tight business. There is very little margin of error. The person getting squeezed is going to be the high-cost operator. As a low-cost operator we have the ability to pick up those high-cost operators." At Beverly Enterprises corporate officials could spot a facility that was exceeding corporate limits on expenses instantly. "The computer will flag a facility the moment it starts moving into an area of high labor, high food, whatever it might be," Van Tuyle said. "So with the techniques and tools that we have available, the alert bell will ring quickly." In effect, the alert sounded when homes were endangering corporate profits by spending too much on patient care.

Beverly also reaped advantages from the crackdown on nursing homes by state regulators. While the industry continued to be shaken by reports of horrendous conditions, a series of fires swept through nursing homes in the early 1970s, killing or seriously injuring residents. Almost all these homes were mom-and-pop operations with a pattern of building code violations. The fires received widespread publicity, forcing the homes to comply with more stringent codes. Rather than spend money to install sprinklers and other safety measures, many mom-and-pop facilities sold out to chains. To take just one example, Ohio had the sorry distinction of leading the United States in the number of deaths from nursing home fires in the 1970s. After a decade of shameful headlines, the state adopted a new fire code, and over one hundred nursing homes closed during the following three years, only to be replaced by chain-owned facilities. When state regulators clamped down on nursing homes, Beverly, perversely, thrived. As analyst Jonathan Frank noted, it became a recognizable name, promising a McBeverly brand of care that sounded familiar even if the quality was unknown.

Moreover, like the supermeds in general, Beverly's growth was boosted by the capital reimbursment policies of Medicare and Medicaid. When Beverly acquired new facilities, mortgage interest and depreciation were charged off to the taxpayers, allowing corporate expansion with limited investment of corporate dollars. Then Beverly received an additional bonanza from the federal government. Under the Economic Recovery Tax Act of 1981, Beverly was permitted to write off part of its investment in nursing homes from its taxes. It could also depreciate its facilities at an accelerated rate, thus further lowering its tax liabilities. Under these provisions many nursing home operators—particularly independent and nonprofit ones—found that it was more profitable to sell than to own. Over the next few years Beverly bought out three other chains, ranging in size from eight to twenty-one nursing homes apiece.

At the same time, state and local governments were helping the construction of new facilities through tax-exempt industrial development bonds. Beverly kept its corporate funds intact by borrowing from its bondholders. Meanwhile, the buyers escaped paying taxes on the interest while Beverly deducted the payment of interest from its taxes. Beverly exploited this tax loophole in the mid-1980s so successfully that it managed to raise $19.3 million in a single year. Almost 25 percent of its long-term debt was being financed through industrial development bonds. The impact on both federal and state governments that approved the bond issues was substantial. When Beverly applied for $15.5 million in industrial development bonds in Massachusetts, the bonds were estimated to cost the federal and state governments almost $700,000 and $180,390 a year, respectively, in lost revenues. Eventually Americans would be paying higher taxes to compensate for this subsidy.

Taxpayers are not the only ones who have underwritten Beverly Enterprises' growth; employees have contributed, too. The situation that nursing aide Mark Turns encountered in Pennsylvania is not unique in Beverly Enterprises facilities. The corporation has been cited frequently for insufficient and inadequately trained staff. In Arkansas, for example, where the company has extensive holdings, 82 percent of its homes were cited repeatedly in 1980 for inadequate staffing, according to the AFL-CIO. During that year Beverly facilities in Arkansas averaged close to four citations apiece. The following year Beverly facilities compiled an even worse record. Eighty-eight percent were cited every four months on the average for failing to meet the minimum licensing requirements on staffing. AFL-CIO organizers claim that Beverly has hired inexperienced staff to whom they offered little or no training. State regulators cited each Beverly facility approximately 3.5 times in 1980 for insufficient training; the next year they issued an average of 3.5 citations to 97 percent of Beverly homes.

An inadequate and untrained staff can't help but affect the quality of patient care, especially when the nurses' aides who provide the bulk of care are required to attend helpless patients under conditions that inevitably result in patient neglect. Testifying in 1983 before the U.S. House Select Committee on Aging, a representative of the Service Employees International Union stated, "Health care workers and patient care issues are inextricably tied together. Poor staffing conditions mean patients lack care, and workers suffer stress and constant pressure to work faster regardless of the impact on their patients. Low wages and inadequate benefits produce high turnover and little continuity of care for long-term patients and a constant state of retraining and putting new staff on patient units with little experience in hospitals."

In summing up the relationship between staff and nursing home supermeds like Beverly Enterprises, the union official said, "Health care workers directly pay for the impressive profits of the corporate health industry with rock-bottom wages, poor or nonexistent benefits, and stressful working conditions." In fact, Beverly Enterprises pays an hourly wage scarcely more than McDonald's pays workers who grill Big Macs. At Beverly Enterprises facilities, nurses' aides feed, wash, clothe, and toilet patients. In addition, because of inadequate nursing staff, the aides, not the nurses themselves, are often required to ensure that doctors' orders are being followed. For all this nurses' aides earn an average weekly wage that is substantially less than workers with considerably less responsibility. Pest exterminators, janitors, hair dressers and elevator operators, according to the Bureau of Labor Statistics, earn more per hour than nurses' aides at Beverly Enterprise facilities.

In April 1986, Beverly president David Banks told *The New York Times* that the company "would love" to pay its employees $7 an hour, approximately twice the minimum wage, to reduce turnover and attract a qualified staff, a tacit admission that staffing problems exist. But Banks said the company couldn't afford to because of low profit margins.[11] Apparently Banks conveniently forgot that at the time of the interview Beverly Enterprises earned a before-tax profit of 16.2 percent, substantially higher than that of many corporations. Beverly didn't lack the money but the will to staff its facilities properly. Beverly spends 66 percent of its total budget on labor. Through its staffing policies, Beverly Enterprises substantially reduces its costs. And every dollar that is not spent on wages can be churned into profits.

In the 1980s Beverly began to look for ways to reduce its reliance on Medicaid patients. If it could attract self-sufficient private patients, Beverly could set rates for them far above the reimbursement levels allowed by Medicaid and dramatically increase its revenues. As David Grant, director of acquisitions for Beverly Enterprises, explained this new policy, "The key determinant [in deciding to buy a nursing home] is going to be the number of private pays. A facility that is primarily Medicaid is not going to do well for us. . . . We also want to look at some of the ancillary income related to physical therapy, occupational therapy, a beauty shop, and other services. . . . We want to see how a seller's averages compare to ours in the dietary and laundry areas and so forth. We try to make savings in areas that are not going to produce a bad reputation for us and in a way that is not going to drastically reduce our operating reimbursement in subsequent years."

Beverly was following this new policy in 1983 when it decided to construct a new 180-bed facility, Beverly Manor Convalescent Hospital, in Irvine, California, not far south of Disneyland. Under state law Beverly Enterprises was required to devote 69.4 percent of its beds to patients on Medicare or California's version of Medicaid, Medi-Cal. But Beverly insisted that it couldn't make money under those circumstances. "The inability of the Medi-Cal program to meet the ever-rising costs of operating skilled nursing facilities similar to the project is a primary factor in this situation," Charles Van Gunst, director of development, told the state health planning agency. With so few private patients Beverly claimed that it would lose $1 million a year for four years and $1.5 million in the fifth year.

Instead, Beverly proposed to reverse the state requirement and construct a home with 65 percent private and only 35 percent Medicare and Medi-Cal patients.[12] The financial difference was substantial. While it would receive between $37 and $39 a day for each Medi-Cal patient and between $83 and $109 a day for each Medicare patient, Beverly intended to charge private patients $73 a day initially. When Beverly Manor was fully occupied, the rates would go up to $97 a day, over two and a half times the Medi-Cal rate. Private patients would be subjected to steady increases totaling 27 percent over four years. Under those circumstances it is little wonder that the U.S. House Select Committee on Aging found that most nursing home residents, those well-screened private patients so dear to Wall Street analysts, are drained of all assets and reduced to bankruptcy within two years.

Along with its request for permission to build the new facility, Beverly Enterprises submitted a remarkable budget that specified the allocation of its projected revenues. With private rates rising regularly, Beverly Manor would increase its revenues by $1.65 million during its first three years. Patients would receive few benefits from this expanding income. Instead, Beverly Enterprises itself was to be the major beneficiary. The corporation would receive an additional $116,830 in annual management fees from Beverly Manor. While the revenues expanded, management fees were the fastest-growing budget expense. The fees went toward the operation of the corporate headquarters in Pasadena, the Western Division headquarters in Fresno, California, and its central computer center in Virginia Beach, Virginia. By contrast, Beverly Manor anticipated spending $68,293 more on medical supplies and $51,702 extra for food annually.

Beverly Enterprises drafted the budget for Beverly Manor after studying the costs and expenses at its Escondido, Seal Beach, and Laguna Hills facilities. Their 1982 budgets had been dissected thoroughly, passed up and down the corporate chain of command, reviewed by employees determined to ferret out the tiniest savings. As it stated, "Beverly Enterprises is concerned about the costs of providing long-term-care services. . . . Each cost center is scrutinized from operational and programmatic points of view. . . . From the administrator to the Western Division President, the budgeting process is screened at all levels to achieve the desired facility program."

Nursing home patients depend heavily on drugs, both prescription and over-the-counter, and on medical supplies ranging from bedpans to wheelchairs. At the three California facilities selected to be the models for Beverly Manor, spending on pharmaceutical and medical items averaged $1.94 a patient a day, although Seal Beach spent only $0.13 for medical supplies. Spending was low, too, for food supplies. Beverly facilities were spending an average of $1.90 per patient per day for food. Even with the savings from bulk buying, the figure was remarkably small. In a survey of nursing home spending patterns reported by the Institute of Medicine, for example, Ohio nursing homes that participated in Medicaid reported spending more on food four years earlier. Beverly Manor estimated it would spend $3.44 per patient a day in 1988 to supply all a patient's medical needs, an amount that is less than the cost of a single bottle of cough syrup. It also forecast expenses of $3.02 per patient a day on food in 1988, less than the cost of a McDonald's meal, although many residents require special diets.

The California homes spent equally low amounts on other essential items. Aside from drugs and food, they budgeted $2.16 per patient per day to cover all nursing supplies, crafts, housekeeping, personal items, physical therapy, laboratory tests, radiology, and oxygen. Despite these budgets, however, homes sometimes spent little or nothing on care that is essential to patients' well-being. The Seal Beach facility spent not one penny on physical therapy during one six-month period in 1982, an omission that could have jeopardized some patients' ability to become self-sufficient and leave. The Escondido home spent only $0.05 per patient per day on physical therapy, while the Laguna Hills home spent $0.03 per patient per day. The facilities were penurious on other items, too. The Laguna Hills home reduced its spending to the absolute minimum, spending $0.01 per patient per day on crafts, $0.02 per patient on personal items, and nothing at all on beauty care. The Escondido facility reported expenses of $0.05 per patient per day on personal items.

But Beverly Enterprises didn't demand that its facilities stint on one essential item. While the homes were averaging $0.27 cents per patient per day on housekeeping supplies to keep facilities clean and sanitary, they were spending $2.25 per patient per day on management fees. Beverly Manor projected it would spend $5.50 per patient per day on management fees, $2.48 more than it estimated spending on food.

Beverly Enterprises didn't break down all operating costs on a per-patient per-day basis but lumped staff training, required to qualify for Medicare funds, under miscellaneous, discretionary expenses. The three facilities together spent less on an estimated annual basis to train their staff, $2,864 a year, than they did on postage, $6,059 a year, or professional dues and subscriptions, $5,817.

The corporation also offered a breakdown of staff hours that would be devoted to patient care at Beverly Manor. As the facility was filled, the staff would spend less time on individual patient care. When Beverly Manor opened, 10 patients were expected, and by Beverly Enterprises' estimates each staff member would spend almost 6½ hours a day on nursing care. But when the facility was fully occupied with 180 patients, each employee would spend only 3 hours a day on such care. In the beginning skilled nurses were expected to spend 34 minutes a day with each patient; later they would spend only 11 minutes. It was assumed that other Beverly Enterprises employees, too, would spend less time with patients as their numbers increased. The kitchen staff would take over 1½ hours to fix meals per patient per day for 10 patients but only 23 minutes per patient per day to prepare for 180 patients. Housekeepers would spend 48 minutes per patient a day cleaning initially, but with 180 ill and often incontinent patients they would spend only 15 minutes per patient per day. Beverly Manor didn't intend to employ a physical therapist until there were 100 patients. Then the therapist was expected to spend 3.6 minutes per patient per day; with 80 more residents the time per patient would be halved, to 1.8 minutes. The social service worker could spend 1.8 minutes per patient per day with 100 residents but only 1.2 minutes with 180. Overall staffing dropped swiftly from 12.45 hours per patient per day to 4.41 hours. As the private patients saw their charges raised $32 a day, they actually received less attention. During those years revenues were supposed to rise extravagantly, a 600 percent increase in 5 years; yet the patients who were contributing to that increase were getting less for their money.

At Beverly Manor Convalescent Hospital the corporation revealed its profitmaking secret. Beverly Enterprises' formula is to maximize profits by minimizing services. In May 1982 Van Tuyle told the *Los Angeles Times*, in a graphic example, that every penny not spent on food for the elderly saves Beverly Enterprises $600,000.[13] Beverly Enterprises employs this formula in newly acquired facilities, too, but it takes a little longer. In the mid-1980s the company bought out numerous facilities, increasing the number of patients under its care by 51 percent. Despite this growth, its before-tax profits dropped slightly. Beverly reassured stockholders that the decline was caused by new nursing homes that had yet to be imprinted with its corporate style: "Management anticipates that newly acquired facilities will continue to yield lower pretax returns in the initial operating period [of three years] than in subsequent years."

Sometimes it didn't take that long. In 1982, when Beverly bought out the Michigan-based Provincial House chain, it immediately and dramatically raised its administrative charges to Medicaid. After the acquisition, Michigan taxpayers were charged 20 percent extra to administer the very same facilities. Not even the names had changed. Half of this Medicaid money was siphoned off to corporate headquarters. In effect, Beverly was forcing Michigan residents to pay more to boost the cash flow to Pasadena. Some Michigan Medicaid funds trickled into the $426,954-a-year salary paid to Van Tuyle and the $319,580 annual salary earned by David Banks. By then Beverly was the largest single provider of long-term care in Michigan. In ten of the twenty-four counties it controlled 75 to 100 percent of the nursing home beds. In twelve other counties it operated more than half.[14] Under those circumstances Beverly Enterprises was difficult to challenge. Without Beverly the elderly might be unable to find beds.

Beverly was increasingly free to do as it liked. Even while Beverly was making more money in Michigan, it was reducing services. On their visits state inspectors found that the elderly were neglected more frequently in homes that had been bought out by Beverly Enterprises. A heavy dose of Valium ordered for one patient was passed out to other residents "as if it were a stock drug," an inspector noted. The nursing staff fell below the minimum requirements. When patients were injured in accidents, their families were not notified, and no records were kept of the incidents. The head of a dietary staff had no training in nutrition. The elderly who needed special diabetic or salt-free diets didn't get them. Filthy linen was kept near the dining room where the patients ate. Bedridden patients weren't receiving proper care to avoid bed sores. Patients were served "unsafe and unappetizing" meals of puréed bologna and warm milk, according to an inspector.

In general, the Provincial House facilities bought out by Beverly deteriorated to the level of care in existing Beverly Enterprises homes. Conditions were so serious in the 360-bed Beverly Manor Convalescent Center in Pontiac, for instance, that inspectors nearly closed it. The elderly did not receive the drugs and medical care ordered by their doctors. Thirty-two patients weren't given blankets for their beds, and fourteen had no pillows. Elderly residents were found tied in restraints. Over 23 percent of Beverly homes, judged on a state rating scale of "better," "average," or "worse," fell into the "worse" category.

The National Council of Health Centers, a trade association of for-profit nursing homes, offers a convincing explanation for Beverly Enterprises' corporate style. "The reasons for the efficiency of the proprietary homes are simple: the profit motive and the rigors of the market place," it said in a report extolling the virtues of investor-owned nursing homes. "In fact, although profit and nonprofit homes face many of the same obstacles—inflation, overregulation, and so on—for-profit homes have one clear advantage: an incentive to fiscal accountability to restrain costs."[15]

At Beverly Enterprises money is shifted from patient services to corporate profit. The government pays Beverly Enterprises to care for the nation's elderly, but taxpayers' dollars buy little in terms of comfort, dignity, or security. Corporate staffing and spending policies inevitably cause patient abuse. If such nursing facilities have shed their Dickensian past, as *Forbes* claimed, they are still far from "homes" for the elderly. Even Van Tuyle paused once when asked if he would be happy to place his mother at Beverly facilities. "As far as I'm personally concerned the patient is number one. It's a thankless business. You're going to get criticism—there's a lot of emotion involved—and we do make mistakes," he admitted. But Van Tuyle's avowed belief that "the patient is number one" is belied by the conditions within his nursing home empire. In fact, its record, particularly in Texas, where it controls fifteen thousand beds, helped persuade Institute of Medicine investigators that "Excellent facilities are found in each category [investor-owned and nonprofit nursing homes] but truly awful ones are almost always proprietary."

Texas illustrated the linkage between inadequate budgets and poor patient care. In 1983, for example, Beverly spent 12 percent less on patient care than other nursing homes in the state, and it showed. Although Beverly operated 12.7 percent of Texas nursing homes, it received 18.2 percent of all citations from the state Department of Human Resources. The violations included wet and soiled linens on beds, mattresses spotted with urine and feces, human excrement on the floors of patient rooms, and inadequate staffing. Not only are Beverly Enterprises facilities cited more frequently for neglecting patients but also for failure to correct violations. Because of the lack of response the state penalized facilities by stopping Medicaid payments. Beverly Enterprises received 17 percent of all holds that were placed on nursing home payments. Some facilities that fail to rectify violations are dropped from the Medicaid program. Beverly facilities were overrepresented among these homes, too, receiving 14.3 percent of all program terminations. One of every eleven Beverly facilities has been denied Medicaid funds in comparison to one of every twenty homes statewide.[16]

Van Tuyle says that Beverly Enterprises likes to operate in states where health inspectors have a positive attitude, where, as he put it, "they're not out to function like a police force."[17] In short, where state officials are unlikely to fret overly about the quality of care in Beverly facilities. In Florida Beverly Enterprises found such a hospitable environment.

Beverly began its drive to dominate the long-term-care market in Florida in the early 1980s. In 1982 alone it increased its capacity from 29 homes with 2,672 beds to 34 homes with 4,193 beds. Beverly Enterprises gained control of 10 percent of all nursing-home beds in Florida, a significant share in itself but even more significant in a state where there is little corporate ownership. Only Beverly possessed the sophistication and cash to sweep in boldly and become the largest single provider of nursing home care. At the same time that Beverly was buying out Florida mom-and-pop facilities, it also was budgeting close to $50 million to build new facilities. Moreover, Beverly's rising power was enhanced further by its cozy relationship with Hospital Corporation of America, then the owner of 18 percent of its stock. HCA then operated 38 hospitals in Florida, ready sources of patients to nearby Beverly facilities.

Beverly eventually attracted the official notice of the U.S. Department of Justice. The Justice Department intervened after Beverly, in the middle of its Florida shopping, announced that it was acquiring Mississippi-based Mediplex, with twelve nursing homes the second-largest chain in Florida. Attorneys from the Justice

Department warned that in acquiring such a large market share Beverly might violate federal antitrust statutes. To eliminate that danger, the two companies restructured the sale.

State officials seemed supremely indifferent to the magnitude of Beverly's ambitions or the threat they might pose for Florida's elderly. While Beverly was still in the midst of its Mediplex acquisition, it asked permission to build a 120-bed home in Titusville. With that certificate of need approved plus the two facilities owned by Mediplex, Beverly would control 48 percent of the nursing-home beds in Brevard County. Even after the Justice Department required new terms for the Mediplex sale, Beverly would operate 36 percent of the beds in the county. With such a large market share Beverly would be in a position to dictate the quality and cost of long-term care. The elderly would be a captive market; the few remaining choices would largely vanish. Nursing home patients have little freedom to move. When more than one of every three nearby facilities is under the same management, such patients face nearly insurmountable odds. Moreover, Beverly would be in a position to ration long-term care to prospective patients. State regulators had been parsimonious with their certificate of need permits. As a result they managed to make Florida, the state with the largest percentage of elderly population, also the state with the lowest number of nursing home beds per capita. If Beverly decided to pursue private patients, what would happen to the large number of impoverished elderly? If it picked only the most profitable patients, what about the elderly who were sicker but more expensive to treat?

State regulators, seemingly oblivious to such questions, granted permission for the Titusville facility. The Florida AFL-CIO and the Brevard County health planning council immediately challenged the certificate of need. At a new hearing in 1982, the AFL-CIO raised numerous questions about Beverly's record—frequent citations for patient neglect, chronic staff shortages, numerous wrongful-death lawsuits by families of former patients—but the permit was upheld. The administrative hearing officer construed Florida statutes narrowly and ruled that if patient neglect existed, it was not "relevant, significant information," unimportant to Beverly's expansion, meaningless to the Brevard County residents.

While state regulators were approving the Titusville facility, Beverly Enterprises was settling a wrongful-death suit for $100,000 in Tampa. Mildred Burnside was fifty-three years old when she entered Tampa Health Care Center in 1982. Several months later she was dead. She died, according to the pathologist's report, from an "overwhelming" blood infection, a frequent complication of untreated bed sores. If conditions then were like those found later, Mrs. Burnside spent the last few months of her life amid filthy walls, cockroaches, and ceilings festooned with cobwebs.

If Titusville residents had been able to scan the state licensure files, they might have concluded that patient care was "relevant" and "significant" to the certificate of need. Based on those records, they might very well have concluded that Beverly Enterprises shouldn't be allowed to dominate the long-term care in their county. The violations didn't occur in just one home, an "orphan," as Van Tuyle referred to a facility with a history of violations, or in just one part of Florida. They occurred so often they could only have resulted from willful lack of corporate oversight. They ranged from cockroaches in the kitchens to bare mattresses. Patients were tied up and left unattended. Similar violations were cited throughout the Florida facilities—helpless, incontinent patients left to lie in their own wastes, surrounded by the stench of unclean linen and unwashed bodies. There was another pattern, too: When inspectors returned to a facility, nothing had changed.

During the year that Beverly Enterprises with its "the patient as number one" philosophy was becoming the number one operator of nursing homes in Florida, the pattern emerged clearly. In 1981 at Jacksonville Convalescent Center they issued a citation for cockroaches in May, in June, in July, and again in August. The Dade City Geriatric Center was cited for cockroach infestation in January, and fresh larvae were still hatching in the kitchen in March. At Walton County Convalescent Center the elderly lay in their own urine, men had stubble on their cheeks, and the stench of urine and filth was widespread. The unsanitary conditions ranged from unwashed denture containers to dirty water trays. At Community Convalescent Center, nine bedridden patients were left to lie unattended until they'd developed substantial bed sores. Sometimes the elderly lay on stripped-down mattresses while flies buzzed overhead. Cockroaches scurried around unchecked; the air was putrid. At Ocala Healthcare Center the elderly lay unwashed and unshaven in their wastes. Bedpans were left casually stacked on wheelchairs. At Clewiston Health Care Center elderly patients were tied in restraints but inspectors couldn't find the physician's orders that were required for their use. At Tarpon Health Care Facility there were no records to account for the use of patients' trust funds. At Spanish Gardens Nursing Center in Dunedin the elderly were served puréed food that had been watered down and minced meat patties from leftovers that had been scraped off plates and ground up.

Patients were mistreated for years at Beverly Manor Convalescent Center in St. Petersburg before the state interceded. Conditions were so horrendous that the Veterans Administration had temporarily stopped sending patients to the nursing home in 1979, but two years later, when inspectors arrived, they found feces smeared on the walls, uncovered bedpans deposited on bedside tables, and dirty wheelchairs obstructing hallways. Van Tuyle admitted the home had been mismanaged but claimed that was before Beverly Enterprises spent $200,000 on improvements. Yet the elderly saw little change in their surroundings. In fact, inspectors reported early in 1982, "The facility failed to provide a sanitary and comfortable environment for patients and personnel." Patients were discovered with their wrists tied together. Roaches raced across the kitchen floor. Patients received drugs that weren't ordered by their doctors or weren't given prescribed medications. Inspectors returned five months later and found the facility, if anything, worse. Patients still weren't receiving correct medications and treatments. There were new problems, too. Elderly patients were dressed only in hospital gowns. Soap and towels were not supplied. The facility smelled; bandages and other infectious wastes were disposed of improperly. Not enough nurses were on duty during both day and night shifts to meet licensing requirements. After repeated evidence that patients were endangered by these conditions, the state finally called a moratorium at the 262-bed facility and refused to permit further admissions until violations were corrected. Eventually they were.[18]

Beverly Enterprises has compiled one of its longest and worst records in its home state of California. Beverly Enterprises and the California State Department of Health Services agreed early in 1981 to settle outstanding violations of the health code and pending fines for a total of $25,000. The violations, which dated back to 1977, included thirteen instances of "imminent danger" when conditions created a "substantial probability" that residents would die or suffer serious injury. They also included twenty-two citations for serious but less immediately life-threatening circumstances. It paid another $5,000 so the state would drop a suit that sought permanent revocation of the licenses of two facilities where patients were ill treated. As penalties were being negotiated, the California Health Facilities Commission was releasing a 1982 report that helped to explain their frequency. According to figures supplied by the company, Beverly was spending below the state average on almost all measures of patient care, including nursing services, housekeeping, linen, and food. Assessing these data, the Institute of Medicine concluded, "The performance of Beverly Enterprises, one of the major chains operating facilities in California, was particularly poor."

Many patients continued to be endangered at its California facilities. Eleven percent of Beverly homes were fined in 1983 for jeopardizing patients' lives, for example, while the state average of all facilities was only 7 percent. California officials issued citations although nursing homes could—and usually did—appeal alleged violations to hearing officers and then the courts. When fines were finally imposed they were so small—$4,000 for negligence that nearly cost a patient his leg—that they were hardly deterrents. In 1985, however, the state legislature passed a package of tough nursing home regulations. For the first time inspectors were working with laws and penalties that nursing home operators could be forced to take seriously. Inspectors began to tackle violations at Beverly Enterprises. After four patients died at Beverly Manor in Los Gatos, the state levied a record fine of $197,000, the largest penalty in California history and far more than Beverly could have expected in the past. The fine exceeded by $35,000 the total amount of all fines levied against its eighty-two California facilities between 1981 and 1982. More sanctions followed.

Edith Hyde Sears, eighty-one years old, was a patient at Julia

Convalescent Hospital, a Beverly Enterprises facility in Mountain View on the night of June 12, 1985, when she began to vomit and cried out for nurses. Seventy-five minutes later she felt chest pains and gasped for breath. The nurses contacted her doctor, who ordered a transfer to a nearby hospital, but an ambulance was not summoned immediately. Ten minutes after Sears arrived at the emergency room of Kaiser Hospital, her heart stopped. Two days later, she died. A state investigator reported, "More than forty-five minutes passed from the time the patient exhibited classic symptoms of acute myocardial infarction [heart attack] until the ambulance was called." Sears wasn't the only patient whose death at Julia Convalescent Hospital was probed in 1985. Virginia Glissmeyer, sixty-three years old, had been striken with pneumonia once when she started running a high temperature and developed lung problems. Still, the staff waited eight days to transfer her to a local hospital. She died of pneumonia twenty-four hours after being admitted to Kaiser Hospital in Santa Clara. An investigator found, "The facility staff failed to inform the attending [staff] physician of [high] temperatures in a patient with a known history of pneumonia, failed to report green oral secretions and the development of two decubitus ulcers (bed sores)." Three other patients died allegedly as a result of improperly treated bed sores, according to the state.

The California Department of Health Services ordered a seven-member team into the facility after receiving an anonymous list of thirty-one alleged violations. Investigators discovered that in three instances nurses calculated dosages of medicine incorrectly and administered up to seven and a half times the maximum amount of prescribed morphine. They also found that a twenty-two-year-old woman who was injured in a car crash never received the wheelchair or oxygen ordered by her doctors. Another car accident victim fell two and a half feet while she was being moved from a whirlpool bath. Four patients deteriorated rapidly, losing six to nineteen pounds in a month, but their doctors were never notified. After the team spent two weeks probing conditions at the home, the state charged Julia Convalescent Center with twenty-two violations of the health code.

In 1986 the California Health Department levied fines of $800,000 against Beverly Enterprises' facilities on charges that nine patients had died because of improper care. The state, however, didn't stop with fines. Action was begun to revoke the licenses of Beverly Manor, Julia Convalescent Hospital, and Beverly Manor in Santa Cruz, which was cited for allegedly failing to consult a doctor after an elderly woman with a history of breathing problems developed new symptoms. The state also denied seven pending licenses for new Beverly homes until these cases were resolved. To settle the charges, Beverly agreed to pay more than $600,000 in fines, the largest fines in California history. The three facilities were put on probation for four years, and while the Health Department agreed to issue the pending licenses provisionally, it refused to grant any new licenses to Beverly Enterprises for fourteen months. Moreover, the state said that it would revoke the licenses of both the facilities on probation and the new homes if Beverly homes couldn't match the statewide compliance record. Beverly also agreed to submit and modify, if requested, all policies and procedures of its facilities to the state Department of Health Services. The state health director said, "This settlement will send a clear signal to other nursing homes that poor-quality patient care will not be tolerated by this department." After the settlement was announced, Van Tuyle said, "I don't think the effect is going to be dramatic. We operate in forty-six states and we think that we do a good job." But he refused to comment on the Health Department's comments, claiming that he hadn't read them.[19]

Beverly Enterprises is a dramatic illustration of the dangers of for-profit medicine. Barbara Frank of the National Citizens Coalition for Nursing Home Reform, based in Washington, D.C., said, "They have a crummy reputation and they are notorious for their spending. They take a lot off the top in administrative expenses and off the bottom in patient care." Their record stands out. At Beverly Enterprises homes, history tends to repeat itself. In Michigan, in Florida, in Texas, in California, and in other states, the pattern is clear. The lust for profit predominates.

Many of its violations are reprehensible. It is difficult to understand that a nursing home operator, even on a stringent budget, could watch idly while patients lie in their own wastes or are denied sheets and blankets. It is difficult to comprehend that an administrator would want to work in a filthy, stench-ridden home. Yet in the Beverly Enterprise system they do. In their corporate headquarters, tucked away in Pasadena, Van Tuyle and other Beverly Enterprises officials are isolated from the the day-to-day consequences of their policies. Moreover, they can't be concerned merely about the elderly in their facilities. They must worry, too, about stockholders, and if those interests conflict, their duty is clear: The stockholders should win.

Beverly Enterprises may herald the future of for-profit medical care. The Institute of Medicine, summarizing its analysis of the long-term-care industry and applying it to the supermeds, concluded, "Throughout the American health care system, there is an increasing trend toward corporatization. The emergence of the large, multisystem corporate health care providers seems to herald a new era in American health care. These developments are altering not only the structure of decision-making and locus of power but perhaps the structure and performance of the health care system as well."

CHAPTER EIGHT

No-Frills Medicine

THROUGH government subsidies and political connections, Miguel Recarey, Jr., leveraged a $4,000 investment in a Miami hospital into a multimillion-dollar for-profit health care empire, International Medical Centers (IMC). Recarey, who arrived in the United States as a penniless refugee from Fidel Castro's Cuba in 1961, told the *Miami Herald* in 1984, "This is a fantastic country. It provides opportunities to everyone and I hope that I can be somewhat of an inspiration to people to work hard and accomplish goals."

Recarey's own accomplishments were considerable. His International Medical Centers was the largest and most profitable health maintenance organization in Florida, enrolling nearly 200,000 patients in 140 offices. Its revenues approached $405 million a year and its profits reached $1.2 million a month, a substantial portion of which came from the Medicare program. The federal government paid the premiums for 75 percent of its enrollees, pumping approximately $360 million a year into IMC, and the company's monthly profits on its Medicare beneficiaries were ten times the national average.

Recarey lived flamboyantly. He drove a fleet of flashy cars that included a Maserati, a Jaguar, and a $69,200 Mercedes-Benz. He lived in a million-dollar waterfront estate, relaxed aboard a forty-two-foot yacht, and escaped from business pressures at the exclusive, members-only Bahamian island of Cat Cay. He hobnobbed with influential politicians, socialized with Princess Yasmin Khan, hired George Burns and Barbara Mandrell to promote IMC, and shuttled between Miami and Washington, D.C., with a phalanx of aides. He earned over $1.3 million in 1985.

Two years later Recarey was a broken man and his empire was in shambles. On April 22, 1987, Recarey was indicted by a federal grand jury on labor racketeering charges. He was accused of paying $115,000 in kickbacks to secure a health care contract with the South Florida Hotel and Culinary Employees Welfare Fund. The union contract was thought to be essential to his empire-building. Without it IMC would have lacked sufficient private patients to meet the federal government's conditions for participation in Medicare. Recarey was also charged with one count of obstruction of justice and one count of bribing a potential government witness.* He resigned as IMC's president immediately. (Ironically, on the same day Recarey was indicted, the Florida Department of Insurance charged IMC with twenty-three counts of fraudulent and dishonest enrollment practices. The instances allegedly occurred over a three-year period throughout the state of Florida.) A few days later, Dr. William L. Roper, head of the Health Care Financing Administration, announced that Medicare intended to cancel its $36-million-a-month contract with IMC because of serious financial and managerial deficiencies.[1]

The Florida Department of Insurance assumed control of IMC's operations following an audit by Touche Ross that revealed the health maintenance organization lost $18.6 million in 1986 despite its lucrative Medicare contract. The audit revealed a company that was distinguished by careless management and runaway expenses. IMC spent nearly $86 million or about 21 percent of its total revenues on general and administrative expenses, including salaries, marketing, and advertising costs, up sharply from the $54.84 million spent on such expenses in 1985. By contrast, Maxicare/Health America, a for-profit HMO chain, spent 9.1 percent on administrative expenses. Meanwhile, IMC was keeping a tight grip on medical expenses for its enrollees. According to Touche

*The federal government later added a wiretapping charge to the indictment, but by October 1987 Recarey had disappeared.

Ross, although IMC received an additional $48 million from Medicare in 1986, it spent only $21 million more on medical expenses. Despite the audit, much of IMC's spending remained a mystery. Touche Ross couldn't explain fully the $18.6 million loss, although part might be attributed to remunerative consulting fees to Recarey Enterprises, IMC's holding company. In 1986 IMC paid $3.9 million in management fees to Recarey Enterprises, about $1 million more than in 1985. At the beginning of 1987 IMC signed new contracts that would pay three Recarey Enterprises employees/stockholders $4.2 million over five years.

Moments before a Leon County Circuit Court judge was to begin a hearing at which IMC creditors sought to place the health maintenance organization under state receivership, IMC's attorney announced that the HMO had been sold. D. H. Blair, a privately held New York brokerage and investment banking firm, agreed to purchase IMC. Under the contract terms D. H. Blair would acquire IMC's remaining assets and assume all liabilities. The purchase guaranteed that enrollees would continue to receive medical care after weeks of being refused treatment from unpaid doctors and hospitals. This contract eventually fell through and IMC was bought by Humana.

Although Recarey managed to hide the magnitude of IMC's financial difficulties for years, the federal government had been aware that there were problems at the health maintenance organization. Kevin Moley, a Medicare official who oversees health maintenance organizations, told Ken Cummins of the *Fort Lauderdale News/Sun-Sentinel* that IMC had been a continuing problem for the federal government. "IMC has been nothing but a thorn in the side of this program since April 1985," he said. At that time, through Recarey's political contacts, IMC was exempted from the Medicare requirement that private patients comprise at least half of its enrollees. Also in 1985 South Florida newspapers began reporting regularly on financial irregularities and questionable care at IMC. Yet the federal government refused to confront IMC's problems because it feared that by doing so, the Medicare-sponsored health maintenance program might be jeopardized. About 20 percent of all senior citizens who signed up for the HMO program nationwide were IMC enrollees. If IMC's problems were an aberration, the federal government could have disowned Recarey, jettisoned IMC, and never looked back. It wasn't that easy. The federal government was afraid to renounce IMC because the bad publicity might reveal the fundamental weakness of HMOs that lie in the financial incentives to withhold medical treatment in order to increase profits.

In May 1985, less than a year before IMC's collapse, Secretary of Health and Human Services Otis Bowen convened a summit meeting of key members of Congress and federal officials to discuss IMC. So many government agencies were then investigating or trying to resolve IMC's problems that Bowen moved the meeting from his personal office to an adjacent conference room to accommodate all the people who needed to attend. They included five House members and two dozen representatives of the General Accounting Office, the Health Care Financing Administration, and the U.S. Department of Labor.

IMC's strongest critic, Congressman Dan Mica, Democrat of Florida, who called the HMO "the biggest mistake we've ever made in this country," outlined the situation in West Palm Beach, his hometown. According to Mica, an attorney in Palm Beach County was preparing fifty-one major malpractice suits against IMC. At the Palm Beach County consumer advocate agency, between five hundred and one thousand complaints were lodged against the HMO. Mica also believed that IMC was in worse shape than its officials were admitting. He had been told privately by IMC officials that fifty thousand insurance claims had been lost. Mica suspected it was done intentionally. Moreover, he was told that, if promised immunity from prosecution, IMC officials would disclose problems that went far beyond those yet known.

Although federal officials were reluctant to charge IMC publicly with wrongdoing, almost no one bothered to defend IMC or Recarey in private. Not a single person in the conference room once questioned Mica's appraisal of IMC during the three-hour discussion. But if Mica expected to persuade the government to intervene, he had come to the wrong meeting. While he stressed the need to protect IMC patients, the others talked policy. More precisely, they were talking public relations. Congressman Hal Daub, a member of the House Health Subcommittee, complained,

"Irreparable harm could occur if the HMO industry is tarnished. I'm concerned about the public image of HMOs in the new world of health care that we've embarked on."

The federal investigators sat around the granite conference table and waited for instructions. When the meeting ended, they knew they were expected to do remarkably little. They weren't told explicitly that the investigations shouldn't be pursued. Instead they were asked to be as thorough as possible in their inquiries. It was clear, however, that if so much time was spent investigating that the press lost interest, they would not be penalized. As Daub said, "There's no need to become rambunctious. A steady hand on the tiller is what's needed now."

Bowen, a physician appointed to his position only two months earlier, scarcely commented until the very end of the meeting, then neatly summarized their dilemma. "If IMC gives a bad image, the future is not good because IMC is the largest HMO program in the country," he said. "The HMO program is at stake. We don't have many choices. We have the authority to either approve them or close them down. We can't slap them on the wrist."

Closing IMC was never considered. Aside from the damaging publicity this would cause, its enrollees would be without health care. That left only approval. Another eleven months would elapse before the Department of Health and Human Services would be pressured by events to terminate the contract between IMC and Medicare.

The federal government began its promotion of HMOs in the 1970s, when President Richard Nixon endorsed prepaid medical care in an effort to deflect a drive to pass national health insurance. Pressured by mounting health costs and deep inequities in access to medical care, Congress came close to enactment of a national health insurance program. There was broad support among both Democrats and Republicans, liberals and conservatives. Senator Edward Kennedy, Democrat of Massachusetts, was holding hearings around the country on the health care crisis and leading a nationwide campaign on behalf of a massive new government program that would insure all Americans. Senator Russell Long, Democrat of Louisiana, who chaired the Finance Committee, was lobbying his colleagues on behalf of catastrophic health care insurance. Led by Governor Nelson Rockefeller of New York, many Republicans were also calling for national health care.

To seize control of the national debate, President Nixon announced "a new national health strategy" on February 18, 1971. Nixon said that the existing health care system "operates episodically" on "illogical incentives," enabling doctors and hospitals to profit from sickness rather than health. In the future, Nixon said, the United States would do something it had never done before: The government would promote and financially reward good health by its support of health maintenance organizations. The principle was simple. HMO enrollees partially surrender their freedom to select a personal physician in order to receive all their medical care for one flat fee paid in advance.

It was the first time that a majority of Americans had heard of health maintenance organizations, although prepaid health plans had existed in California since the 1930s. They began when the Los Angeles Department of Water and Power contracted with two doctors to provide medical and hospital care for a flat fee to its two thousand workers and their families. Then, during World War II, industrialist Henry J. Kaiser set up similar plans for the workers at his shipyards and steel mills on the West Coast. With a missionary's fervor, Kaiser worked to develop a program of prepaid medicine that would provide low-cost, comprehensive care. He established a special foundation to promote his Kaiser-Permanente plans, which expanded beyond his wildest expectations, eventually enrolling five million Americans thoughout the United States.

Nixon presented an audacious plan that would revolutionize the delivery of health care in the United States. He was an unusual revolutionary, but his approach was not as unlikely as it first appeared. Like other presidents before and since, Nixon adopted a seemingly radical concept, stamped a conservative *imprimatur* on it, and used it to defeat far more fundamental changes. There was another irony, too. Doctors adamantly opposed to national health insurance as socialized medicine didn't foresee the potential dangers of losing their control of health care to health maintenance organizations. As Sanford C. Bernstein & Co. pointed out, "As health maintenance organizations (HMOs) . . . proliferate, the current anarchic and uncontrolled fee-for-service system will be displaced by what could be called competitive socialized medicine." Ironically, physicians received their comeuppance not from the liberal left but from the conservative right.

Congress took a full two years to approve Nixon's ambitious health care strategy. Under the Health Maintenance Organization Act of 1973, the federal government began a campaign to enroll Americans into prepaid health plans. It would take an enormous effort. While the government was convinced that HMOs would control costs, few people seemed willing to sign up. They had to be convinced to abandon the American ideal of unlimited quality and access to health care that was embedded in fee-for-service medicine. The federal government tried to conquer that resistance in two ways. First, under the new law, businesses that hired more than twenty-five workers and offered traditional health insurance were required to offer at least two HMO plans. The HMOs had to be approved by the federal government and meet certain financial standards.

Second, the HMO Act set up a financial assistance program so that HMOs could attract the interest of business and the financial community. The federal government took on the role of health care entrepreneur, bankrolling fledgling HMOs with venture capital supplied by the taxpayers. Like most venture capitalists, the federal government didn't always invest wisely. Many HMOs promptly went bankrupt with taxpayers' money. Fourteen HMOs alone declared bankruptcy in 1981. Still, the government would spend some $145 million on grants and $219 million in loans to set up HMOs.

Frank Seubold, director of the HMO office, told the Group Health Institute, "We have pursued vigorously the task of bringing solid information on HMOs and their financial performance to the attention of leading organizations in the financial community through conferences in Washington, Chicago, and New York.

"And we have produced best sellers: *The Investors' Guide to HMOs* and *Profiles in Private Funding of HMOs*. I won't say that the financial floodgates have opened but I do believe your position will be well understood when you choose to present your case for financing."[2]

The HMO program was phenomenally successful. Only four million Americans were members of HMOs in 1973, but the *Health Market Survey,* a newsletter covering HMOs, estimated that enrollment surged to 28 million in 1987. The number of HMOs has grown exponentially, expanding from 39 in 1971 to 654 in 1987. Some 33 cities have five HMOs apiece; 6 cities have more than 10 apiece. Chicago is the most heavily contested city, with 30 health maintenance organizations, followed by Los Angeles with 20, Miami with 16, and San Francisco with 13. In the first six months of 1986, Interstudy, an Excelsior, Minnesota, health care consulting firm, reported that HMO enrollment had grown by 12 percent while 118 new plans began operations. And Sanford C. Bernstein & Co. forecasts wildly optimistic projections of future growth. Its research predicts that 75 million people, one of every three Americans, will be enrolled in HMOs by 1990.

In addition, another 15 million Americans were enrolled in the increasingly popular preferred provider organizations. PPOs are a hybrid of HMOs and fee-for-service medicine. Enrollees pay a predetermined rate but are given more freedom to select a doctor. The number of PPOs grew from 33 in 1982 to 343 in 1985.

Sanford C. Bernstein & Co. projected that altogether close to 70 percent of Americans may be enrolled in some type of prepaid medical plan by 1990. The federal government has wrought an extraordinary transformation of the health care system in an amazingly short time. Little wonder that Kevin Moley rhapsodized, "The fee-for-service sector is the past."

By 1981 the federal government announced it was phasing out its financial support of HMOs. It took another two years to shut the money-lending window. The last loan was made to a Rugby, North Dakota, HMO in August 1983. The government claimed federal funds were no longer needed because private investors were now ready to take over. In effect, the federal government did with HMOs what it had done with Medicare: It set up a program and then created an industry to profit from it.

Encouraged by the growing popularity of HMOs among working Americans, the federal government next decided to promote prepaid health plans to its Medicare beneficiaries. Under the Tax Equity and Fiscal Responsibility Act of 1982, Medicare launched a $1 billion test of senior citizens HMOs. The federal government signed contracts with a limited number of HMOs, primarily in Florida and California, to provide health care to the elderly. Under its contracts the HMOs agreed to provide a full range of benefits to senior citizen beneficiaries at a fixed rate that would be 95 percent of Medicare's average cost. Medicare paid approximately $300 monthly for each Medicare enrollee. If their costs were lower than the Medicare payment, the HMO could keep the difference; if their costs were higher, the HMO agreed to absorb the loss. The government intended to expand prepaid health plans for senior citizens throughout the United States if these HMOs reduced Medicare costs. Medicare awarded twenty-seven demonstration contracts in twenty-one cities. One of the first went to International Medical Centers. Under IMC's Gold Plus plan, typical of the new HMOs, senior citizens were given free doctor visits, prescription drugs, hospitalizations, eyeglasses, routine dental care, and hearing aids. Other Medicare beneficiaries had to pay part or all the costs of these services. The HMOs provided substantial new benefits to senior citizens, but to survive financially they had to offer these services and still make a profit.

Mike Recarey knew opportunity when it pounded on the door. With Medicare financing, his clinic, which held a state contract to provide health care to Cuban Americans, might multiply into a chain that twined across the state of Florida. Recarey launched IMC's Gold Plus plan with a full-scale media blitz that never stopped. IMC assembled a cadre of marketing, advertising, and public-relations experts. It printed slick four-color promotional brochures and twenty-four-page newspaper supplements. In one full-page newspaper ad George Burns waved a cigar, flashed a grin, and told senior citizens, "If you want to find out how to live longer, save thousands, and feel like a million, stop by any of these [IMC] locations for more information." Other ads featured singer Barbara Mandrell saying, "I think the IMC Gold Plus Plan is really great" and actor Glenn Ford affirming, "I'm proud to be part of the largest HMO in Florida and the fastest-growing in the United States."

IMC recruited senior citizens aggressively. A sales force worked the hallways of condominiums and senior citizen centers. Some sales representatives were in effect bounty hunters who were paid a $50 commission on each enrollee. Before long there were charges that IMC's representatives were sometimes signing up senior citizens without their knowledge or consent. In a typical instance a Miami Beach physician complained that one of his patients, a ninety-eight-year-old man, was sitting in front of his retirement hotel when a young IMC representative offered him and his neighbors free blood pressure tests. The elderly man agreed and was taken to an IMC clinic. After his blood pressure was taken, he asked for a copy of the reading to show his doctor. An IMC representative said that he would have to sign for the report and also provide his Medicare number. In fact, the man was being unwittingly duped into signing an IMC membership application and contract, which was completed by IMC personnel. Two days later, when his son heard about the incident, the man returned to the clinic and demanded the cancellation of his application. The doctor said, "The lack of honesty and truth demonstrated by this incident I find to be very disturbing. To me it is no wonder that the IMC-HMO is the largest in the state of Florida when they have recruiting practices as unscrupulous as the one I've just described. He is not the only patient I have who has been signed up with IMC-HMO in this manner only to come to see me and then be shocked to discover they have no Medicare benefits."

The Department of Health and Human Services hadn't reckoned with a Mike Recarey when it started its experiment. Most HMOs were small, but Recarey seemed determined to enroll Florida's entire elderly population. A year after the program started, 222,703 senior citizens were members of five South Florida HMOs. Over 100,000 of those were signed up for Gold Plus. IMC was a medical McDonald's, franchising its clinics to independent operators in six counties. IMC took in the Medicare fees, deducted administrative costs, and passed the remaining payments on to its franchisees. At sales meetings IMC's marketing representatives promised that physicians could earn profits of 10 to 40 percent from their Medicare patients. Experienced medical administrators, however, cautioned that such high profits were possible only if costs were cut by denying patients care.

Medicare, however, was anxious to restrain its costs and unconcerned about the quality of care. While the federal government was investing billions—over $1.1 billion in the first ten months alone—to set up the HMOs, virtually nothing was spent to ensure that patients were cared for properly. Theodore Weinberg, compliance director for the HMO program, said, "We do not make assessments of quality. We make no judgments because we don't know how to do that and the law recognizes that." Medicare undertook no monitoring of the quality of care at the HMOs and established no procedures to investigate or respond to patients' complaints.

South Florida physicians were soon complaining about the care at IMC facilities. A former president of the Palm Beach County Medical Society, Dr. Lee Fischer, said, "Quality of care is an area of tremendous concern which can have devastating consequences. . . . Because most HMOs receive a capitation payment for each individual enrolled, they have a built-in financial incentive to deliberately underutilize medical care. . . . I am worried that a large number of people who know nothing about health care, but a lot about making a profit, are forming their own HMOs so they, too, can get a piece of the pie. The public needs protection from unscrupulous businessmen who will be enjoying the good life in Europe while their former HMO members hunt for a new health care provider."[3]

The doctors, however, were not considered uninterested observers. IMC was taking away their private patients. Doctors who already faced vigorous competition among themselves confronted a new rival in the federal government. By subsidizing the HMOs, the government was helping the prepaid plans to mass-market cut-rate medical care. The senior citizens who joined the HMOs received almost all their medical care free, while those who continued with private doctors were billed for charges above Medicare's payment. Disgruntled doctors in Palm Beach County raised over $100,000 to air anti-HMO television commercials. While the doctors were hard-pressed to beat the federal government's prices, they could attack the quality of care.

At IMC franchises physicians were given incentives to undertreat patients. Out of their share of the Medicare payment physicians were required to pay for all the medical care of Gold Plus members. If patients needed to be sent to a hospital or referred to a specialist, the clinics were responsible for the bills. A former head of IMC's quality assurance committee, Dr. Lee A. Bricker of Miami Beach, pointed out, "The thing that makes IMC attractive to a doctor is that he gets discretion over how funds are spent. It is strictly the doctor's sense of honor that governs how much he keeps and how much he spends on his patients." Under those conditions the less care doctors delivered, the more money they could earn. Some doctors found the mingling of fiscal and medical control of their patients too great a temptation. They cashed out their Hippocratic Oath.

Soon members of Congress from South Florida were receiving disturbing letters from constituents about IMC operations. In 1986 Congressman Dan Mica chaired hearings of the U.S. House Select Committee on Aging in Palm Beach and Broward counties on IMC. The hearings revealed that IMC was in serious disarray. Enrollees claimed that they were being refused treatment or dunned by hospitals and doctors whose bills weren't paid by IMC.

Katheen Moyer's testimony was typical of the complaints about IMC. Moyer described her sixty-five-year-old mother's treatment in Palm Spring. Her mother enrolled late in 1984 and in December began a series of appointments with HMO doctors who treated her for emphysema and an ulcer. She didn't improve, and in August 1985 she was bedridden and in acute pain. Moyer said, "We couldn't believe what was going on—we did not understand any methods that the HMO worked by. My mother by now had seen her doctors seven times and gone to emergency three times in eight months and they still wouldn't help her." Moyer then took her mother to a specialist who examined her and called her HMO doctor to request a biopsy of her left breast and stomach and a bone scan. Moyer said, "My mother had been there since late 1984 and it was not until August 1985 that she first saw a specialist—and for months she was bedridden and still they could not find anything. They came up with acute arthritis, she did have emphysema, and it was an ulcer, stomach ulcer, created her pain, but cancer was not mentioned once."

On September 5 Moyer and her mother returned to the surgeon who performed the biopsy. "It was through him that we learned she had cancer and the reason for all her pain—the cancer had spread from her breast to her ribs and spine," Moyer said. They went to a cancer specialist who scheduled chemotherapy for the following week, but when the time came, her mother was too weak to undergo the treatments. She was hospitalized for eight days to build up her blood count, then discharged on October 3. She was given an appointment to begin chemotherapy on October 17. "Again we couldn't understand this wait—we didn't think Mom could get worse but she did," Moyer said. By October 6 her mother was readmitted to the hospital. "It was then that we . . . found out that the cancer had spread to her liver, kidney, and lungs and it was too late for any treatments," Moyer said. Moyer brought her mother home on October 17, the day she was finally supposed to start chemotherapy. She died on October 20.[4]

The committee also heard from doctors and hospital representatives who testified about IMC's poor care and their inability to get paid when they treated IMC patients. James Rogers, assistant administrator of Northwest Regional Hospital in Margate, said, "Another concern we have about HMOs is that the acuity levels of illnesses are increased perhaps due to patients [being] delayed the care that they should promptly receive. . . . We do see patients that arrive on death's doorstep because they have been denied initial essential care. Once we get them up into the intensive care unit, it takes a greater amount of services to get them back to where they were than if the HMO had just admitted them in the first place. . . . The physicians on our staff do not resist or object to caring for indigent patients—that is part of the responsibility that comes with being on our medical staff. What they do resent is taking care of a patient on a Good Samaritan basis and have someone else make money on their Good Samaritan act." Northwest Regional Hospital was then overdue payment on $408,000 by IMC, and it wasn't alone. IMC also owed doctors who were beginning to refuse to treat IMC patients. Rogers said, "What does concern us, though, is when I am up until 3:00 A.M. in the morning and we have a physician that is on call saying, 'I do not want to take another HMO patient, they owe me $40,000 as it is.' "[5]

Another Northwest Regional Hospital witness, Dr. Neil Schultz, charged that IMC had tried to pressure the hospital to release patients prematurely. "You usually get phone calls from either a secretary in one of the HMO clinics or possibly a physician who works for that clinic, putting strong pressure on you that the patient has to be discharged," he said. "Not really paying much attention as to how critically ill the patient is or anything like that, they just start putting pressure on you saying that the patient has to—either 'You have to send the patient out, you are keeping him in there too long.' . . . And if you tell them that the patient's condition really does not warrant discharge at this time, they say, 'Well, the patient has really been there too long and you are just keeping him in the hospital for an excessive period of time.' " Schultz said that he would then receive calls daily until the patient was finally released.[6]

Some IMC members who were discharged by hospitals were too sick to return home and were released to long-term-care facilities. Nursing homes, too, were distressed by the condition of these patients. Druid Hills, a Clearwater, Florida, nursing home, compiled dozens of instances of IMC patients who received inferior medical treatment. According to a typical chart, an IMC patient was "discharged from hospital . . . in deplorable condition. Required nasopharyngeal suctioning constantly, moaning in terrible pain—had morphine around the clock . . . expired within eighteen hours of admission in agony." An outraged Druid Hills executive director wrote the Florida Association of Home Health Agencies, "If nursing facilities were operating in this manner, state or federal agencies would close their doors."[7]

In a precedent-setting case in 1985, the state of Florida charged an IMC doctor, Dr. Leon Shore of Davie, with medical malpractice in the death of Lawrence Schubert, an eighty-two-year-old Gold Plus member. The Florida Department of Professional Regulation charged that Schubert was prematurely discharged from Humana Hospital of South Broward. The complaint alleged "gross and repeated malpractice." It also alleged that he exploited his patient for his own financial gain.

Schubert was admitted to Humana Hospital with a diagnosis of cerebrovascular accident. His X rays indicated pneumonia, congestive heart failure, or both. Schubert continued to deteriorate until he needed a bladder catheter and a nasogastric tube for feeding. He couldn't swallow or eat but Shore ordered the feeding tube removed. Shore then arranged for Schubert to be transferred to Sunrise Retirement Home in Fort Lauderdale, which provided no medical services. Hospital doctors and nurses vigorously opposed the transfer, insisting that the patient required continuous hospital care. Schubert's daughter, Joan Murray of Cooper City, also objected strenuously. "I told Shore that I totally objected," she said in a sworn statement. "It was no place for my father to go because of his condition." But according to the complaint, Shore stood to profit from the discharge. Shore had a financial interest in Transflorida Group HMO, an IMC affiliate. The HMO was financially responsible for Schubert's care in the hospital but not at the retirement home. The day after the transfer Murray visited Schubert, who was feverish and very ill. She arranged for her father to be readmitted to the hospital, where doctors diagnosed pneumonia. He died less than a month later.

William Furlow, an attorney for the Department of Professional Regulation, said, "We have received complaints alleging that an HMO doctor has done something inappropriate and the reason he/she did it was because of financial interest as opposed to the best thing for the patient. To the best of my knowledge and recollection, the Leon Shore case is the first case where the probable cause panel of either one of the medical boards [Board of Medical Examiners and Board of Osteopathic Medical Examiners] has decided that the case was sufficiently strong to find probable cause and proceed."[8] In the end, however, the physicians who compose the Board of Medical Examiners decided to drop the charges after their investigating attorney advised he "no longer felt confident" that Shore acted improperly.

Under federal government pressure IMC created a quality assurance committee that met weekly to review the performance of its clinics. According to Bricker, about 15 percent were given A's but another 20 percent got D's and F's. "About 20 percent of the centers really did unacceptable or marginal work," he said. After the committee was created, the federal government didn't follow up. It exerted no pressure to improve the quality of care at the facilities that received failing marks. In fact, it didn't even review the reports. The federal government was satisfied when IMC set up the committee. It was then able to continue to receive Medicare funds while the inadequate care persisted.

IMC has not been the only troubled HMO. Problems have surfaced at prepaid plans throughout the country. Although complaints have centered on the Medicare-sponsored HMOs, that may well be because they are the only ones under scrutiny. Congress has paid close attention to the senior citizen HMOs while the quality of care at HMOs generally has not been reviewed by any government agency. Yet prepaid plans operate on the same principles, and the deficiencies at IMC and other Medicare HMOs provide ample reason to be concerned about no-frills medicine.

In 1987 Senator John Heinz, Republican of Pennsylvania, the ranking minority member of the U.S. Senate Special Committee on Aging, released a report on Medicare HMOs that found "flagrant violations of sound medical practice" throughout the United States. Heinz said, "With HMOs, like DRGs, we find beneficiaries falling victim to unscrupulous health providers, who would squeeze out the last cent of profit at the cost of high-quality care."[9]

Senate investigators found that the struggle between cost and quality was not always resolved in the patient's favor. "The pressures to save money can outweigh the HMO's regard for quality and access and, in some cases, its physicians' responsibilities to provide the necessary services," the report stated. Among the examples were:

- A California HMO told physicians that Medicare beneficiaries were using too many services and no more should be enrolled. "Physicians should ensure that their office staffs do not actively encourage existing patients in the practice to join these plans, as they naturally produce an adverse selection," its letter cautioned. "The marketing of these plans should be left to the Health Plan professionals to ensure a balanced profile of patients." The HMO also warned physicians, "Contracts are for a one-year term and may be renewed annually contingent upon satisfactory utilization practices."

- An elderly woman in California discovered a lump in her breast. After mammography three HMO doctors said there was no evidence of cancer. Surgery was performed, however, to remove the lump. Afterward the surgeon said that a radical mastectomy should have been performed. Frantic, she arranged an appointment with a second surgeon who was not associated with an HMO. The surgeon agreed that she needed immediate surgery for a radical mastectomy. During the operation the surgeon discovered the cancer had metastasized to her lymph nodes and spread to her lungs. She wrote, "At seventy-six I felt the little money I had left would sustain me for the rest of my life. Instead it all went out, and more from relatives, for all the doctor and hospital bills."
- A Minnesota woman visited her HMO with stomach complaints. She was tested for cancer of the bowel, a procedure that gives inaccurate results frequently, according to the American Cancer Society. Although her symptoms persisted, the test was not repeated after the initial negative findings. On two occasions she was treated for a spastic colon. Three months after her initial visit she required emergency surgery for a perforated colon. The surgeon indicated that if her colon had not perforated, she would not have required a colostomy and her survival chances would have been substantially higher. The woman started chemotherapy but died a little over a year later. Adequate testing might have saved her life.
- A New Jersey woman who had crippling arthritis found that her HMO delayed treatment. She was ping-ponged from one doctor to another and told that nothing more could be done for her pain. She was then informed that the doctors were no longer associated with the HMO and referred to still another doctor, who wanted to repeat the complete series of medical tests. Discouraged, she saw a private physician who performed a hip replacement operation and additional surgery so she could remain mobile.

Despite evidence of inadequate medical care, business is bullish on HMOs. After the federal government discontinued its HMO loans in 1981, the financial community started to invest heavily. In the next two years over $480 million, more than the federal government had spent on HMOs in a decade, flowed into the HMO market. Investor financing became a major source of HMO funds. To get access to private capital, HMOs began going public. U.S. Health Care Systems converted from a nonprofit to a for-profit health plan and issued the first stock in 1983. In six months it raised $44 million. Its stock split twice and soared from $8.90 to $22.50. Its success was not lost on other HMOs. A few months later, Maxicare Health Plans and Health America also issued stock, raising a total of $36 million. Within a year later seven other investor-owned HMO chains were operating in more than one state.

In the 1970s so few for-profit HMOs existed that statistics on them were not even kept. Since then their growth has been nothing less than phenomenal. In 1981 only 18 percent of all HMOs were for-profit, but by 1985 their share climbed to 36 percent. Many were new plans, but between 25 and 33 percent were formed by plans that had converted from nonprofit to for-profit operations. The for-profits enrolled 26 percent of HMO members in 1985, compared to 12 percent in 1981. Before the decade ends the for-profits could control the market. Nearly half of new HMO members join for-profit plans.

The era when Henry Kaiser looked to prepaid plans to offer low-cost medical care to his workers has vanished. Gone, too, are the days when HMOs were considered nominally altruistic organizations indifferent to growth and profitability. Today HMO managers keep one eye on costs and revenues and the other on the Dow Jones Industrial Average. The for-profit boom is simply understood. Investors will put their money only where they have a reasonable expectation of hefty returns.

HMOs are growing, as the hospital chains did, by taking over financially troubled plans and linking them into national chains. Between 1985 and 1987 at least one HMO a month was being bought out. In the mid-1980s the chains were growing by 22 percent a year. Half a dozen national chains were in the midst of a bidding war over the HMOs that were put on the market. Acquisition-hungry HMOs bid the buyout price up to $1,000 per enrollee. Medicare enrollees were worth up to $3,600 each. As Donald W. Moran and Theresa E. Savela of ICF Incorporated, a Washington-based consulting firm, pointed out, "The business of building HMOs to sell them down the road to eager investors can be a spectacularly profitable one. One would expect every venture capitalist with $200,000 to burn to rush into the market to cash in on the expected windfalls. For if building one HMO and selling out at these prices is a good idea, building ten HMOs and taking them public for $150 million within three years looks like a great idea."

Among the more promising investor-owned HMOs was Maxicare Health Plans, a nonprofit plan that converted to for-profit. In 1972 Fred Wasserman, a medical management consultant, recruited 10 Los Angeles doctors to found Maxicare. By 1986 Maxicare was operating in 14 states and 15 of the 30 largest markets in the United States. More than 200 physician groups were offering care to an estimated 850,000 members. Wall Street analysts tagged it the "West Coast wonder"; the press plugged its success in articles titled "Maxicare, Maxiprofits." In three years, after its initial public offering in 1983, Maxicare expanded meteorically, increasing revenues by 500 percent, its earnings per share by 600 percent, and profits by 700 percent. Even doctors viewed the company favorably because they often got a share of the profits. Wasserman said, "We've learned that people with equity tend to have a greater commitment to perform."

Since Maxicare went public, the competition has gotten tougher. HMOs were a spectacular growth industry in 1987, and the profit potential has enticed dozens of companies into the fray. In addition to Humana and Hospital Corporation of America, a handful of publicly traded HMOs such as U.S. Health Care and United HealthCare are fighting for market share. Major insurance companies, including Aetna Life Insurance, Metropolitan Life Insurance, Prudential Life Insurance, and Travelers Corporation were selling—or on the brink of marketing—HMO plans in 1987. The stakes were high. Metropolitan Life alone has committed $100 million to the development of its HMO plan.

Most of the insurance companies are newcomers who have

been forced to offer prepaid health plans to survive. HMOs have already devoured 10 percent of the private health insurance market, and the percentage is expected to grow. When 1986 began, Lincoln National Corporation, the nation's ninth-largest group health insurance company, had never written an HMO policy. Then it underwent an amazing transformation. In one year Lincoln National had formed fourteen joint ventures and acquisitions that included Fireman's Fund Employers Insurance Company. By 1987 it had 400,000 members in its HMO plans and announced an ambitious strategy to shift 70 percent of its indemnity customers to prepaid health plans. Stephen H. Berkey, president of Alternative Care Technologies, a division of Lincoln National, said, "Our business is managed health care. We don't consider our business to be in the group health and life business anymore. There are a number of new players—hospitals and hospital chains—that are getting into the HMO business. PPOs, HMOs, and the whole dramatic change of how health care is being delivered, managed, and paid for has turned 180 degrees in the last two and a half years."

The competition keeps getting tougher. In mid-1986 Maxicare launched preemptive strikes against its rivals. It announced early in July that it was spending $64 million to purchase HealthCare USA, a money-losing HMO with operations in four states. Before the month ended Maxicare startled Wall Street by announcing plans to acquire the nation's largest HMO, HealthAmerica Corporation, paying $400 million for its nine hundred thousand members. It was a bold move; some analysts felt it was rash, but it put Maxicare far ahead of its competitors. With its new acquisitions Maxicare became the first for-profit chain to operate nationwide. It was also the largest, with $1.6 billion in annual revenues and two million members in thirty-two states. Wasserman said, "The combined company will clearly be able to serve more markets than any other HMO in the nation with the immediate capability to service employers in twenty-four of the thirty largest markets in the United States." Maxicare was no longer merely a West Coast wonder. David L. Goldsmith of Robertson, Colman & Stephens said, "They've raised the stake for everybody else. Everybody else has talked about going nationwide and going to GM and saying,

'We're your HMO.' No one truly has had the locations to be able to do this."

To complete the purchases, however, Maxicare had to increase its debt, and the acquisitions hurt the company's profits. At the end of 1986 it reported a fourth-quarter net loss of $22.1 million despite a 143 percent rise in revenues, from $149.2 million to $362.4 million. The dismal fourth-quarter results also hurt its annual results. Earnings per share plunged 83 percent, to $0.13 in 1986 from $0.75 a share in 1985, while net income slid 79 percent, to $4.3 million from $20.4 million. Revenues, however, climbed 75 percent, to $914.4 million from $523.3 million. Some analysts believed that despite the disappointing 1986 results—which continued into 1987—Maxicare would be strengthened through the acquisitions. Larry Selwitz of Bateman Eichler, Hill Richards, Inc., forecast, "Maxicare will become such an awesome, dominant force among HMOs that it should be able to dictate prices."

Big business is a potent new force behind the growth of HMOs' brand of discount medicine. By controlling billions of dollars in health care benefits, big business has the ability to reshape the health care system. In the mid-1980s many corporations began to exercise that power. As Jack Myers, a health policy expert at the American Enterprise Institute in Washington, D.C., told a gathering of doctors, "It's not just the government who is coming after you. It's the boardrooms of the country that are going after you. They're mad, they're big, and they have a lot of dollars." Corporations awoke to the virtues of HMOs when they discovered that their health care spending nearly doubled between 1980 and 1985, to $90 billion a year. They were spending close to $125 billion a year, slightly in excess of 50 percent of their pretax profits, on health care.

One of those companies, as its chairman, Roger Smith, told the American Medical Association, was General Motors, which insures 2.1 million employees and retirees, almost 1 percent of the entire United States population. Between 1973 and 1984 its health care expenses rose 14 percent a year, faster than the national average, adding roughly $483 per car to its production costs. GM's largest supplier of goods and services was Blue Cross and Blue Shield of

Michigan. By the mid-1980s General Motors was spending 40 percent of its total benefit package, $2.3 billion a year, on health care. Moreover, it anticipated that unless costs were restrained, spending would double in five years. Smith said, "Most people I know agree that the quality of health care in this country is unsurpassed, but unfortunately so is the cost. In fact, some people have suggested that our hospitals need a second recovery room—right next to the cash register."

At that point General Motors commissioned a study of its health care spending. The results startled company officials. GM, which pays all the health care costs for its insurees, found that it was providing equally generous benefits to health care providers near its plants. In New Jersey the company learned that some 30 percent of its total spending was considered of "questionable" necessity. In Michigan employees who gave birth were hospitalized a day longer than the national average. Smith said, "It's just hard for us to understand why GM mothers in Michigan need a day more in the hospital than mothers in Ohio or California for a normal delivery. Imagine the effect if all eighteen thousand of our deliveries required an extra day's hospitalization."

In 1985, determined to restrain costs, General Motors added prepaid health care to its benefit package. After vigorous promotion, the company convinced 130,000 people to switch to prepaid plans. The results appeared on corporate balance sheets immediately. For the first time in a quarter century General Motors decreased its overall health care costs. Less than two years after General Motors first introduced prepaid plans some 600,000 employees and retirees were enrolled in 68 HMOs and dozens of PPOs. GM has been so pleased by the results that when its Saturn plant opens in Tennessee, employees will be offered only HMO coverage. The company will no longer pay for visits to fee-for-service doctors. Smith said, "Inefficient practices on the part of health care providers contribute to excessive costs. . . . A 10 percent reduction in costs could be achieved through these programs even as the quality of health care is improved."

Some large corporations like Lockheed and Rockwell International are requiring new employees to join HMOs, while others, like Walt Disney World, are organizing their own prepaid plans. After reviewing the cost of insuring Mickey Mouse and his friends through traditional group health plans, Walt Disney decided it could save money through direct negotiations with hospitals. As central Florida's major employer, Walt Disney World exercised considerable clout. It organized its own preferred provider organization, signed up over sixteen thousand workers, and began pressing for discounts. Orlando was small enough that hospitals could expect a substantial increase in patients if they captured only a small fraction of the enrollees in Walt Disney's preferred provider organization. To win their allegiance, hospitals were willing to cut their rates. The discounts were large enough that PPO members who went elsewhere were required to pay an extra $500 a day at other hospitals for the privilege.

It was a devastating blow to hospitals that weren't selected. Winter Park Memorial Hospital, long popular with Disney employees, immediately lost 8 percent of its maternity patients. It wasn't only hospitals that were endangered; physicians were threatened, too. Although Walt Disney was bartering with hospitals, it was helping to choose the physicians who would be eligible to treat PPO members. Doctors who couldn't admit patients to the chosen hospitals would be disadvantaged, too. PPO members could be treated by those doctors, but if they needed to be hospitalized, they had to pay more.

Despite their corporate popularity, many employers who have adopted prepaid plans are souring on HMOs, wondering if the supposed savings are more mythical than real. Sales representatives hawk the prepaid plans aggressively with promises of reductions in health care costs. But after the marketing blitz ends, not all companies fare as well as General Motors. At Texas Instruments, for instance, HMO premiums exceed those charged for indemnity insurance. Over half the officers of 320 companies in the nonprofit Kaiser-Permanente plan said their health costs weren't reduced, while 8 percent said their costs went up. Less than a third, only 30 percent, reported reduced health care spending. Over two hundred major national corporations surveyed by the Washington Business Group on Health found that HMOs were considered only "somewhat effective" at lowering costs. Its vice president Rick Lee said, "The system hasn't had as great a savings as anticipated."

Minneapolis and St. Paul, Minnesota, offer a preview of the future of no-frills medicine. It's scarcely encouraging for employers or consumers who hoped for savings. More Twin Cities residents, almost half the entire population, are enrolled in HMOs than in any other city in the United States. Ten HMOs and five PPOs vie fiercely to capture the loyalty of the remaining five hundred thousand residents. Moreover, the doctor glut hit there early, producing a patient-to-physician ratio that is one third higher than the national average. As a result, 90 percent of the physicians have been driven into HMOs to generate business.

Tom Hoban, executive vice president of the Hennepin County Medical Society, says that the HMOs are skimming patients from doctors who practice traditional, fee-for-service medicine. "Private doctors simply can't increase their practices," he said. "Most Twin Cities physicians would be happy if they could just maintain their practices. But they can't. The collegial atmosphere in medicine is rapidly disappearing."

Twin Cities doctors formed their own prepaid plan, called an independent practice association, to compete with HMO entrepreneurs. Initially many doctors resisted, then realized they were losing patients to participating physicians. The HMOs marketed their services to businesses and enrolled their employees before they needed medical care. Hoban said, "Doctors in the Twin Cities said, 'Our patients will never leave us, and if they do, they will come crawling back.' We told them they would leave. We thought patients would leave if the prepaid plans could offer care for one dollar less. We were wrong. They left for fifty cents—and they didn't come back."

The stiff competition should reduce health care costs; at least that theory has generated enthusiasm for prepaid care. The plans are in a position to negotiate cut rates with doctors and hospitals and pass those savings along to consumers and employers. In the Twin Cities it hasn't happened. Money that might have been returned is being spent lavishly to woo new patients. Millions have been flung into advertising and promotional campaigns. In this battle the biggest beneficiary may be advertising agencies and public-relations firms. *The Minneapolis Star and Tribune* watched its health-related advertising soar from 11,000 inches in 1982 to 46 million inches in 1985. More than $15 million was spent on media and direct-mail campaigns in that year alone.

Meanwhile, many enrollees were paying nearly as much for HMO plans as for idemnity insurance that offered a broader choice of services and providers. Instead of undercutting traditional insurers, the HMOs raised their rates to match. Fosten Boyle, a Honeywell vice president and member of the Minnesota Coalition on Health Care Costs, said, "Rather than providing true price competition, HMOs have used the price umbrella of fee-for-service as a target. They've been healthy in terms of interjecting an element of cost consideration that would otherwise not be there. However, when you look at the history of how we've applied HMOs—offering them all early on, with many cases of the healthy going to the HMOs and the HMOs pricing just under indemnity insurers—they have not necessarily brought us cost savings."[10]

At Honeywell healthy employees whose medical costs were low tended to join HMOs, while workers who saw their doctors more frequently stayed with the Blue Cross and Blue Shield plans. As a result, Blue Cross and Blue Shield had higher expenses and raised its premiums. After a three-year study the company calculated that HMOs raised its overall medical costs for its Minneapolis employees by $5 million.

In 1986 HMO enrollment dipped in Minneapolis-St. Paul after the state government solicited closed bids on its health care contracts. Minnesota Blue Cross/Blue Shield underbid HMOs with its Aware Gold plan, offering comprehensive care, low premiums, and a choice of doctors and hospitals. When the new rates were announced, the HMOs lost 2,559 members, reducing their share of state workers from 46 to 42 percent.

Prepaid health plans are an emerging fourth force in medicine beside doctors, hospitals, and insurers and are becoming the power brokers in health care, wheeling and dealing between purchasers and providers of health care. They are the bargaining agents who squeeze providers for the biggest price concessions. Medicine, once marketed retail, is being sold wholesale with increasing frequency.

In hotly contested markets, so many discounts are offered that the bargain price becomes the going rate. Then, as Michael McCullough, president of Baylor Physician Associates, pointed out, "If you bring everyone in, who will you be preferred over? If you bring everyone in, who will you compete with?" Wholesale buyers may find the savings largely illusory.

Government and big business have been able to promote HMOs successfully largely because of the doctor glut. Gary Janko, president of Bay State Health Care in Cambridge, Massachusetts, said, "In the beginning a doctor working for an HMO had to do it under cover of darkness. Now there are doctors always looking for patients."[11] Solo practitioners find that economic survival is difficult in the 1980s. Between 1980 and 1984 physicians in group practices grew by 44 percent and groups with more than one hundred doctors doubled, according to the American Medical Association. By 1986 nearly half of the doctors under age forty were in group practices. Doctors found that if they huddled together, they could lower costs, get referrals, and make a profit. Ironically, however, group practices were ready targets for health maintenance organizations. They could sign up doctors in groups more quickly than they could go door-to-door negotiating with individual physicians. By the mid-1980s over 175,000 physicians, 43 percent of all doctors, had contracted with at least one HMO. Some signed with far more. In California, for example, doctors routinely contracted with fifty prepaid plans, in some instances agreeing to provide medical care for a flat rate of only $10 per month per enrollee.

Doctors are signing contracts because they can't pay their bills without them. Doctors are losing patients in droves. The American Medical Association reports that some doctors are losing twenty families a month from their practices and no replacements are to be found in the waiting rooms. In a single year some doctors have seen HMOs recruit 25 to 33 percent of their patients. And in places like California the rate is higher. The California Medical Association found in a 1986 membership survey that over 70 percent of doctors reported losing patients to prepaid plans. Some specialists reported even bigger losses. Over 87 percent of the obstetrician/gynecologists and 91 percent of the pediatricians said their patients are switching to HMOs. Over 40 percent of the doctors said that they had been asked by patients to join a prepaid plan. The California poll discovered that 75 percent of its sample had signed up with at least one prepaid plan but they weren't necessarily happy about the arrangement. Some 56 percent said they were moderately to severely dissatisfied with their contracts. Only 6 percent said they were very satisfied. Nearly 75 percent said they were seeing more patients but, because of mandatory discounts, weren't earning more. Four times as many doctors reported decreased revenues as indicated increases.[12]

Belatedly, doctors are entering the battle for bodies, forming their own independent practice associations. In Georgia, for instance, six health maintenance organizations were already active in the Atlanta area, where they had enrolled 170,000 members by 1984. Another 10,000 to 20,000 Georgians were members of preferred provider organizations. In 1984 the Medical Association of Georgia projected that in two years one third of the state's population would have joined a prepaid plan. That would mean a lot of physicians with empty appointment books. In October of that year the state medical society, alarmed by its own projections, summoned an emergency meeting of its membership. As Michael Fowler, executive director of the state society, recalled, "Our real goal, the major purpose of the meeting, was to try to maintain doctors' control of health care in Georgia." The medical leadership believed Georgia doctors had two choices: They could go to work for an HMO sponsored by a for-profit company, or they could start their own.

It wasn't easy convincing Georgia doctors that a physician-sponsored HMO was wise. The medical society had to coax doctors to invest in something they didn't like and didn't want. Yet, there were those projections. While HMOs were still concentrated in Atlanta, their future growth could come only in small cities and towns throughout the state. In the end, physicians succumbed to reality. Members voted reluctantly to create the prepaid plan, one of ten physician-sponsored HMOs that now exist in the United States. More than 2,500 doctors joined and contributed $3.5 million in start-up capital through direct contributions and stock purchases. Eighteen months later, the Georgia Health Network, the first HMO to be created, owned, and controlled by a state medical society, was ready to enroll its first member. Fowler said, "Physicians signed contracts rapidly even though they didn't want to. It was a matter of survival and marketplace pressures offsetting philosophical objections."

The Georgia Health Network and similar HMOs reveal the medical profession's rampant sense of desperation. By capitalizing on their vulnerability, discount medical plans threaten to subvert the historic relationship between doctors and patients. Traditionally doctors are their patients' allies, but HMOs contain an omnipresent threat that doctors will be turned into their adversaries, that physicians will become the collaborators of business managers and restrict care to increase the HMOs' and their own profits. A doctor who has been in private practice for forty years said, "What's everything about now? It's about money. Who has to be against the good care of the patient a certain amount? It's the doctor. He has to restrain many things. Finally the patient is suffering. The patient-doctor relationship is suffering. We have a conflict right now."

Dr. Robert A. Berenson, a Washington, D.C., internist who writes about health policy, explains the quandary that confronts HMO doctors. In many HMOs, he says, primary care physicians are paid a flat $20 to $25 a month to treat patients. At the end of the year doctors can earn a bonus if the HMO has spent less than the budgeted amount for specialists and hospital services. Under those contract terms doctors will earn the most money if the HMO signs up healthy patients and shuns patients who are likely to drive up costs. But Berenson says, "The physician's financial interest clearly requires him to encourage only his relatively healthy patients to sign up for the HMO. Yet the physician's trustee responsibility to this patient's well-being may require him to actively encourage his sickest patients to join the HMO. The ethical dilemma is not theoretical but real, largely because the potential effect on physician income of who joins the HMO is not trivial."

Berenson points out that HMO doctors are exposed to pressure from colleagues as well as business managers. Doctors who make referrals to specialists, order extra tests, or hospitalize patients reduce the amount of money that can be distributed in annual bonuses. He says, "The physician with consistently poor performance . . . would be seen as responsible for disproportionately using up pools intended for distribution to fellow IPA physicians. Possibly, although less likely, the physician would be dropped by the IPA for being a high-cost provider, contributing negatively to the group's bottom line."[13]

HMOs have set up administrative and financial hurdles to discourage such poor fiscal performance. A primary care physician is a "gatekeeper" who sees patients initially and decides if they should be referred to specialists or hospitalized. Even when the gatekeeper decides a patient needs to be hospitalized, HMOs routinely require a second opinion from a review panel hired to hold down hospital admissions. In fact, HMOs have achieved their greatest success in rationing hospital care. The Group Health Association, an HMO trade group, said in 1987 that HMOs averaged 427 days of hospital care per 1,000 members compared with the national average of 920 days. HMOs were particularly adept at reducing hospital admissions among the elderly. The total number of inpatient care for senior citizens in HMOs was 1,905 a year while the national average was 3,339 a year. HMOs may also require second opinions before certain tests or procedures can be ordered. Some HMOs also employ physicians who review the gatekeeper's services and are authorized to deny payment if they disagree with the treatment. A silent conspiracy to deny care can be the result.

In 1987 family practitioners and specialists fought bitterly about HMO policies in Huntsville, Texas, a small town between Houston and Dallas. The dispute arose when Maxicare signed a contract with the Family Practice & Surgery Clinic. Its director, Dr. C. Alvin Jones, said the contract was signed "as a matter of survival" so the HMO wouldn't open its own clinics and steal clinic patients. The clinic doctors and the specialists fought over fees, but they disagreed even more about referrals. While the family physicians wanted to be the ultimate authority, the specialists distrusted that power and insisted on a contract that would set up a three-member panel of specialists and the clinic's medical director to arbitrate conflicts about referrals. Dr. James M. Hanna, a dermatologist, said, "The guy with the most expertise and training should be calling the shots." Another physician, Dr. Michael deBerardinis, a urologist who refused to sign with Maxicare, said that despite the loss of patients and money he would not submit to the clinic's demand for control. "I feel like Custer," he said. "If I'm going to make a stand, I'm going to make a stand here. And if a million Indians mow me down, the Indians win."[14]

The specialists insisted that the clinic had an economic incentive to do as little as possible for patients once it received its $50,000-a-month HMO payment. In a brochure distributed to an estimated twenty thousand households, eighteen physicians said, "We have not joined an HMO because it is our belief that contracting with an HMO at this time may diminish the quality of health care we are committed to providing." Wasserman, however, dismissed the concern about patient care. He contended that the specialists refused to accept clinic physicians as gatekeepers because they wanted to earn more money by rendering more services. "You are in Texas and you still carry guns in Texas," he said. "Doctors still consider themselves independent." But Huntsville specialists had reason to worry about Maxicare's intentions. In a 1986 interview with *Business and Health,* Wasserman said, "People tend to forget that utilization is part of quality. Too much care usually means poor care."

As the fight continued, the clinic began referring Maxicare patients to specialists in Conroe, thirty miles to the south, or Houston, sixty-five miles south. Some specialists reported that they were losing over $25,000 a year because of the lack of referrals. But the specialists far outnumbered clinic doctors on the staff of the county's only hospital, Huntsville Memorial Hospital. Its medical staff revised the hospital bylaws to require the board certification of all department chiefs who have the power to grant and renew admitting privileges. As a result, none of the clinic doctors would be eligible to head a hospital department. They believed that the change was a not-so-subtle threat to their staff privileges.

In another controversy about care versus cash, forty obstetrician-gynecologists quit Maryland's MD-IPA after the HMO tried to make the doctors financially responsible for the costs of most prenatal tests. The doctors said that the reimbursement plan was "economic blackmail" that would reduce the quality of care for their patients. Under the reimbursement policy MD-IPA would pay a fixed rate for obstetrical patients; any tests that the doctors ordered would have to come out of the flat fee. Rockville ob-gyn

Craig Dickman said, "I don't care how much of a purist you are, there's always the knowledge that the cost for the test is coming out of your pocket." Added Dr. Thomas Ein of Silver Spring, "Giving incentives not to do tests that ensure the well-being of my patient isn't the way to stop [unnecessary tests]." Andrea Stillman, the plan's communications director, said that the reimbursement schedule was necessary to cut costs and stay competitive in the Washington, D.C., market. She said, "Women look forward to having a sonogram whether it has medical utility or not—there is a real question mark there. . . . We can't afford to pay for tests just because it has become customary to do them."[15]

Traditional medicine has its flaws. Doctors determine if services are needed and also set their fees. This poses the danger of excessive care. Doctors may order additional tests, for example, to be "safe" even though they have every reason to believe that the results will be negative. Such marginal services have contributed to the overall rise in health care costs. Yet, in general, patients are less likely to be injured by too many procedures than by too few. HMOs assure consumers all the care they need, but they determine what that need is. In the end patients get the amount of care that can be delivered for the fixed price. As Stuart H. Altman, dean of the Heller School at Brandeis University, pointed out, "It's very easy for an HMO to make big bucks by and large for doing very little." In general, HMOs operate by doing very little. That poses a threat to the health of all patients but particularly low-income members who may be the most attracted by their promises and the least capable of evaluating the quality of care. This danger is one disturbing result of a major HMO study by the Rand Corporation. The think tank has been evaluating the operations of the Group Health Cooperative of Puget Sound since 1976, in the largest study ever conducted of an HMO and its members. The study, the first to compare no-frills and fee-for-service medicine, contradicts claims that HMOs deliver equal care at significant savings. Its findings are particularly bothersome since Group Health is a nonprofit HMO. Most Americans who have enrolled in prepaid health plans in the past decade are joining HMOs that are operated for a profit and therefore have a far greater incentive to underserve members.

The Group Health Cooperative of Puget Sound claims it saves members about 25 percent in health care costs, but in 1986 the Rand Corporation attributed those savings to its reductions in hospital admissions. HMO enrollees were hospitalized at a rate that was 40 percent below that of fee-for-service patients. Low-income people in particular were significantly worse off in the HMO. They had higher death rates, more serious symptoms, and were hospitalized more often. About 35 percent of HMO members reported serious symptoms, compared to 22 percent of the fee-for-service patients. HMO members also averaged ten days a year in a hospital compared with only six days a year for non-HMO members. The authors concluded, "HMOs in general may be predisposed to underserve and the poor may be less likely to overcome this obstacle."

Patients in the study preferred fee-for-service medicine. The Rand Corporation reported, "In answer to questions designed to measure satisfaction, 15 percent of the group assigned to the HMO had nothing good to say about their medical care compared to 10 percent of the fee-for-service group." The HMO users were especially upset by long waits for appointments and the reduced availability of hospital care and specialists. "Among the features that participants liked least," noted Allyson Ross Davies, the principal author of the Rand study, "are those that appear to be most responsible for lower medical care in the HMOs, such as appointment queues and the reduced availability of hospital care."

Group Health patients may have suffered because of HMOs' assembly line medicine. The only group whose health improved were patients with average incomes above $43,668 a year, about twice the national average. They may be educated and articulate enough to summarize their problems succinctly, while low-income people needed to spend more time talking to their physician than the in-and-out HMO visits allowed.

More evidence that HMOs offer substandard care comes from insurance companies, which are discovering that a likely consequence of no-frills medicine is an increase in lawsuits. Noah D. Rosenberg, a Los Angeles attorney who specializes in health law, warned the Risk and Insurance Management Society that employees will hold corporations offering prepaid health care liable for inadequate care. He projects that patients will sue not only their doctor, hospital, and health maintenance organization but also their employer. Rosenberg said that so far employers have not recognized the hazards that are involved in the promotion of HMOs. He advised, "The [HMO] contract is going to affect the quality of care you provide. Less quality, less care is probably going to be the situation."[16]

The Physicians Insurance Company of Michigan (PICOM), a major issuer of malpractice insurance, also believes that HMOs may generate lawsuits and has begun penalizing physicians who contract with prepaid plans. When it sets insurance rates PICOM hands out penalty points to physicians who seem likely to be sued for malpractice. With two points a physician is required to pay a 25 percent surcharge. The penalty is substantial, amounting to $10,116 a year extra for a typical orthopedist or neurosurgeon in the Detroit area, for example. In 1985 PICOM started to give one penalty point automatically to HMO physicians. PICOM Vice President Tom Nixon said the company believed its policy was realistic. Since HMOs stress reduced costs, he said, physicians may provide substandard care, raising the risk of malpractice suits. "When there is an economic incentive to provide fewer services than you might provide in a traditional practice, you've got to consider the higher costs of providing insurance to providers who practice in such a setting," Nixon said.

To date HMOs have been a shell game that promises much but delivers far less. HMOs shuffle costs through the health care system but pass along few of those savings and provide little reassurance that quality of care will be protected. As Jay Plotkin, a Winter Park, Florida, obstetrician, said, "The one that ultimately suffers is the patient. We doctors are only human and we're going to think, 'Here comes the discount patient.' "

CHAPTER NINE

•

Taming the Corporation

DR. JACOB J. KATZOW, a George Washington Medical School professor, speculates, "Just as war is too important to be left to generals, medicine may have become too important to be left to the experts." Yet precisely that has happened. Medicine has been relegated to the experts, and it is time that stopped. Americans deserve better medical care than they are getting and at a lower cost than they have been paying. Both objectives are possible, but only if consumers seize far more control than they have exercised in the past. Consumers who have the most to gain or lose have had minimal impact on the quality and variety of health care services that are available.

The medical world operates for the sake of insiders. It has produced superbly for them, generating ample revenues for the supermeds and handsome incomes for physicians. It has performed substantially less well for consumers. There is shockingly little evidence that patients benefit from a large number of commonly prescribed treatments. They have endured expensive treatments that don't heal or cure but often harm. Yet this can change. Less costly and more effective health care is possible. It doesn't necessarily require passage of new government programs or multibillion-dollar expenditures. It may require a revolution in attitudes, however. Consumers must apply the same standards of accountability to health care corporations that are used to monitor industry in general. They need to demand information, some of which already exists in government files but is not publicly available, so they can judge the quality of supermed hospitals and the doctors who practice in them. Consumers need to develop allies, too, so the marketplace can be forced to work for them instead of against them. This is not an easy undertaking, but the stakes—quite literally life and death—are high indeed.

The strategy is simply stated. Consumers should reward outcomes. They should pay hospitals and doctors for results. Consumers and their representatives in business, labor unions, and government should provide incentives for excellence even if it means paying more. The extra money that is spent here can be saved through the elimination of unnecessary services.

While this may seem obvious, it represents a radical, new perspective on health care. Medicine has always emphasized the delivery of care, not the results of services. Patients may think that they are being treated, but it is actually their illness that is receiving attention. Hospitals and doctors intervene to alter the course of a specific illness. If patients also improve their overall well-being as a result, it is coincidental. It is a subtle but vast difference with enormous implications for health care. It has put the focus on process rather than results. It is the genesis of the classic statement that the operation succeeded but the patient died. Medicine in 1988 is still operating on a piecework basis. Under the current system consumers don't reward excellence; perversely, they must reward poor care. If their health deteriorates, their cost rises as they pay for more frequent, more sophisticated, and more expensive treatments. The sicker the patients, the greater the potential for financial rewards for supermeds and physicians. It is an irrational set of incentives.

In the 1980s consumers have a rare opportunity to shape health care. Consumers can exert influence because the health care industry is changing and power has yet to solidify. Consumers have much to gain from the competitive hustle. They are being courted through sheer financial necessity. With the excess hospital capacity and a doctor surplus consumers can demand attention. These conditions are unlikely to last, however. In the marketplace, surplus is replaced rapidly by dearth. In fact, the American Medical

Association reports that medical school applications are falling because of fear that the financial rewards of becoming a physician are dwindling. And supermeds are seeking new uses for empty beds and finding them, for example, in the elderly who need extended nursing care and patients who require rehabilitation therapy. After the health care system adapts economically, consumers will have lost their leverage.

The time may be right, but it is also short. Consumers have another advantage in the 1980s that must not be allowed to slip away. Until now supermeds have not translated their economic power into political power. That, too, is likely to change. For years the supermeds have pursued financial gain without government regulation. That changed abruptly when Congress passed prospective payment. While the supermeds were unleashed economically by prospective payment, at the same time the federal government was embarking on the most massive regulation of an industry since it began to regulate the railroads in 1883. Although the supermeds were freed to seek higher profits, the government began to regulate the practice of medicine itself by establishing diagnostic-related groups. The federal government thought since it could regulate freight rates, it could regulate sickness. If it could determine the rate to haul corn from Des Moines to Los Angeles, it could set payment for heart attacks. In the process it totally ignored patients' idiosyncrasies. A malnourished eighty-year-old woman who develops a respiratory infection after a winter in a poorly heated apartment is unlikely to recover as rapidly as a seventy-year-old man who catches a chill when he darts into an air-conditioned clubhouse after a fast-paced set of tennis. Although the government ignored these essential differences, the DRGs will have to be revised eventually to incorporate them. However, the new system will be created in a vastly different environment. Through the DRGs the government has politicized illness and invited the supermeds into politics. Scholar Peter Woll of Brandeis University points out in *American Bureaucracy* that whenever the federal government has tried to regulate an industry, the industry has seized control and dominated the regulatory process. In the end the regulation preserves the economic power of the industry.[1] Consumers have no reason to think that the federal government or the health care industry will respond differently. In fact, Hospital Corporation of America has been compiling statistics on its money-losing DRGs to prove that rates should be raised. Consumers must act before supermeds forge this alliance with their regulators.

For consumers to stand up to the supermeds, they must stand up for themselves first. Their assertiveness will not always be welcomed. Hospitals are run primarily for the convenience of their real constituents—doctors, not patients. Doctors may feel personally challenged by their patients' questions. A forty-year-old urologist in Greenbelt, Maryland, said, "When my father was practicing, when he said something, that was that. When I say something, it's, 'Why, doctor?' If patients want to practice medicine, they can do what I did and go to medical school." Consumers can expect to encounter the natural resistance of people unwilling to relinquish their power just as the supermeds have been fought by the university-based medical elite.

Investor-owned corporations like the supermeds spend inordinate time, money, and energy promoting public confidence through good public relations. Goodwill may be elusive, but it is extremely valuable. Supermeds try to appear public-spirited even if their products are endangering customers. They loathe negative publicity, understandably, since it is bad for business. Unfavorable media coverage can plunge stocks to instant lows, erode revenues and profits, and stunt future growth if moneylenders, losing confidence in management, refuse to provide financing for new acquisitions. Supermeds are especially sensitive to negative headlines because of their product. Front-page newspaper articles about high death rates or unnecessary surgery can spin occupancy levels in their hospitals into a downward spiral that may require years to reverse. Publicity is a little-used but potentially powerful tactic in the effort to impose accountability on publicly held corporations.

The AFL-CIO's Food and Allied Service Trades (FAST) discovered this in its drive against Beverly Enterprises. In the 1980s FAST began to organize service employees at Beverly nursing homes throughout the United States. It quickly encountered well-financed, well-organized corporate resistance. In response FAST adroitly used the local and national media to expose conditions at Beverly Enterprises facilities. The labor union was well prepared.

It spent a year researching Beverly Enterprises before it began its publicity campaign. FAST sent researchers to states where Beverly owned nursing homes to gather data on health care violations. FAST organizers probably knew as much about Beverly as its corporate officers. Before they finished, organizers had amassed an entire room of files of newspaper clippings, company reports, and Security and Exchange Commission filings. Organizers slipped reporters copies of reports detailing violations of state health and safety statutes. FAST generated well-placed articles about patient abuse and newspaper editorials deploring the conditions and calling for change. The newspaper publicity helped build public support for the organizing drive because FAST was able to link the plight of the workers and the elderly, publicizing both as victims of a highly profitable corporation. The union argued that if Beverly increased its staff, paid a decent wage, and provided proper training, the elderly would receive better care.

FAST didn't rely simply on press releases to create a media blitz. It bought Beverly stock, stormed annual meetings after alerting the media, and peppered Robert Van Tuyle with repeated questions. Reviving tactics of the 1960s protests, FAST organizers staged sit-ins at corporate headquarters. It challenged certificate of need filings and industrial revenue bond applications. The union went to Wall Street and launched a campaign to turn institutional investors, major holders of Beverly stock, against the company. FAST persuaded Beverly's second-largest shareholder, Chase Manhattan Bank, to vote against the company and in favor of a union-sponsored resolution to create an outside committee to oversee patient care. The unwelcome publicity and FAST's tenacious exploitation of Beverly's susceptibility to it worked. FAST and Beverly reached an accord. Beverly would cease interfering with union organizing efforts if FAST would stop generating bad publicity about the company in the media.

This multipronged strategy can be employed against the health care conglomerates. As powerful as the supermeds are, they can be surprisingly vulnerable. Since they, too, are publicly traded and widely held by institutional investors, the supermeds can be held accountable for their actions. They hold annual meetings, open to the public and press, where shareholders can raise questions about the management and operation of the corporations, where investors can quiz corporate officers about the quality and delivery of services and demand answers. Consumers can and should use these meetings to expose poor-quality care, to demand that low-income patients are treated, to protest the closing of facilities or elimination of services. The public meetings can launch public campaigns to change supermed corporate policies.

In the past, consumers were powerless because they saw their grievances as personal complaints. They didn't see that their individual problems of high cost, low quality, and inadequate and sometimes unavailable services were not personal dilemmas but a reflection of corporate policy. But if consumers understand that essential fact, they can begin to act together to change those policies. Time and again supermeds have demonstrated a tremendous willingness to adapt to new conditions. As the Institute of Medicine reported, "These findings support the broad conclusion that for-profit institutions respond more precisely to economic incentives than do not-for-profit institutions." The Institute of Medicine concluded that supermeds charged more when insurance policies paid more. They invested more when it produced financial rewards. They bought and sold facilities if those activities were profitable. They raised expenses when those costs were reimbursed and cut them sharply when they weren't. In shifting their corporate strategies, supermeds responded to changing demands from insurance companies, the federal government, and employers. Up until now those groups constituted the supermeds' public. The other public, the consumers who use supermed services, has not spoken out or furnished management with the incentives to improve the quality of their care.[2]

A publicity campaign requires sophistication and skill more than money. Even so, it can be extremely effective in industries like health care that are highly competitive. FAST won the right to organize Beverly because so much trouble was created for management that officers became convinced it would be easier to give in than to keep fighting. The same strategy, aimed at supermeds like National Medical Enterprises or American Medical International, would work, too. As FAST discovered, supermeds are sensitive to the pressure of their institutional shareholders. Supermeds that don't respond to consumers may change when their largest shareholders begin to raise questions about bad publicity and its likely impact on stock prices. Among the largest investors in supermed stock are public and nonprofit institutions that are sensitive to public pressure. In 1986, for example, College Retirement Equities, which manages the pension funds for university professors, maintained one of the ten largest holdings in Humana and American Medical International, while the Michigan State treasurer was the single largest holder of AMI stock. Other supermed investors included Harvard College, the Ford Foundation, Rockefeller University, the University of Texas, the University of Delaware, Cornell University and General Electric's pension and medical care trusts. Such investors may provide a point of leverage for concerns about supermeds' quality of care.

The hospital industry has been forced to take the quality of patient care more seriously by even the little publicity that has focused so far on performance. When the media obtained information on hospital mortality rates through Freedom of Information Act requests in 1987, the hospital industry was outraged. Hospital spokesmen claimed that the public could not interpret the statistics correctly. The industry argued that the public would assume that high death rates meant poor quality, yet the figures could also indicate only that the hospital treated a large number of very ill patients. Although the industry might be right, consumers might not want to accept that risk. If a patient can choose between a hospital where there is a zero death rate for a scheduled procedure and a hospital with a mortality rate of 33 percent, for instance, he may be unwilling to risk his life on the one-out-of-three chance that the industry is correct. And the hospitals know it.

In 1987 consumers won a valuable ally in the Joint Commission on Accreditation of Hospitals, a private group that accredits five thousand of the sixty-one hundred hospitals in the United States. Its president, Dr. Dennis O'Leary, dean of clinical affairs at the George Washington University Medical School, promised that in the future the group would revise its accreditation standards to stress quality of care as much as well-equipped surgical suites in its hospital ratings. At a press conference O'Leary said this was a "historic agenda for change" and conceded that publicity about hospital mortality rates influenced the commission's decision to change. "We now have the fundamental knowledge and methodology to begin to define and measure the quality of care that hospitals provide," he said. "If we don't do this others will and the probability that they will misinterpret the results of their efforts is too high." O'Leary said that the JCAH would begin developing standards that are oriented to results rather than procedures. "In the past we could only ask the question, 'Can the hospital provide quality care?' Now we can ask, 'Did it provide quality care?' " O'Leary admitted that hospitals are likely to resist, but he said, "There has been a psychological breakthrough that is important —the acceptance within the professional community that it is maybe okay to set professional performance standards and expected criteria for performance." O'Leary said that the Joint Commission of Accreditation of Hospitals would begin to incorporate these standards into hospital reviews in 1990.[3]

Publicity campaigns may curb the more voracious "less care, more profit" appetites of the supermeds. Alone, however, they cannot ensure that excellence will replace profit-seeking excesses. Consumers have lacked power over health care in large measure because of their unfamiliarity with the private world of medicine. Yet consumers don't have to understand the intricacies of brain surgery to select a superior hospital and a well-qualified surgeon to perform the operation. That is the kind of information that consumers need. The federal government possesses this information through the data on the Medicare program but refuses to release all of it except through Freedom of Information requests filed by newspapers. Consumers should write their representatives to demand that the government that spends over $6 billion a year on research also budgets money to distribute the results to the public that paid for it.

Consumers need to discard notions, often encouraged by hospitals and doctors who benefit from them, that medicine is a mysterious calling. Medicine is a business, which like all industries conforms to underlying patterns of the marketplace with reassuring inevitability. If consumers realize that health care is an industry and learn its economic laws, they will improve their ability to evaluate medical advice and to determine if it is likely to improve their health or simply the doctors' financial well-being. Some of these economic rules follow:

- Surgical patients fare better if their hospital performs a given procedure frequently. They are likely to be endangered, however, by the proliferation of heart transplant centers, which became a hospital status symbol in the 1980s. Five Washington, D.C., area hospitals were vying to open heart transplant facilities in 1988, although health planning experts said that the community needed three at the most. They warned that without sufficient patients all five surgical teams would not be able to perform the operation often enough to ensure their competency. In addition, researchers have found a strong relationship between the surgical volume and results in coronary bypass operations. Jonathan A. Showstack of the University of California-San Francisco reported in *Journal of the American Medical Association* in 1987 that high-risk patients were more likely to survive surgery at hospitals where a given operation was performed frequently. Showstack analyzed the results of 19,000 bypass procedures at 77 California hospitals. Patients who needed emergency surgery had a death rate of nearly 8 percent at hospitals performing 100 or fewer operations a year compared to 4.6 percent at hospitals with over 351 operations annually. At the high-volume hospitals patients also recovered faster after surgery. Showstack said that 12 lives might have been saved if procedures had been done in hospitals where at least 200 operations a year were performed.[4] The National Center for Health Services Research and Health Care Technology Assessment has reported similar relationships for cardiac catheterization, total hip replacements, and respiratory distress syndrome.
- Patients increase their survival rates if they hire busy surgeons. A growing number of general surgeons don't have enough cases to polish their skills. Dr. Ira Rutkow, a Freehold, New Jersey, surgeon, said, "Surgeons do well what they do most often." As a result, he told a symposium sponsored by the American Medical Association and Johns Hopkins Medical Institutions, the surgeon glut poses "a crippling and tragic effect" on the future

quality of surgery in the United States. He projected that consumers would be presented a choice—a group of "splendid technicians" who operate frequently and a "dispirited and deprived" group that doesn't operate frequently enough to maintain their skills.[5]

- Consumers are more likely to be treated surgically than medically if they live in a community with a high number of surgical specialists. In a single year an American is twice as likely to be operated on as a Briton, a figure that correlates precisely with the number of surgeons in the two countries, according to Dr. John P. Bunker, a researcher in medical practice variations at Stanford University. The United States has twice as many surgeons as Great Britain, and the U.S. surgeons performed twice as many operations.
- Consumers are more likely to be treated in a hospital and to pay more for their stay if they live in a community that has a large number of hospital beds and medical personnel. For instance, residents of New Haven and Boston have enormously different hospitalization rates even though the communities are very similar in many respects. They are both major medical centers with highly regarded medical schools and many teaching hospitals. Yet Boston residents are 50 percent more likely to be admitted to a university hospital than New Haven residents are. Moreover, they will pay twice as much for their care. Dr. John E. Wennberg, an epidemiologist researcher at Dartmouth Medical School, finds only one explanation that accounts for these differences: Boston has twice as many hospital beds and medical staff for its population as New Haven does. "It is not as if you are dealing here with a finite amount of need, as if care were rationed in markets with low beds per capita," Wennberg told a U.S. Senate Appropriations panel. "As beds are added cases are admitted which in other areas . . . many physicians believe can be done in the outpatient department or perhaps not done at all in the case of certain discretionary operations."[6]
- Consumers who want to avoid unnecessary trips to the doctor should avoid recent medical school graduates and doctors who are new to a community. Both are more likely to suggest return

visits, according to the National Center for Health Services Research and Health Care Technology Assessment.

- Doctors are likely to ask well-insured consumers to return more often, and such patients will be subjected to more tests and procedures in both doctors' offices and hospitals. Dr. John Marshall, director of the National Center for Health Services Research and Health Care Technology Assessment, said, "The less the individual pays for medical care directly, the more likely is the physician to initiate visits and related expenditures."[7]
- Consumers who live in cities and communities that attract a high number of doctors will pay more for health care. Consumers would get instant relief from the high cost of medical care if it were possible to restrict the number of doctors in their communities. Physicians seem invariably to drive costs up. Marshall reported that when Medicare reduced reimbursement rates for doctors in Denver by 10 percent, for instance, doctors quickly managed to circumvent the cuts. They performed more operations, offered more services, and ordered more diagnostic tests. Altogether, the physicians managed to increase their billings by 10 percent, precisely the amount required to offset the reduction in reimbursement rates.
- A pregnant woman who prefers natural childbirth should shun doctors who are solo practitioners or who were trained in foreign medical schools. Both groups have higher rates of Cesarean deliveries. Women also are more likely to have Cesarean births if they are well insured or live in communities with a high proportion of obstetrician-gynecologists, according to the National Center for Health Services Research and Health Care Technology Assessment.[8]
- Emotionally disturbed individuals are more likely to be hospitalized now than they were in the past. While public hospitals are releasing psychotic patients to fend for themselves on the streets, less seriously ill individuals are being hospitalized in large numbers. A 1987 report by the U.S. Office of Technology Assessment found, for instance, that over a hundred thousand emotionally disturbed children are being hospitalized annually. Yet James Eagan, chairman of the psychiatry department at Children's Hospital National Medical Center in Washington,

D.C., says, "Some of them don't deserve to be in the hospital, clearly. The question is: Why are they there if they really don't need to be there?"[9]

In large measure psychiatric hospitalizations are increasing because of growth in capacity and expanding insurance coverage. Since 1980 four major chains—Hospital Corporation of America; National Medical Enterprises; Community Psychiatric Centers in Santa Ana, California; and Charter Medical Corporation, based in Macon, Georgia—have nearly tripled the number of their facilities with psychiatric programs. By 1987 psychiatric facilities represented over half of NME's hospitals, and fifteen more were under construction. Charter operated a chain of fifty-eight psychiatric hospitals, up from eleven in 1980. Insurance companies have helped to fuel this expansion by their willingness to provide better benefits for inpatient than outpatient care. In Massachusetts, for example, Blue Cross/Blue Shield typically pays for sixty days of inpatient psychiatric care, which can total $100,000 or more a year, but only $500 a year for outpatient care. Yet Dr. Charles Kiesler, Vanderbilt University provost and former executive of the American Psychological Association, says sweepingly, "Traditional inpatient care for mental disorders is neither the most effective nor the most cost-effective method of treatment. . . . In no case [studied] has mental hospitalization produced better treatment outcomes than any alternative care."[10]

While these rules of the medical marketplace are fascinating, they are troubling, too. They indicate that consumers may receive a variety and quality of care that has nothing to do with their medical conditions. Instead, health care often seems to be determined as much by the provider's personality and training as by the patient's needs. Consequently, consumers may be paying for unnecessary and even injurious care.

Epidemiologist Wennberg started studying these variations in health care in 1970 when he directed the state of Vermont's regional medical program. He first looked at surgical and hospitalization rates, then moved on to medical procedures. So far he has conducted studies of hospitals and physicians in Iowa, Maine, Massachusetts, Rhode Island, and Vermont and has studied health maintenance organizations throughout the United States. His research demonstrates that all too frequently consumers receive medical care based not on need but on happenstance.

Wennberg discovered early that consumers received radically different care for similar medical conditions. Patients were always hospitalized for a few conditions such as strokes, heart attacks, hip fractures, and appendectomies, but these were the exceptions. Many more patients' treatments, including hospitalization and surgery, depended not on their individual conditions but on the community in which they lived. Wennberg found high variations in the frequency with which patients were hospitalized for problems such as peptic ulcers, hypertension, depression, and knee operations. In one Vermont town 60 percent of the children had their tonsils removed before age fifteen, but in another town the rate was only 8 percent. In Maine 70 percent of the elderly women had undergone hysterectomies before age seventy-five in one community, while in another the rate was only 25 percent. In Iowa over 50 percent of men in one city had prostatectomies, while only 15 percent did in another city. Wennberg could find only one explanation to account for these variations satisfactorily. Physicians who lived in different communities had widely different practice patterns. Wennberg's research contains a clear warning for consumers. They should listen to medical advice with a healthy dose of skepticism, since even routine procedures carry medical risks. The more times a given operation is performed, the more deaths there will be from it. Between fifteen hundred and seven thousand men will die annually as a result of prostatectomies, depending on the operation's frequency. As Wennberg points out, "That's a lot of deaths."

Analyzing his research, Wennberg said, "Medicine is as much art as it is science and will always be so. An enterprise as large as medical care will always produce variations in approach. Rather, the goal should be to reduce variations that are highly aberrant, that reflect supply factors rather than scientific knowledge, or that reflect idiosyncrasies of physicians rather than the values, needs, or wants of their patients."[11]

Consumers should know, too, that physicians and hospitals often treat patients on the basis of subjective intuition rather than quantitative knowledge. David M. Eddy, a Duke University physician-mathematician, is developing formulas whose use will enable analysis for the first time of the clinical effectiveness of medical technologies. This research could have been done long ago. Eddy says the appropriate mathematical formulas have been known for centuries but were never before used to correlate procedures and outcomes. Eddy explained, "We have developed quantitative methods that allow us to analyze existing information from randomized controlled trials and case control studies, adjust the evidence for various biases that affect their results, and statistically combine the evidence from separate studies to get a quantitative estimate of the effect of the technology on important health outcomes such as mortality, radiation hazard, biopsy rates, and costs. These quantitative methods enable us to go much farther than the usual technology assessment method of convening a group of experts and asking them to arrive subjectively at a consensus." Until Eddy completes his work, however, consumers will be treated by procedures that cause, at the very least, unnecessary pain and disability.[12]

For half a century women with breast cancer were subjected to needless disfigurement and disability as a result of radical mastectomies in which the entire breast, lymph nodes, and the underlying chest muscle were removed. Radical mastectomies, known as the Halsted procedure, became the standard treatment for breast cancer because of the prestige of the doctor who pioneered the treatment. Dr. Robert Gordon, special assistant to the director of research at the National Institutes of Health, said the treatment was supported by "very, very limited data." After World War II, new research suggested that certain women would survive equally long, perhaps even longer, with less physical impairment and psychological trauma, if only the breast were removed and surgery were followed by radiation treatment. However, the research was never followed up. In 1972, over a quarter century later, almost 50 percent of breast cancer victims underwent the mutilating Halsted procedure. It wasn't until the National Cancer Institute convened a conference on breast cancer in 1979 that less radical surgery became standard. As late as 1981, however, radical mastectomies were performed on 4.5 percent of women who underwent surgery for breast cancer. Commenting on the demise of the Halsted treatment, Gordon said, "These figures indicate the end of more than a half century of standardized treatment of totally inappropriate therapy."[13]

Other patients continue to receive medical treatment just as unnecessary as the Halsted procedure. Potential stroke victims are being harmed more often than helped by surgeons who perform a virtually untested procedure that became widespread in the mid-1980s. The procedure, called carotid endarterectomy, is designed to clear out fatty plaque that has accumulated in the carotid artery, the brain's main source of oxygen. During the operation a diagonal incision is made in the left side of the neck and the carotid artery clamped above and below the fatty plaque. Surgeons then slice open the artery and, using scalpels and other instruments, remove the plaque. The number of operations has risen from about 15,000 in 1971 to 103,000 in 1988. With the operation's growing popularity, even patients who showed no physical symptoms of blocked arteries began receiving the operation. The American Heart Association says only a third of those operations are medically indicated and warns that up to 11,000 patients die or suffer strokes needlessly as a result of surgical complications. Dr. Mark Dyken, professor of neurology at the Indiana University School of Medicine, told an American Heart Association conference, "People who didn't come into the hospital wouldn't have died—at least in the short term." The only major study of the procedure showed that twice as many people died and seven times as many suffered strokes following the operation as might have been expected. Dyken said, "If I had a narrowed artery that isn't causing trouble, nobody's cutting on me."

This isn't the only operation that is more popular than useful. Coronary bypass surgery is performed far too often. Some 90 percent of the patients who undergo this operation receive no benefits from the surgery, according to the National Institutes of Health. A seven-year study of 780 patients with heart disease indicated that patients who were treated medically lived just as long as those who had surgery. Moreover, patients who didn't have the procedure avoided the risk and pain inherent in all operations. According to Robert Gordon, the 10 percent who can benefit from bypass surgery share two precise characteristics: They have triple vessel disease and a poorly functioning left ventricle. He said all other heart disease patients, including those who have had heart attacks or mild to moderate angina, can safely defer bypass surgery. Yet many are operated on.

Patients also undergo gall bladder surgery too frequently. Patients with gallstones are referred to surgery even if they have no pain. Although surgeons routinely prescribe cholecystectomies, the removal of the gall bladder, in these cases, patients have little to gain from the procedure. Dr. John Bunker of Stanford University, who evaluated the effectiveness of cholecystectomies for asymptomatic gallstones, concluded it would increase life expectancy "by no more than a week or two—and perhaps even decrease it."

Unlike many doctors, Bunker evaluates medicine from the neglected perspective of expected benefits versus comparative risks. He suggests that by avoiding hospitals consumers can improve their health and save money. He believes that too many operations are performed and that "many, perhaps most" medical procedures are overused. Bunker said, "It is generally assumed that more care leads to better outcomes, even though the improvement in outcomes may be quite small. Let me suggest, to the contrary, as utilization rates are progressively increased, as they are in areas of higher operation and high hospitalization rates, that more care may lead to 'negative benefits,' that the risks may actually exceed the benefits." Directing his harshest criticisms at unnecessary operations, Bunker claims that only 10 to 15 percent are intended to save lives. The remainder are done for the relief of discomfort, disability, or disfigurement, and are better avoided. "While such surgery is not intended to prolong life, it may nevertheless shorten it, since all surgery carries some risk of death," he said. "The net impact of such surgery is, therefore, to shorten life expectancy of the population as a whole." Humana's Dr. David Rollo shares this jaundiced opinion of his colleagues' medical effectiveness. Rollo says flatly, "I don't even go to a doctor if I have a problem." Rollo estimates that only 10 percent of patients improve because of medical attention. Even without medical advice he said that consumers would recover fully from 80 to 85 percent of their health problems. The remaining patients are treated by physicians whose knowledge is obsolete and techniques are outdated. "As doctors stay in practice, doctors become more dependent on the knowledge they already have," he said. "It's a painful experience to go to medical meetings, to sit and listen, to take notes, to absorb. There's a tendency to say, 'I know everything.' "

Bunker and Rollo hold theories that might be considered radical in medical circles, but they are supported by experiments set up by doctors themselves to eliminate unnecessary medical treatment. With the help of epidemiologist John Wennberg, Maine physicians collected statistics on the frequency of medical procedures and hospital admission rates in communities throughout the state. They studied them with his small area analysis techniques. When the differences were documented, the doctors began to use the statistics to pressure colleagues to reduce variations. The organizers of the Maine Medical Assessment Program believed that if doctors were shown that their practice styles were different, they would change. Standardized treatment would emerge. In the process consumers would be saved from unnecessary and inappropriate treatment. The project organizers discovered, for example, that children were being hospitalized for common illnesses such as bronchitis and pneumonia at widely varying rates. There was a 250 percent difference in hospitalization rates across the state. In a community where doctors admitted patients freely, the hospital chief of staff posted the individual hospitalization rates for his pediatricians in the physicians' lounge. That one thumbtack dropped hospital admission rates by 47 percent in three years. When the chief of staff retired, the postings stopped and the admission rates rose.

By shunning hospitals except when admission is absolutely necessary, consumers can avoid another danger that is more common than might be supposed. Over a third of hospital patients studied develop iatrogenic illnesses as a result of medical treatment, according to testimony before a U.S. Senate Appropriations Committee panel. Almost 10 percent of the patients contacted seriously disabling or life-threatening iatrogenic illnesses. Some fifty thousand Americans a year die from infections and diseases caught in hospitals. As many patients are dying each year from hospitalizations as from automobile accidents.

Obviously, consumers must insist that the effectiveness of medical treatments be studied quickly. Obviously, too, they need to demand the disclosure of existing information. The medical establishment, however, has opposed its release. At a conference on small area analysis, sponsored by Dartmouth University and the American Medical Association, doctors urged that the research be kept from the public. Dr. Robert E. McAfee of Portland, Maine, told the conference, "We must control the data, we must be in charge of the data, and we must interpret the data." Otherwise, warned Dr. Paul Rohlf, a Davenport, Iowa, urologist, "You could have surgical rates on the front page of the newspaper."

Jim Firman, a health policy analyst, is convinced that consumers possess unexercised power in the medical marketplace. Firman believes that consumers suffer because they lack sufficient information to judge health care and then discriminate wisely among practitioners. If information were available, consumers could promote competition on the basis of quality, price, convenience, and coverage. Consumers spend enormous sums on health care but their spending too often has enriched providers more than it has improved health care. "My feeling is the power is there for the taking. So it is really a question not of seizing the power, because it's already there; people just have to learn how to wield it," he said.

As a health researcher at the Robert Wood Johnson Foundation, Firman grew increasingly worried about the paucity of consumer information. The longer he thought about it, the more certain he became of the solution. If business management techniques and computer software were combined, he reasoned that enough information could be generated to help consumers select health care more rationally. Too often, he believed, consumers put up with less than satisfactory care because they felt, rightly, that the search for better care would be costly, time-consuming, and, perhaps, unsuccessful in the end. And he thought if an up-to-date information system could be merged with a consumer co-op, members might be able to use the strength of numbers to purchase a better quality of health care at a lower cost. In 1984 he left the foundation and began to test his theory. "There were several trends working together," he said. "It was obvious that the cost of health care was going up. The government was cutting back on its benefits and services and the competition in the health care community was heating up. All of those conditions combined made it clearer that it wasn't wise for consumers to rely solely on government or health care providers. To rectify the situation, consumers needed to organize and take matters into their own hands."

Firman secured grants from numerous foundations and formed a board composed of well-known consumer advocates including Esther Peterson, former presidential adviser, and Arthur Flemming, former secretary of the Department of Health, Education, and Welfare. The United Seniors Consumer Cooperative was organized in Washington, D.C., in 1986. Despite its name, members don't have to be senior citizens to get a variety of benefits for a relatively modest annual fee. It negotiates discounts with hospitals and doctors, publishes a newsletter, sells medical supplies such as eyeglasses at bargain prices, and operates referral services. Other groups provide similar services, but the cooperative's strength lies in its data bank, which tailors information precisely for members. They won't just get names of physicians, for example; they can call up for a board-certified neurologist in Alexandria, Virginia, near a subway stop and with handicapped-accessible parking who agrees to accept Medicare reimbursement for full payment. If they want to switch insurance policies, they can get a computer printout analyzing the similarities and differences in coverage. "We don't make decisions for people or even recommendations," Firman said. "Our job is to provide people with the information they need to be better consumers."

Firman is trying to ensure that the co-op reflects members' needs. They helped to design the computer software system; they participate on the bargaining committees that negotiate contracts with hospitals and doctors. He envisions a future when the computer data bank will include consumer ratings of doctors. "The real issues are qualitative things," he said. "How well can this person communicate with you? Do they make you feel at ease? Do they explain things to you? Are they accessible at different hours? These are the kinds of things which really make the difference between the adequate doctor and the good doctor in my view. That's why I think consumers can evaluate and rate those kinds of things. We can help encourage consumers to identify and use those kinds of doctors."

If the United Seniors Consumer Cooperative can succeed, if it can become the prototype for local consumer organizations, it will supply the missing element in the medical marketplace. Consumers who have been left out of the economic warfare will be able to climb into the trenches. The ramifications are far-reaching. Consumers would be able to exercise more control over health care than they have ever had; they would possess more power over medicine than they have ever known. American medicine has never encountered consumer power before. Ironically, consumers may end up empowered not in spite of the supermeds but because of them. Corporations that sell health care as if it were hamburgers may listen to consumers before medical providers who believe that patients need only to follow doctors' orders. In 1986 the supermeds believed the public wanted cheap medical care even if quality had to be sacrificed. In trying to meet that demand, they often provided neither. All too frequently they delivered care that was poor and expensive. But corporate agendas can change.

In the decade of the 1980s medicine has discarded its bedside manner. The supermeds have revolutionized health care. As medicine looks ahead to the 1990s, it is clear that health care, like other necessities of life, will be a commodity to be bought and sold. As David Jones said, "Here at Humana we treat health care like the serious undertaking it is. Profit is the cost of doing business, and any institution that doesn't cover all the cost of doing business doesn't continue in business." The medical establishment claims that the supermeds are destroying the fundamental mission of medicine, that of a higher calling that places the patient ahead of greed. Yet if those inchoate values are so deeply embedded in the practice of medicine, they could not have been uprooted so easily. The supermeds exposed the fundamental nature of medicine, that it is a business, that doctors expect to be compensated—and well—for their care, that hospitals will offer services that make a profit, and that in the end someone must pay.

NOTES

CHAPTER ONE

1. Martha Barnette, "Hospital Primed for World Renown," *The Washington Post,* November 27, 1984, p. A14.

2. "AMA Critical of 'Commercialization' of Heart Transplants," *The Miami News,* December 6, 1984, p. 18A, and Dennis L. Breo, "Ethical Issues Debated After Successful Implant of Second Artificial Heart," *American Medical News,* December 7, 1984, p. 1.

3. Quoted in Rick Atkinson, "Humana, Inc., Provokes Strong Feelings at Home," *The Washington Post,* January 13, 1985, p. A7.

CHAPTER TWO

1. Michael Specter, "Health Bill Seen at 15% of GNP by Year 2000," *The Washington Post,* p. A1.

2. Arnold Relman, "The New Medical-Industrial Complex," *New England Journal of Medicine,* August 11, 1980, p. 963.

3. John K. Iglehart, "Kaiser, HMOs and the Public Interest: A Conversation with James A. Vohs," *Health Affairs,* Spring 1986, p. 49.

4. Edward M. Kerschner and Thomas M. Doeflinger, "Back to the Future: America's Second Great Restructuring" (New York: Paine Webber, February 11, 1985), p. 4.

5. Cynthia Wallace, "AMI's Weisman Aims to Build Integrated Healthcare Networks," *Modern Healthcare,* August 16, 1985, p. 40.

6. "NME Tried to Buy Clout: Documents," *Modern Healthcare,* March 29, 1985; Mark Tatge, "HHS Approves Reimbursement of Costs for Proposed NME Las Cruces Facility," *Modern Healthcare,* May 24, 1985.

CHAPTER THREE

1. Paul Starr, *The Social Transformation of American Medicine* (New York: Basic Books, 1982), pp. 118–20.

2. Joseph A. Califano, Jr., *America's Health Care Revolution: Who Lives? Who Dies? Who Pays?* (New York: Random House, 1986), p. 52.

3. "Investor-Owned Industry and Federation: David Williamson Looks at Past, Future," *Federation of American Health Systems Review,* March–April 1986, p. 23.

4. Figures from the inspector general's *Semiannual Report to the Congress, April 1, 1985–September 30, 1985,* p. 10.

5. *Hospital Merger Increased Medicare and Medicaid Payments for Capital Costs* (Washington, D.C.: U.S. General Accounting Office, December 22, 1983).

6. *Public Hospitals: Sales Lead to Better Facilities but Increased Patient Costs* (Washington, D.C.: U.S. General Accounting Office, 1986), p. 24.

7. *Proceedings of the Conference on the Future of Medicine* (Washington, D.C.: U.S. House of Representatives, Committee on Ways and Means, February 1, 1984), p. 18.

8. "Pricing Revolution Aids the Big Guys," *Business Week*, January 9, 1984, p. 56.

9. Anne Bagamery, "Health Care," *Forbes*, January 2, 1984, p. 94.

10. Information on profits in memorandum from HHS Inspector General Richard P. Kusserow to Lawrence DeNardis, Acting Secretary for Legislation, July 11, 1986.

11. *Semiannual Report to the Congress, April 1, 1985, to September 30, 1985*, p. 19.

12. *Cataract Surgery: Fraud, Waste and Abuse* (Washington, D.C.: U.S. House Subcommittee on Health and Long-Term Care, July 19, 1985), p. viii.

13. Seth Shaw, "The Compelling Issue of Access to Capital," *Business and Health*, January–February 1985, p. 17.

14. Barbara J. Culliton, "University Hospitals for Sale," *Science*, March 2, 1984, p. 119.

15. Kenneth Abramowitz, "New Health Service Economics," *Bulletin of the New York Academy of Medicine*, January–February 1985, p. 35.

CHAPTER FOUR

1. *Forecast of Physician Supply and Requirements* (Washington, D.C.: Office of Technology Assessment, 1980), p. 115.

2. *Payment for Physician Services: Strategies for Medicare* (Washington, D.C.: Office of Technology Assessment, 1986), p. 46.

3. Lauren LeRoy, Deborah A. Ellwood, and John K. Iglehart, "Trends in Health Manpower," *Health Affairs*, Winter 1985, p. 95.

4. David Hilfiker, "A Doctor's View of Modern Medicine," *The New York Times Magazine*, February 16, 1986, p. 44.

5. Carol Brierly Golin, "Physicians Altering Expectations of Future," *American Medical News*, November 22, 1985, p. 20.

6. Joseph D. Wassersug, "Medical Schools Preach Long-Gone Fantasy," *American Medical News*, April 10, 1987, p. 32.

7. *Health Care Competition Week*, August 1985.

8. Carol Brierly Golin, "Hospitals Woo M.D.'s to Attract Patients," *American Medical News*, April 11, 1986, p. 1.

9. *Payment for Physician Services: Strategies for Medicare*, p. 119.

10. M. Lawrence Podolsky, "Give Your Patients More Than They Bargain For," *Private Practice*, March 1985, p. 67.

11. Dr. Jack Hyman, "Our Rendezvous with Destiny," *American Medical News*, November 9, 1984, p. 34.

12. Elizabeth Willson, "To Advertise or Not to Advertise: Why Doctors Are Divided," *Florida Trend*, November 1985, p. 107.

13. Dr. Richard J. Feinstein, "A View from the 21st Century," *American Medical News*, March 21, 1986, p. 18.

14. Thomas J. Billitteri, "Bringing Innovation to Florida's Medical Market," *Florida Trend*, January 1985, p. 110; Paul Saltzman, "State's Doctors Take On Mayo Clinic Staff," *The Miami Herald*, May 5, 1985, p. 70.

15. Donna Crossed Bodewes, "New Outpatient Center Gives Rise to Turf Battle Among Physicians," *American Medical News*, October 4, 1985, p. 17.

16. Karen Sandrick, "Doctors Turn to Unions," *Private Practice*, November 1985, p. 12.

17. Interview, February 1985.

18. *Variations in Medical Practice* (Washington, D.C.: Senate Appropriations Subcommittee on Labor, Health and Human Services, Education, and Related Agencies, 1985), p. 88.

CHAPTER FIVE

1. McKenzie testified before the Senate Special Committee on Aging on September 26, 1985.

2. Data on Maine PRO published in Volume II of September 26, 1985, hearing record, pp. 323–25.

3. Avery quoted in *Los Angeles Times,* April 14, 1985.

4. AMA study published under title *AMA's DRG Monitoring Project and the Prospective Payment System* in 1984.

5. Kellawan testified on September 26, 1985.

6. Barbaccia testified before the Senate Special Committee on Aging on January 7, 1986.

7. Byrnes and Jones testified on September 26, 1985.

8. Greenberg testified on September 26, 1985.

9. "Hospital Payment Plan Stirs Debate on TV Show," *American Medical News,* November 22–29, 1985, p. 39.

10. *Medicare: Physician Incentive Payments by Hospitals Could Lead to Abuse* (Washington, D.C.: U.S. General Accounting Office, 1986).

11. AMA report is titled *Diagnosis-Related Groups and the Prospective Payment System;* American Society of Internal Medicine report is titled *The Impact of DRGs on Patient Care.*

12. Kenneth E. John, "Poll Finds Widespread Concern About Early Release from Hospital," *The Washington Post,* Health Section, October 28, 1986, p. 5.

13. Kratt testified on September 26, 1985.

14. Dorothy Seeley testified before the House of Representatives Select Committee on Aging on April 10, 1986.

15. David Lothson, *Trick-or-Treat: Industry at a Crossroads* (New York: Paine Webber, October 31, 1986), p. 14.

16. Creston Nelson, "Detailed Medicare DRG Data Offer Inside Look at Hospitals," *South Florida Medical Review,* September 24, 1985.

17. Robert Steinbrook, "Hospital Death Rates of Medicare Patients Released," *Los Angeles Times,* April 25, 1987.

18. Bradford Gray, ed., *For-Profit Enterprise in Health Care* (Washington, D.C.: National Academy Press, 1986), p. 398.

19. Carol Cancila, "M.D.: Court Victory May Aid Others Unfairly Dismissed," *American Medical News,* September 12, 1986, p. 20.

20. Robert V. Pattison and Hallie M. Katz, "Investor-Owned and Not-for-Profit Hospitals," *New England Journal of Medicine,* August 11, 1983, pp. 347–53.

21. *For-Profit Hospital Care: Who Profits? Who Cares?* (Washington, D.C.: National Council of Senior Citizens, March 1986), pp. 32–38.

22. Florida Hospital Cost Containment Board, *1984–85 Annual Report* (Tallahassee, Fla.: Florida Hospital Cost Containment Board), p. 17.

23. Pricing information in Charles L. Stallings and Marcus P. Zillman, *Florida Hospital Index: A Consumer's Guide to Cost and Services.* (Jefferson, N.C.: McFarland & Company, Inc., 1986).

CHAPTER SIX

1. Helen King Cummings and James P. King, "Financing Indigent Care: Public Problems, Private Responsibilities," *FAH Review,* March/April 1985.

2. Speech by John C. Bedrosian to the Rotary Club, Los Angeles, California, 1985.

3. Testimony before the National Citizens' Board of Inquiry, published by the National Council on the Aging, *Health Care USA*, p. 16.

4. Vicky Cahan, "When the Patient Can't Pay the Medical Bill," *Business Week,* February 18, 1985, p. 39.

5. Carol Cancila, "Lack of Health Care Access Big Problem," *American Medical News,* June 20, 1986, p. 27.

6. Bradford L. Kirkman-Liff, "Refusal of Care: Evidence from Arizona," *Health Affairs,* Winter 1986, pp. 16–24.

7. Harris Meyer, "New Yorkers Have Trouble Getting Care," *American Medical News,* June 20, 1986, p. 18.

8. Harry Nelson and Anne C. Roark, "Health Care Crisis: Less for More," *Los Angeles Times,* April 7, 1985, p. 1.

9. *New England Journal of Medicine,* February 27, 1986, pp. 552–57.

10. Florida Hospital Cost Containment Board annual reports for 1983, 1984, and 1985.

CHAPTER SEVEN

1. Transcript of hearing before State of Pennsylvania Unemployment Compensation Board of Review, January 21, 1983, regarding the claim of Mark A. Turns.

2. Jeff Blyskal, "Gray Gold," *Forbes,* November 23, 1981, p. 80.

3. Kathryn M. Welling, "Really Rocking: Nursing Homes Are the Healthiest Thing in Health Care," *Barron's,* June 2, 1986, p. 13.

4. *Beverly Enterprises: Patient Care Record* (Washington, D.C.: The Food and Beverage Trades Department, AFL-CIO, 1983).

5. Jonathan M. Frank, *The Value Line Investment Survey,* May 16, 1986, p. 1275.

6. Steven Greenhouse, "Super Star of Nursing Homes," *The New York Times,* April 14, 1986, p. D1.

7. *Rights of the Institutionalized Elderly: Lost in Confinement,* briefing paper by the U.S. House Subcommittee on Health and Long-Term Care, September 18, 1985.

8. Quoted in Welling, op. cit.

9. Richard Elliott, Jr., "No Tired Blood: Nursing Home Operators Are Long on Enthusiasm, Short on Experience," *Barron's,* March 24, 1969.

10. Information on the history of the nursing home industry from Catherine Hawes and Charles D. Phillips, "The Changing Structure of the Nursing Home Industry and the Impact of Ownership on Quality, Cost, and Access" in Bradford Gray, ed., *For-Profit Enterprise in Health Care,* pp. 492–541.

11. Greenhouse, op. cit. p. D14.

12. See *Rights of the Institutionalized Elderly* and Beverly Enterprise Certificate of Need application submitted to Office of Statewide Health Planning and Development, Sacramento, California.

13. *Los Angeles Times,* May 25, 1982.

14. *Beverly Enterprises in Michigan: A Case Study of Corporate Take-over of Health Care Resources* (Washington, D.C.: The Food and Beverage Trades Department, AFL-CIO, 1983).

15. *Long-Term Care for the Elderly: Investor-Owned Nursing Homes,* undated paper prepared by the National Council of Health Centers, Washington, D.C.

16. Information on violations in Texas homes from Bradford Gray, ed., *For-Profit Enterprise in Health Care,* p. 520.

17. Peter Dammann, "Big Nursing Home Chain Picks Oregon," *Willamette Week,* December 1–7, 1981, p. 1.

18. Information on Florida violations from the files of the Florida Department of Health and Rehabilitative Services.

19. Information on California violations from Phyllis Gapen's "Beverly Sues for Nursing Home Licenses," *American Medical News,* September 12, 1986; "Calif. Nursing Home

Faces Loss of Licenses," *American Medical News,* January 12, 1986; and David B. Hilder, "Fine of $600,000 Is Set for Beverly Enterprises, Inc.," *The Wall Street Journal,* October 17, 1986.

CHAPTER EIGHT

1. Sources include conversations with William L. Roper, Rosemary Goudreau, and Rosalind Resnick, "Politics Blamed in Demise of IMC," *The Miami Herald,* May 11, 1987, p. 1B, and Rosalind Resnick, "State Takes Control of IMC's Operations," *The Miami Herald,* May 5, 1987, p. 1A.

2. John K. Iglehart, "HMOs (For-Profit and Not-for-Profit) on the Move," *New England Journal of Medicine,* May 3, 1984, pp. 1204–5.

3. Fischer testified before the House of Representatives Select Committee on Aging on April 1, 1986.

4. Moyer testified on April 1, 1986.

5. Rogers testified on April 1, 1986.

6. Schultz testified on April 1, 1986.

7. Steve Sternberg, "IMC Favors Cash over Medicine, Some Say," *The Miami Herald,* May 22, 1986, p. 1.

8. Steve Albert, "DO Charged with Releasing HMO Patient Prematurely," *South Florida Medical Review,* October 22, 1985, p. 4.

9. *Medicare and HMOs: A First Look, with Disturbing Findings* (Washington, D.C.: U.S. Senate Special Committee on Aging, Minority Staff Report, April 7, 1987).

10. James B. Kenney, "Using Competition to Develop a Buyer-Driven Market," *Business and Health,* November 1985, p. 39.

11. Mark F. Baldwin, "Boston HMOs Ready for Stepped-up Battle," *Modern Healthcare,* May 10, 1985, p. 46.

12. "Many Calif. M.D.s Dissatisfied with Contracts," *American Medical News,* June 12, 1986, p. 15.

13. Robert A. Berenson, "Capitation and Conflict of Interest," *Health Affairs,* Spring 1986, p. 55.

14. Paul R. McGinn, "Contract Dispute Splits Specialists, Family M.D.s," *American Medical News,* May 8, 1987, p. 23.

15. Harris Meyer, "Ob-Gyns Quit Md. HMO to Protest Payment Plan," *American Medical News,* March 13, 1987, p. 1.

16. Pamela Russell, "Employers Face Challenge of Selecting Health-Care Plans in Complex Market," *Investor's Daily,* April 7, 1986, p. 25.

CHAPTER NINE

1. Peter Woll, *American Bureaucracy* (New York: W. W. Norton & Company, Inc., 1977).

2. Bradford Gray, ed., *For-Profit Enterprise in Health Care,* p. 142.

3. Carol Cancila, "JCAH to Review Clinical Outcomes," *American Medical News,* September 19, 1986, p. 1.

4. "Bypass 'Regionalization' Offers Better Outcome Chances for Patients: Study," *American Medical News,* February 13, 1987, p. 46.

5. "Surplus of Surgeons Seen as a Threat to Quality of Operations," *The Washington Post,* Health Section, October 21, 1986, p. 6.

6. *Variations in Medical Practice* (Washington, D.C.: U.S. Senate Appropriations

Subcommittee on Departments of Labor, Health and Human Services, Education, and Related Agencies, 1985), p. 34.

7. Ibid., p. 56.

8. Ibid., p. 56.

9. Laurent Belsie, "Psychiatric Services for Children Grow," *The Christian Science Monitor*, May 14, 1987, p. 37.

10. *Variations in Medical Practice*, p. 141.

11. Ibid., p. 9.

12. Jane Stein, "Quantifying Medical Outcomes for More Effective Delivery," *Business and Health*, September 1986, p. 47.

13. *Variations in Medical Practice*, p. 74.

BIBLIOGRAPHY

I have divided this bibliography into two parts: general articles and books on the subject of changes in the health care industry, and specific material that relates to individual chapter topics. In addition, I drew on corporate annual reports and Security and Exchange Commission filings of the major supermed corporations.

GENERAL SOURCES

Abramowitz, Kenneth. "New Health Service Economics," *Bulletin of the New York Academy of Medicine,* January–February 1985.

Califano, Joseph A., Jr. *America's Health Care Revolution: Who Lives? Who Dies? Who Pays?* New York: Random House, 1986.

Ehrenreich, Barbara, and Ehrenreich, John. *The American Health Care Empire.* New York: Random House, 1970.

The Future of Health Care Delivery in America. New York: Sanford C. Bernstein & Co., 1985.

Ginzberg, Eli. "The Grand Illusion of Competition in Health Care," *Journal of the American Medical Association,* April 8, 1983.

———. "The Monetization of Medical Care," *New England Journal of Medicine,* May 4, 1984.

Gray, Bradford H. "Overview: Origins and Trends," *Bulletin of the New York Academy of Medicine,* January–February 1985.

———, ed. *For-Profit Enterprise in Health Care.* Washington, D.C.: National Academy Press, 1986.

Health Care: How to Improve It and Pay for It. Washington, D.C.: Center for National Policy, 1985.

Health Care in the 1990s: Trends and Strategies. Report by Arthur Andersen & Co. and the American College of Hospital Administrators, 1984.

Health United States 1984. Washington, D.C.: U.S. Department of Health and Human Services, December 1984.

Health United States 1985. Washington, D.C.: U.S. Department of Health and Human Services, December 1985.

Health United States 1986 and Prevention Profile. Washington, D.C.: U.S. Department of Health and Human Services, December 1986.

Hospital Statistics. Chicago: American Hospital Association, 1985.

Kosterlitz, Julie. "The Hospital Business," *National Journal,* September 28, 1985.

Lothson, David J. *Hospital Management Industry*. New York: Paine Webber, March 27, 1985.

Medicare Prospective Payment and the American Health Care System. Washington, D.C.: Prospective Payment Assessment Commission, 1987.

Medicare's Prospective Payment System: Strategies for Evaluating Cost, Quality, and Medical Technology. Washington, D.C.: U.S. Congress, Office of Technology Assessment, 1985.

Starr, Paul. *The Social Transformation of American Medicine*. New York: Basic Books, 1982.

"Summary of Views Presented to the Committee on the Implications of the Growth of For-Profit Enterprises in Health Care," Institute of Medicine Conference, Washington, D.C., March 15, 1984.

Variations in Medical Practice. Washington, D.C.: U.S. Senate Appropriations Subcommittee on Labor, Health and Human Services, Education, and Related Agencies, 1985.

REFERENCES

CHAPTER ONE

Atkinson, Rick. "Humana, Inc., Provokes Strong Feelings at Home," *The Washington Post*, January 13, 1985.

Barnette, Martha. "Hospital Primed for World Renown," *The Washington Post*, November 27, 1984.

Breo, Dennis L. "Ethical Issues Debated After Successful Implant of Second Artificial Heart," *American Medical News*, December 7, 1984.

Russell, Christine. "Artificial Heart Is Implanted," *The Washington Post*, November 26, 1984.

Sternberg, Steve. "Artificial Hearts Pay Off in Publicity," *The Miami Herald*, February 24, 1985.

CHAPTER TWO

Annual Report. Washington, D.C.: Federation of American Health Systems, 1984.

———. Washington, D.C.: Federation of American Health Systems, 1985.

Bromberg, Michael D. "The Medical-Industrial Complex: Our National Defense," *New England Journal of Medicine*, November 24, 1983.

Deveny, Kathleen, and Power, Christopher. "How Humana Got a Painful Black Eye," *Business Week*, July 21, 1986.

Economic Trends. Chicago: American Hospital Association, 1986.

"Hospitals Restructure for New Markets in Move to Establish Health Systems," *Federation of American Hospital Systems Review*, November/December 1984.

Iglehart, John K. "Kaiser, HMOs, and the Public Interest: A Conversation with James A. Vohs," *Health Affairs,* Spring 1986.

Jones, David A. "Access, Quality, Affordability Dominate Health Care Issues," *Frontier,* March 1986.

Lefton, Doug. "Public Hospital Limits Care to Tampa's Poor," *American Medical News,* April 20, 1984.

Lothson, David J. *Trick or Treat: Industry at a Crossroads.* New York: Paine Webber, October 31, 1986.

Moore, Francis A. "Who Should Profit from Your Illness?," *Harvard Magazine,* November–December 1985.

"NME Tried to Buy Clout: Documents," *Modern Healthcare,* March 29, 1985.

O'Rourke, Kevin. "An Ethical Perspective on Investor-Owned Medical Care Corporations," *Frontiers of Health Services Management,* September 1984.

Relman, Arnold. "The New Medical-Industrial Complex," *New England Journal of Medicine,* August 11, 1980.

Rosett, Richard N. "Doing Well by Doing Good: Investor-Owned Hospitals," *Frontiers of Health Service Management,* September 1984.

Schlender, Brenton R. "Health Care Firm to Report 2nd-Period Loss," *The Wall Street Journal,* March 17, 1986.

Statistical Profile of the Investor-Owned Hospital Industry 1984. Washington, D.C.: Federation of American Hospitals, 1985.

Talbot, David. "Hospitals," *Bulletin of the New York Academy of Medicine,* January–February 1985.

Tatge, Mark. "For-Profits' Inpatient Occupancy Drops in Quarter; Outpatient Visits Are Rising," *Modern Healthcare,* May 10, 1985.

———. "HHS Approves Reimbursement of Costs for Proposed NME Las Cruces Facility," *Modern Healthcare,* May 24, 1985.

Wallace, Cynthia. "AMI's Weisman Aims to Build Integrated Healthcare Networks," *Modern Healthcare,* August 16, 1985.

Werronen, Henry J. "Integration: A Formula for Hospitals' Survival," *Business and Health,* January–February 1986.

Wikler, Daniel. "Forming an Ethical Response to For-Profit Health Care," *Business and Health,* January–February 1985.

Williamson, David G., Jr. "Investor-Owned Versus Not-For-Profit Hospitals—What Are the Issues?," *Frontiers of Health Services Management,* September 1984.

CHAPTER THREE

Annual Report of the Board of Trustees of the Federal Hospital Insurance Trust Fund. Washington, D.C.: U.S. Government Printing Office, 1984.

Bagamery, Anne. "Health Care," *Forbes,* January 2, 1984.

Berki, S. E. "DRG's, Incentives, Hospitals, and Physicians," *Health Affairs,* Winter 1985.

Bishop, Christine E. "Health Employment and the Nation's Health," *Current History,* May–June 1977.

Cataract Surgery: Fraud, Waste, and Abuse. Washington, D.C.: U.S. House Subcommittee on Health and Long-Term Care, 1985.

Culliton, Barbara J. "University Hospitals for Sale," *Science,* March 2, 1984.

Cunningham, M., Jr. "Changing Philosophies in Medical Care and the Rise of the Investor-Owned Hospital," *New England Journal of Medicine,* September 23, 1982.

Desmaris, Henry R. Testimony Before the U.S. House Special Committee on Aging, April 10, 1986.

Hospital Merger Increased Medicare and Medicaid Payments for Capital Costs. Washington, D.C.: U.S. General Accounting Office, December 22, 1983.

Hull, Jennifer Bingham. "Hospital Nightmare: Cuts in Staff Demoralize Nurses as Care Suffers," *The Wall Street Journal,* March 14, 1984.

"Investor-Owned Industry and Federation: David Williamson Looks at Past, Future," *Federation of American Hospital Systems Review,* March–April 1986.

Kennedy, Louanne. "The Proprietization of Voluntary Hospitals," *Bulletin of the New York Academy of Medicine,* January–February 1985.

Lothson, David J. *Health Care Perspective: Third-Quarter Performance.* New York: Paine Webber, November 11, 1985.

Medicare Payments of Return on Equity Capital to Proprietary Providers. Washington, D.C.: U.S. Department of Health and Human Services, 1983.

Memorandum from Richard P. Kusserow, Health and Human Services Inspector General, to Lawrence DeNardis, Acting Assistant Secretary for Legislation, July 11, 1986.

Merrill, Jeffrey C., and Wasserman, Richard J. "Growth in National Expenditures," *Health Affairs,* Winter 1985.

National Hospital Panel Survey Report. Chicago: American Hospital Association, 1985.

"National Medical Care Spending," *Health Affairs,* Fall 1985.

Potetz, Lisa, and Buchberger, Thomas. "Medicare's Transition to National Payment Rates: Effects on Hospitals," *Health Affairs,* Winter 1985.

"A Pricing Revolution Aids the Big Guys," *Business Week,* January 9, 1984.

Public Hospitals: Sales Lead to Better Facilities but Increased Patient Cost. Washington, D.C.: U.S. General Accounting Office, 1986.

Schlesinger, Mark. "The Rise of Proprietary Health Care," *Business and Health,* January–February 1985.

Sclar, Elliott D. "A Health Planner's Perspective on For-Profit Medicine," *Bulletin of the New York Academy of Medicine,* January–February 1985.

Semiannual Report to the Congress, April 1, 1985–September 30, 1985. Washington, D.C.: Office of Inspector General, U.S. Department of Health and Human Services, 1985.

Shaw, Seth. "The Compelling Issue of Access to Capital," *Business and Health,* January–February 1985.

Sigmond, M. "A Community Perspective on Hospital Ownership," *Frontiers of Health Services Management,* September 1984.

Stevens, Rosemary. "The Historical Perspective," *Bulletin of the New York Academy of Medicine,* January–February 1985.

CHAPTER FOUR

Billitteri, Thomas J. "Bringing Innovation to Florida's Medical Market," *Florida Trend,* January 1985.

Bodewes, Donna. "New Outpatient Center Gives Rise to Turf Battles Among Physicians," *American Medical News,* October 4, 1985.

Feinstein, Richard J. "A View from the 21st Century: How Medicine Met Its Demise," *Miami Medicine,* September, 1985.

Forecast of Physician Supply and Requirements. Washington, D.C.: Office of Technology Assessment, 1980.

Gapen, Phyllis. "Consultant Offers Tips on Marketing for Physicians," *American Medical News,* February 8, 1985.

Golin, Carol Brierly. "Hospitals Woo M.D.'s to Attract Patients," *American Medical News,* April 11, 1986.

———. "Physicians Altering Expectations of Future," *American Medical News,* November 22, 1985.

Havelick, Penny L., and White, Mary Lou S. *Medical Group Practices.* Chicago: American Medical Association, 1986.

Health Care Competition Week, August 1985.

Hilfiker, David. "A Doctor's View of Modern Medicine," *The New York Times Magazine,* February 22, 1986.

Hyman, Jack. "Our Rendezvous with Destiny," *American Medical News,* November 9, 1984.

LeRoy, Lauren; Ellwood, Deborah; and Iglehart, John K. "Trends in Health Manpower," *Health Affairs,* Winter 1985.

"Lifestyle Is Top Priority for Young M.D.'s," *American Medical News,* December 20, 1985.

Longsdorf, Robert, Jr. "Do-It-Yourself Medicine: Another Challenge for Physicians," *Private Practice,* November 1985.

Moore, Francis D. "The Physicians' Perspective," *Bulletin of the New York Academy of Medicine,* January–February 1985.

National Physician Trends from 1970 to 1983. Chicago: American Medical Association, 1986.

Paris, Ellen. "Hippocrates Meets Adam Smith," *Forbes,* February 10, 1986.

Payment for Physician Services: Strategies for Medicare. Washington, D.C.: Office of Technology Assessment, 1986.

Perl, Peter. "Disciplinary Dispute Damages GHA Talks," *The Washington Post,* March 22, 1986.

———. "Doctors Strike Highlights Pressures on GHA," *The Washington Post*, March 28, 1986.

———. "Health Doctors Extend Contract as Strike Deadline Nears," *The Washington Post*, March 2, 1986.

——— and Weil, Martin. "GHA Physicians Vote Strike Starting Today," *The Washington Post*, March 3, 1986.

Podolsky, M. Lawrence. "Give Your Patients More Than They Bargain For," *Private Practice*, March 1985.

Saltzman, Paul. "State's Doctors Take On Mayo Clinic Staff," *The Miami Herald*, May 5, 1985.

Sandrick, Karen. "Doctors Turn to Unions," *Private Practice*, November 1985.

Socioeconomic Report. Sacramento, Calif.: California Medical Association, January 1985.

Steinwachs, Donald M., et al. "A Comparison of the Requirements for Primary Care Physicians in HMOs with Projections Made by the GMENAC," *New England Journal of Medicine*, January 21, 1986.

Tarlov, Alvin R. "HMO Enrollment Growth and Physicians: The Third Compartment," *Health Affairs*, Spring 1986.

Willson, Elizabeth. "To Advertise or Not to Advertise: Why Doctors Are Divided," *Florida Trend*, November 1985.

CHAPTER FIVE

Cancila, Carol. "M.D.: Court Victory May Aid Others Unfairly Dismissed," *American Medical News*, September 12, 1986.

Davis, Karen, et al. "Is Cost Containment Working?," *Health Affairs*, Fall 1985.

Diagnosis-Related Groups and the Prospective Payment System. Chicago: American Medical Association, 1984.

The Effects of PPS on Quality of Care for Medicare Patients. Washington, D.C.: U.S. Senate Special Committee on Aging, January 7, 1986.

"Hospital Payment Plan Stirs Debate on TV Show," *American Medical News*, November 22–29, 1985.

The Impact of DRGs on Patient Care. Washington, D.C.: American Society of Internal Medicine, March 1984–October 1985.

John, Kenneth E. "Poll Finds Widespread Concern About Early Release from Hospital," *The Washington Post*, Health Section, October 28, 1986.

Lewin, Lawrence S.; Derzon, Robert A.; and Margulies, Rhea. "Investor-Owned and Nonprofits Differ in Economic Performance," *Hospitals*, July 1, 1981.

Luft, Harold. "For-Profit Hospitals: A Cost Problem or Solution," *Business and Health*, January–February 1985.

"M.D. Arrangements with Hospitals Told," *American Medical News*, November 9, 1984.

Medicare: Physician Incentive Payments by Hospitals Could Lead to Abuse. Washington, D.C.: U.S. General Accounting Office, 1986.

Need to Eliminate Payments for Unnecessary Hospital Ancillary Services. Washington, D.C.: U.S. General Accounting Office, September 1983.

Nelson, Creston. "Detailed Medicare DRG Data Offer Inside Look at Hospitals," *South Florida Medical Review,* September 24, 1985.

Pattison, Robert V., and Katz, Hallie M. "Investor-Owned and Not-For-Profit Hospitals," *New England Journal of Medicine,* August 11, 1983.

Quality of Care Under Medicare's Prospective Payment System. Washington, D.C.: U.S. Senate Special Committee on Aging, Vols. I and II, September 26, October 24, and November 12, 1985.

Relman, Arnold. "Cost Control, Doctors' Ethics, and Patient Care," *Issues in Science and Technology,* Winter 1984.

———. "Investor-Owned Hospitals and Health Care Costs," *New England Journal of Medicine,* August 11, 1983.

Report of the American Medical Association's Board of Trustees, AMA'S DRG Monitoring Project and the Prospective Payment System. Chicago: American Medical Association, 1984.

Rosenblatt, Robert A., and Peterson, Jonathan. "Medicare Change Stirs Concern for the Elderly," *Los Angeles Times,* April 14, 1985.

Stallings, Charles L., and Zillman, Marcus P. *Florida Hospital Index: A Consumer's Guide to Costs and Services.* Jefferson, N.C.: McFarland & Company, Inc., 1986.

State of Florida Hospital Cost Containment Board, 1983 Annual Report. Tallahassee, Fla.: Hospital Cost Containment Board, 1984.

State of Florida Hospital Cost Containment Board, 1984 Hospital Financial Data. Tallahassee, Fla.: Hospital Cost Containment Board, 1985.

State of Florida Hospital Cost Containment Board, 1985 Hospital Budget Data. Tallahassee, Fla.: Hospital Cost Containment Board, 1986.

Steinbrook, Robert. "Hospital Death Rates of Medicare Patients Released," *Los Angeles Times,* April 25, 1987.

Watt, J. Michael, et al. "The Comparative Economic Performance of Investor-Owned Chain and Not-For-Profit Hospitals," *New England Journal of Medicine,* January 9, 1986.

CHAPTER SIX

America's Uninsured and Underinsured: A Nation At Risk of Inadequate Health Care and Catastrophic Costs. Washington, D.C.: U.S. House Select Committee on Aging, 1986.

Bedrosian, John C. "New Trends in Health Care Delivery," speech to the Rotary Club of Los Angeles, California, January 13, 1984.

Cahan, Vicky. "When the Patient Can't Pay the Medical Bill," *Business Week,* February 18, 1985.

Cancila, Carol. "Lack of Health Care Access Big Problem," *American Medical News,* June 20, 1986.

"Community Hospitals' Closings Increased in '85, AHA Reports," *American Medical News,* May 9, 1986.

Controlling the Cost of Health Care. Washington, D.C.: Employee Benefit Research Institute, 1983.

Cummings, Helen King, and King, James P. "Financing Indigent Care: Public Problems, Private Responsibilities," *Federation of American Hospital Systems Review,* March–April 1985.

Dalleck, Geri. "For-Profit Hospitals and the Poor," *Clearinghouse Review,* December 1983.

Employer-Sponsored Health Insurance Coverage. Washington, D.C.: Employee Benefit Research Institute, 1986.

The Equitable Health Care Survey: Corporate Initiatives & Employee Attitudes on Cost Containment. New York: The Equitable Life Assurance Society of the United States, February–March 1985.

Feder, Judith. "Falling Through the Cracks: Poverty, Insurance Coverage, and Hospital Care for the Poor, 1980 and 1982," *Milbank Memorial Fund Quarterly/Health and Society,* Fall 1984.

———, and Hadley, Jack. "The Economically Unattractive Patient: Who Cares?," *Bulletin of the New York Academy of Medicine,* January–February 1985.

For-Profit Hospital Care: Who Profits? Who Cares? Washington, D.C.: National Council of Senior Citizens, March 1986.

Gage, Larry S. "Impact on the Public Hospitals," *Bulletin of the New York Academy of Medicine,* January–February 1985.

Gapen, Phyllis. "Hospital Care for Poor at Controversy's Heart," *American Medical News,* January 24–31, 1986.

Hadley, Jack, and Feder, Judith. "Hospital Cost Shifting and Care for the Uninsured," *Health Affairs,* Fall 1985.

Health Care USA. Washington, D.C.: The National Council on the Aging, 1984.

Kirkman-Luff, Bradford L. "Refusal of Care: Evidence from Arizona," *Health Affairs,* Winter 1985.

Martin, Joseph; Dolkart, David; and Freko, Deborah. "Reasons for the Downturn in Under-65 Admissions," *American Hospital Association Policy Brief No. 52.* Chicago: American Hospital Association, 1984.

Meyer, Harris. "New Yorkers Have Trouble Getting Care," *American Medical News,* June 20, 1986.

Nelson Harry, and Roark, Anne C. "Health Care Crisis: Less for More," *Los Angeles Times,* April 7, 1985.

Newhouse, J. P.; Manning, W. G.; and Morris, C. N. "Some Interim Results from a Controlled Trial of Cost-Sharing in Health Insurance," *New England Journal of Medicine,* 1981.

Okie, Susan. " 'Dumping' Patients into Public Hospitals May Shorten Lives, Study Says," *The Washington Post,* February 27, 1986.

Private Initiatives to Contain Health Care Expenditures. Washington, D.C.: Employee Benefit Research Institute, 1986.

Swartz, Katherine. "People Without Health Insurance: How Did Their Characteristics Change Between 1963 and 1983 and Why Has Their Number Increased Since 1980?," paper prepared for the American Health Planning Association's Fifth Annual Conference, March 12, 1985.

Teitelman, Robert, and King, Ralph, Jr. "Insurance Blues," *Forbes*, February 10, 1986.

CHAPTER SEVEN

"Acquisitions Guidelines Reevaluated by Chains," *Today's Nursing Home*, January 1986.

Beverly Enterprises in Michigan: A Case Study of Corporate Takeover of Health Care Resources. Washington, D.C.: AFL-CIO Food and Beverage Trades Department, 1983.

Beverly Enterprises: Patient Care Record. Washington, D.C.: AFL-CIO Food and Beverage Trades Department, January 27, 1983.

Blyskal, Jeff. "Gray Gold," *Forbes*, November 23, 1981.

Certificate of Need Application Submitted by Beverly Enterprises to the Office of Statewide Health Planning and Development, Sacramento, California, undated.

Dammann, Peter. "Big Nursing Home Chain Picks Oregon," *Willamette Week*, December 1–7, 1981.

Elliott, Richard, Jr. "No Tired Blood: Nursing Home Operators Are Long on Enthusiasm, Short on Experience," *Barron's*, March 24, 1969.

Flynn, Julie. "A Nursing Home Company Faces Up to Its Midlife Crisis," *Business Week*, December 29, 1986.

Frank, Jonathan M. "Beverly Enterprises," *The Value Line Investment Survey*, May 16, 1986.

Gapen, Phyllis. "Beverly Sues for Nursing Home Licenses," *American Medical News*, September 12, 1986.

———. "Calif. Nursing Home Faces Loss of License," *American Medical News*, January 17, 1986.

———. "State Stiffens Stance on Nursing Homes," *American Medical News*, November 8, 1985.

Greenhouse, Steven. "Superstar of Nursing Homes," *The New York Times*, April 14, 1986.

Hilder, David B. "Fine of $600,000 Is Set for Beverly Enterprises, Inc.," *The Wall Street Journal*, October 17, 1986.

Keppel, Bruce. "Multihospital Affiliation in Hand, Beverly Aims to Double," *Modern Healthcare*, June 1982.

Long-Term-Care Facility Effectiveness Standards. Sacramento, Cal.: California Health Facilities Commission, June 18, 1982.

Long-Term Care for the Elderly: Investor-Owned Nursing Homes. Washington, D.C.: The National Council of Health Centers, undated.

"Medicare at the Crossroads," testimony prepared by the Service Employees International Union, delivered at hearing of U.S. House Select Committee on Aging, Arlington, Texas, June 1983.

Rights of the Institutionalized Elderly: Lost in Confinement. Washington, D.C.: U.S. House Subcommittee on Health and Long-Term Care, September 18, 1985.

Transcript of hearing before State of Pennsylvania Unemployment Compensation Board regarding the claim of Mark A. Turns, January 21, 1983.

Valiante, John D. "The Capital Requirements for Long-Term-Care Services," *Health Care Financial Management*, April 1984.

Wayne, N. Russell. "Beverly Enterprises." New York: *Value Line Investment Survey*, February 13, 1987.

Welling, Kathyrn M. "Really Rocking: Nursing Homes Are the Healthiest Thing in Health Care," *Barron's*, July 2, 1986.

CHAPTER EIGHT

Abramowitz, Michael. "Maxicare to Purchase HealthAmerica," *The Washington Post*, July 29, 1986.

Albert, Steve. "DO Charged with Releasing HMO Patient Prematurely," *South Florida Medical Review*, October 22, 1985.

Baldwin, Mark. "Boston HMOs Ready for Stepped-up Battle," *Modern Healthcare*, May 10, 1985.

Berenson, Robert A. "Capitation and Conflict of Interest," *Health Affairs*, Spring 1986.

Goldstein, Avram. "Government Seldom Evaluates HMO Care," *The Miami Herald*, November 19, 1984.

———. "HMO Health-Care Empire Was Built on Ads, Political Ties, and $4,000," *The Miami Herald*, September 3, 1984.

———. "HMOs Weighing Cost Against Treatment," *The Miami Herald*, November 18, 1985.

Health Maintenance Organizations and the Elderly: Promises, Problems, and Prospects. Washington, D.C.: U.S. House Select Committee on Aging, April 1, 1986.

Hull, Jennifer Bingham. "HMO Insurance Plans Face Some Threats to Own Good Health," *The Wall Street Journal*, January 16, 1986.

Iglehart, John K. "HMOs (For-Profit and Not-For-Profit) on the Move," *New England Journal of Medicine*, May 3, 1984.

Kenney, James B. "Using Competition to Develop a Buyer-Driven Market," *Business and Health*, November 1985.

Kosterlitz, Julie. "The Government, Health Experts, Wall Street Pinning Their Hopes on HMOs," *National Journal*, November 23, 1985.

Lyons, David. "Chairman, Friends Live High on IMC," *The Miami Herald,* May 11, 1986.

"Many Calif. M.D.s Dissatisfied with Contracts," *American Medical News,* June 12, 1986.

Masso, Anthony. "HMOs in Transition: What the Future Holds," *Business and Health,* January–February 1985.

McGinn, Paul R. "Contract Dispute Splits Specialists, Family M.D.s," *American Medical News,* May 8, 1987.

Medicare and HMOs: A First Look, with Disturbing Findings. Washington, D.C.: U.S. Senate Special Committee on Aging, Minority Staff Report, April 7, 1987.

Meyer, Harris. "Ob-Gyns Quit Md. HMO to Protest Test Payment Plan," *American Medical News,* March 13, 1987.

Moran, Donald W., and Sanela, Theresa E. "HMOs, Finance, and the Hereafter," *Health Affairs,* Spring 1986.

Obrentz, Margery E. *Group Health Insurance: CIGNA's Outlook for the Industry.* New York: Paine Webber, March 24, 1986.

———. *HMO Industry.* New York: Paine Webber, February 12, 1986.

Private Initiatives to Contain Health Care Expenditures. Washington, D.C.: Employee Benefit Research Institute, 1986.

"Record Growth of HMOs," *American Medical News,* August 1, 1986.

Rice, Thomas, et al. "The State of PPOs: Results from a National Survey," *Health Affairs,* Winter 1985.

Russell, Pamela. "Employees Face Challenge of Selecting Health-Care Plans in Complex Markets," *Investor's Daily,* April 7, 1986.

Staver, Sari. "Michigan M.D.'s in HMOs and PPOs Face Higher Liability," *American Medical News,* July 12, 1985.

Stein, Jane. "How HMOs Adapt: A Perspective from the Inside," *Business and Health,* October 1986.

Sternberg, Steve. "IMC Favors Cash over Medicine, Some Say," *The Miami Herald,* May 22, 1985.

Taylor, Humphrey, and Kagay, Michael. "The HMO Report Card: A Closer Look," *Health Affairs,* Spring 1986.

Teitelman, Robert. "Maxicare, Maxiprofits," *Forbes,* December 2, 1985.

———, and King, Ralph, Jr. "Insurance Blues," *Forbes,* February 10, 1986.

Tokarz, Wally. "Florida DO Faces Licensure Hearing," *American Medical News,* November 15, 1985.

———. "Partnership Formed to Develop HMOs, PPOs," *American Medical News,* July 19, 1986.

Watts, Al. "Maxicare to Buy HealthAmerica, Become Nation's Largest HMO," *Investor's Daily,* July 29, 1986.

Wessell, David. "As HMOs Increasingly Become Big Businesses, Many of Them Convert to Profitmaking Status," *The Wall Street Journal,* March 26, 1985.

White, Stephen L., and Rothe, Brent. "The Potential for Hospital Competition and Hospital Costs in Florida in 1983," unpublished, undated paper prepared for the Florida Hospital Cost Containment Board.

Willson, Elizabeth. "Health Care's Newest Wrinkle: Wholesale Medicine," *Florida Trend,* July 1986.

CHAPTER NINE

Belsie, Laurent. "Psychiatric Services for Children Grow," *The Christian Science Monitor,* May 14, 1987.

"Bypass 'Regionalization' Offers Better Outcome Chances for Patients: Study," *American Medical News,* February 13, 1987.

Cancila, Carol. "JCAH to Review Clinical Outcomes," *American Medical News,* September 19, 1986.

Caper, Philip; Keller, Robert; and Rohlf, Paul. "Tracking Physician Practice Patterns for Quality Care," *Business and Health,* September 1986.

Feldstein, Martin. "The High Costs of Hospitals and What to Do About It," *Public Interest,* Summer 1977.

McCracken, Gene, and Bognanni, Sal. "Iowa Employers Use Small Area Analysis in Benefits Reform," *Business and Health,* September 1986.

Past Overuse of Intensive-Care Services Inflates Hospital Payments. Washington, D.C.: U.S. General Accounting Office, September 1983.

Stein, Jane. "Quantifying Medical Outcomes for More Effective Delivery," *Business and Health,* September 1986.

"Surplus of Surgeons Seen as a Threat to Quality of Operations," *The Washington Post,* October 21, 1986.

Ver Berkmoes, Ryan. "Variations Studies Gain Attention, Support," *American Medical News,* April 4, 1986.

Woll, Peter. *American Bureaucracy.* New York: W. W. Norton & Company, 1977.

INDEX

TRAVEL & BUYING GUIDE

Where to find the Oregon in Oregon

1988-89

Bridget Beattie McCarthy

Project Assistant and Editor: Sara Oakland

Logo and Calligraphy: Elizabeth Anderson
Maps: Ann Kendall Taylor and Laurie Causgrove
Symbols: Elizabeth Anderson, Bridget Beattie McCarthy, Lila Braker and Dover Publications.
Typesetting and Mechanicals: Irish Setter
Printing: Artline and Golden Impressions
Cover: Ricki Johnson
Featured Artists: Liza Jones and Paul Miller

Bridget Beattie McCarthy
7277 S.W. Barnes Rd.
Portland, Oregon 97225

Printed in United States of America

ISBN 0-9616696-2-4

Thanks

Thanks and recognition are due: **M. C. McCarthy** for his continued support, good ideas, and patience; **Sara Oakland** for her methodical hard work and consistent good nature; **Larry Hoffman**, **Marcia Lewis**, **Katie Ciuchta** and all the other people at **Action Printers** for their ideas and quick, reliable service; at **Irish Setter**, **Martin White** for typesetting, **Lila Braker** for paste-up and her unflappable organizational talents, and **Carol Davis** for her critical proofreading and paste-up assistance; **Sandra Sato** at **Artline** for her suggestions and commitment to good customer relations; **Alan and Brenda Mitchell** for their comments about the South Coast Regional Notes; **Daryl and Marta Coleman** for their help with the South Central Regional Notes; **Ed Henry** at **EDIT Word Processing** for impeccable manuscript typing; **Portland Mailing Service** for processing our various mailings; **Ann Kendall Taylor** for updating the maps; **David Browne** for photographing Paul and Liza's prints; **Alan Zell** for his suggestions about the cover.

Information from the following sources was used to enhance my own knowledge of the state as I put together the Regional Notes that appear throughout the guide. These are excellent publications which I encourage you to buy and use.

- David D. Alt and Donald W. Hyndman: *Roadside Geology of Oregon*. Missoula, Montana: Mountain Press Publishing Company, 1978.
- Allan P. Bennison: *Geological Highway Map of the Pacific Northwestern Region*. Tulsa, Oklahoma: The American Association of Petroleum Geologists, n.d.
- David E.M. Bucy and Mary C. McCauley: *A Hiker's Guide to the Oregon Coast Trail*. Salem, Oregon: Oregon State Parks and Recreation Branch, circa 1970.
- Joel Connelly: *Twelve Uncommon Trips in the Pacific Northwest*. Seattle, Washington: Pacific Search Publications, 1982.
- Highland Rock and Gift Shop: *The Rockhound's Map of Oregon*. Burns, Oregon: 1982. (See Southeastern Oregon participant listings.)
- Mt. Hood Recreation Association: *Come to Your Senses on the Loop*.
- The Nature Conservancy: miscellaneous brochures.
- Oregon State Parks: *Welcome* brochure, circa 1986.
- Oregon Tourism Division: *The Oregon Book*. Salem, Oregon: Oregon Tourism Division, 1984, 1985, 1986.
- Jordis Schick: *Oregon Blue Book 1985-1986*. Salem, Oregon: Oregon Secretary of State, 1985.
- Earl Thollander: *Back Roads of Oregon*. New York, N.Y.: Clarkson N. Potter, Inc., 1979.
- Antone C. Van Vliet and Alexis J. Panshin: *Identifying Oregon Driftwood*. Corvallis, Oregon: Oregon State University Extension Service, Sea Grant Marine Advisory Program, 1976.

Bridget Beattie McCarthy

Introduction

All across the United States, Americans are looking for ways to distinguish themselves from one another. **People** are searching for things to add individual meaning to their lives now surrounded with high technology and mass production, and they are **beginning again to relate geographically, identifying with their own communities and seeking out the regionally unique in others**.

Even from the earliest times, the arts have helped meet this need. The way people embellish their material culture has always given them regional identity, and we are taking a renewed interest in this now. **As we are getting over the thrill of being able to jet halfway around the world in half a day, we want to see, taste, experience and take home with us that which is regionally interesting.** This guide was designed to respond to both in-state residents' pride and out-of-state visitors' fascination in things that represent the essence of Oregon.

The *Oregon in Oregon* idea stemmed from a handcraft marketing study I did in 1983 supported by grants through the federal and state Economic Development Departments and from the Oregon Arts Commission to find ways to market Oregon's handcrafts. Among other things, it substantiated my belief that there are thousands of people out there looking for **"the real thing"** and that by marketing the work of the hand with other Oregon goods and services through the *Oregon in Oregon* concept, not only craftspeople but the state as a whole, including its visitors, will benefit.

In 1984, Peter Hero of the Oregon Arts Commission was successful in convincing Governor Atiyeh to establish an arts marketing fund that provided the initial seed money to spearhead the *Oregon in Oregon* concept. While the project is still endorsed by the Oregon Arts Commission, it is now supported entirely by the participants themselves.

To be included, **participants have to demonstrate that they make, grow, perform, show, brew, invent or offer an experience that has individual, local or regional character** and be willing to help distribute copies of the guides, thereby cross-selling each other's products and services.

N-M *Where to Find the Oregon in Oregon* (working in conjunction with the Oregon Department of Agriculture) has included in this edition many of the **products selected by Neiman-Marcus** for a special Oregon promotion featured in its stores in the summer of 1988. I am pleased that *Where to Find the Oregon in Oregon* has come to be **recognized as a leading publication promoting regional products and services and the essence of Oregon**.

This is truly a self-help bootstrap project that is meant to be of service to both participants and readers alike. I hope you enjoy this year's edition.

Bridget Beattie McCarthy
April, 1988

Contents

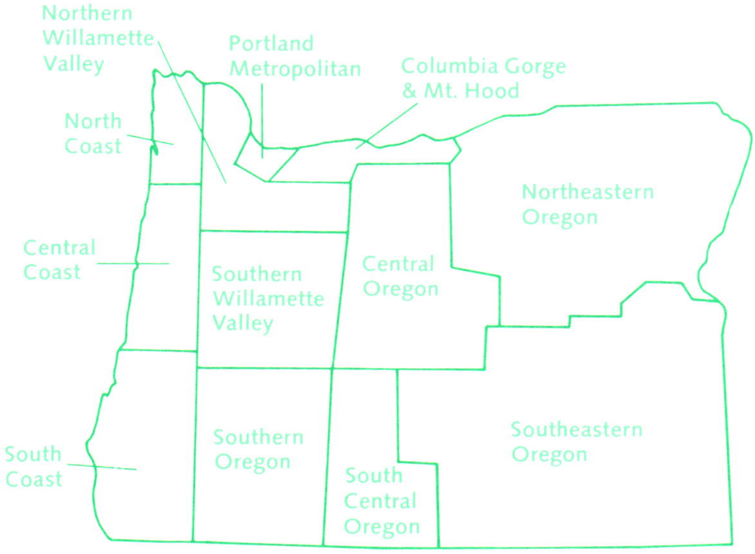

Northern Willamette Valley
Portland Metropolitan
Columbia Gorge & Mt. Hood
North Coast
Northeastern Oregon
Central Coast
Southern Willamette Valley
Central Oregon
Southeastern Oregon
South Coast
Southern Oregon
South Central Oregon

How to Use this Guide

KEY TO SYMBOLS

Each listing in this guide has been coded with one or several symbols as follows:

Individual craftspeople, writers, artists, photographers, inventors, or manufacturers whose studios, workshops, factories, or shops are open to the public or whose products are available by mail order.

Shops, galleries, guilds, co-operatives, art centers, indoor and outdoor markets—basically places where products from more than one Oregon producer, artist, craftsperson, etc., are available.

Wineries, vineyards, distilleries, breweries and brew pubs, tasting rooms.

Restaurants, delicatessens, shops and producers having for sale: Oregon-produced cheese; wine; bread; ice cream; nuts; fresh, dried or canned fruits and vegetables; fresh or smoked seafood; fresh or cured meats; jams; preserves; syrups; dried or fresh herbs; stone-ground flour; et al. Includes: cheese factories, fruit stands, canneries, smoke-houses, jam factories and flour mills, etc. (See separate symbols for wineries, bakeries, candy factories and ice creameries.)

Performing arts, including Shakespearean theater, chamber music, opera, symphony, theater, music, dance and film.

Museums of all kinds, historical societies, environmental demonstration projects, zoos, historic buildings, exhibit centers and educational facilities.

Outdoor experiences, including river outfitters and expeditions, climbing and bicycle guides, gardens, bicycle trails, walking and driving tours, riverboat excursions and helicopter rides.

Country inns and bed and breakfast homes.

Information resources, including visitor and convention bureaus, chambers of commerce and local arts councils.

Events, rodeos, Fourth of July celebrations, festivals, parades, etc.

Bakeries

Ice cream-making establishments.

Places where candies or chocolates are made.

Oregon-grown bulbs, plants, seeds, herbs, shrubs, flowers, ZooDoo and other plant or gardening materials.

Books and bookstores.

Those participants who were chosen by Neiman-Marcus to be part of its 1988 Oregon products promotion.

COMMUNITIES THAT ESPECIALLY WELCOME VISITORS

Scattered throughout this guide you will find a few, larger listings in boxes, printed in color. **Some communities in Oregon are interested in welcoming visitors.** Through their visitor and convention bureaus, chambers of commerce, mayor's offices or even their community centers, they have taken out larger listings that describe their areas in general and list their major events and festivals. For more information about these areas, do not hesitate to contact the sources listed. These communities want to be of service to visitors to their area.

REGIONAL MAPS

Refer to the actual listings following the maps for descriptions, addresses, directions and map-locating numbers. The regional maps show the APPROXIMATE location of each listing. For precise directions, use a road map in conjunction with the addresses and/or instructions given with each listing.

REGIONAL NOTES

The regional notes found at the beginning of each section of this guide are another expression of Bridget McCarthy's interest and concern for what makes one place different from another. It is this particular aspect of regional integrity that is both our most valuable asset and our most vulnerable. Please enjoy Oregon's regional essences and please help us protect them.

1988-89 FEATURED ARTISTS

The arts are one of the best ways to portray an essence of a region; and since the celebration of regionalism is what this publication is all about, *Where to Find the Oregon in Oregon* has incorporated the work of Oregon artists **Liza Jones** and **Paul Miller** into its 1988-9 edition.

Liza Jones is a native of Oregon. She is primarily a printmaker, well known for her etchings of the Oregon Coast. Since 1980 she has been director of Inkling Studio, a print workshop in Portland, which has 20 members working in linoleum, woodblock, mezzotint, engraving, and etching.

Liza received her BFA from Rhode Island School of Design in 1966 and MA from Columbia University Teachers College in 1968. She has taught printmaking at Portland State University and the Museum Art School. From 1977 to 1981 she was chairman of printmaking at the Oregon School of Arts and Crafts. Her prints and large pastels of the Oregon Coast and Eastern Oregon can be seen at several Portland galleries.

For eight years Liza has had her studio at Manzanita, on the Oregon Coast. Much of her imagery comes from the Nehalem Bay area. Her ocean pastels and prints are on display at the Peacock Gallery in nearby Nehalem.

Paul Miller was chairman of photography at the Oregon School of Arts and Crafts for twelve years. He also taught non-silver photography at the Museum Art School from 1986 to 1988 and makes photo-etchings from photos he has taken of Oregon. Paul lives with Liza at Manzanita. Liza and Paul are available by appointment at Inkling Studio in Portland. Tel: 224-2540.

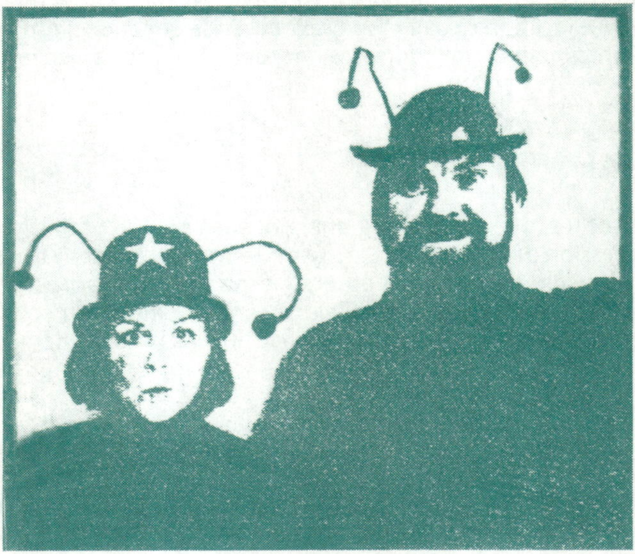

The Humbugs, © *Liza Jones & Paul Miller*

Project Direction

Bridget Beattie McCarthy is a consultant and project developer specializing in regionalism, marketing, facilities development, the arts, tourism and grass roots community development as they relate to supporting the concept of "community" and regional integrity.

Her accomplishments in Oregon include directing a project that furnished the Wy'East Day Lodge at Timberline on Mt. Hood with the work of contemporary Northwest craftsmen (see Columbia Gorge–Mt. Hood Regional Notes and listings) as an arts-tourism promotion that is already attracting articles in national magazines. Her book, *Architectural Crafts*, promotes craftsmen doing architectural-scale work in ten western states to architects and builders throughout the country. She has conducted marketing studies for—among others—Oregon's Economic Development Department, and during the six years that she directed the Oregon School of Arts and Crafts, a seven-acre, ten-building campus was built, which is itself a tourism attraction (see Portland Metro listings).

As well as directing her own company, *Where to Find the Oregon in Oregon*, which has promoted the arts along with other Oregon products and services to the tourism market since 1984, Bridget McCarthy is an experienced fund-raiser and speaker and has served on numerous national boards and juries.

She speaks and consults all over the United States and Canada, helping communities, states, organizations and businesses solve problems through the development of regionally appropriate projects, regional promotions, downtown development plans and the production of "Where to Find the Real Thing" guides. **She is convinced that the celebration and promotion of regionalism with integrity and style is economically, socially and aesthetically sound, and that in the long term quality pays.** For more information contact Bridget Beattie McCarthy, 7277 S.W. Barnes Rd., Portland, Oregon 97225. Tel: 292-4549.

NATIONAL ENDOWMENT FOR THE ARTS, OREGON ARTS COMMISSION and OTHER ENDORSEMENTS

A number of listings mention the Oregon Arts Commission and the National Endowment for the Arts. Grants and funding from these agencies require rigorous application procedures, proof of artistic merit and, in the case of organizations, not-for-profit status, and appropriate arts management practices. Artists' and craftsmen's Fellowship Awards are very competitive and require the submission of slides of current work and other material that is reviewed by panels made up of nationally recognized experts in the field. Other funding sources require equally rigorous application procedures.

STATEWIDE RESOURCES

NW Bed and Breakfast Travel Unlimited

610 S.W. Broadway, Portland, 97205.
Tel: 243-7616
A reservation service, established in 1979, serving 400 bed and breakfast homes and inns in the Northwest, all inspected to meet quality standards. Coastal, mountain, city, or rural accommodations are available. Staying in a B&B home or inn is a special way to see Oregon through the eyes of congenial residents. 9-5 Mon-Fri.

Oregon Elderhostel

Oregon Elderhostel State Office
Western Oregon State College, Administration Bldg., #305, Monmouth, 97361.
Tel: 838-1220, ext. 435 or 800-232-9653 (in-state)
For those who always wanted to know more about the Oregon Trail. . .float the Deschutes or Grande Ronde Rivers. . .or delve into the works of Shakespeare, Oregon Elderhostel offers dynamic, low-cost, week-long study opportunities for persons 60 years and over. Part of an international education program with more than 25 program sites in Oregon. Call or write for additional information.

○ Country Host Registry

See MYRTLE CREEK (Southern Oregon) for listing.

Oregon Arts Commission

835 Summer St. N.E., Salem, 97301.
Tel: 378-3625
State art agency funded by the National Endowment for the arts and the Oregon State Legislature to further the arts in the state. Staff can provide further information on the visual and performing arts in Oregon. The commission provides funds and services to arts organizations and artists of all disciplines throughout the state. It also purchases art work through the states "% for Art" program. It is this agency that provided the initial seed money and support to produce the first edition of this guide in 1984.

Oregon Scenic Waterways Advisory Committee

525 Trade St. S.E., Salem, 97310.
Tel: 378-6500
Exists to protect the natural, aesthetic, scenic, fish and wildlife, scientific, and recreational values of Oregon's rivers. Designated sections of the following rivers are to remain free-flowing, without dams or impoundments: Deschutes, Illinois, John Day, Minam, Owyhee, Rogue, Sandy, North Fork of Middle Fork of Willamette, and Waldo Lake.

Bed and Breakfast Accommodations—Oregon Plus

5733 S.W. Dickinson St., Portland, 97219.
Tel: 245-0642
A reservation service representing over 100 personally inspected homes and inns in the Northwest. Participating hosts are ready to share their homes and knowledge to make guests' visits more enjoyable. Reservations world-wide. Gift certificates for all occasions. "Meeting individual needs with the quality you expect." Visa/MC. 10-4 Mon-Fri.

Advisory Committee on Historic Preservation

State Historic Preservation Office, Parks and Recreation Division, 525 Trade St. S.E., Salem, 97310. Tel: 378-5002
Reviews nominations to the National Register of Historic Places from the State of Oregon, recommends nominations to the State Historic Preservation Officer, and reviews the Statewide Plan for Historic Preservation.

The Historic Preservation League of Oregon

P.O. Box 40053, Portland, 97240.
Tel: 243-1923
The only statewide not-for-profit organization dedicated to the preservation of Oregon's historic resources. Educational workshops available.

Natural Heritage Advisory Council

Division of State Lands
1445 State St., Salem, 97310.
Tel: 378-3805
Advises the State Land Board in the State's Natural Heritage Program and seeks to preserve examples of natural heritage resources and special species in natural areas through the voluntary cooperation of private and public landowners. Maintains data bank of information on natural resources and special species, which is available as time and resources permit through **The Nature Conservancy**.

The Nature Conservancy

1205 N.W. 25th, Portland, 97210.
Tel: 228-9561
The only private not-for-profit land conservation organization dedicated solely to the preservation of natural

diversity. With field offices throughout the country, the conservancy has been able to save over 2,500,000 acres of forests, marshes, prairies, mountains, and islands. In Oregon there are 32 preserves totaling nearly 35,000 acres. All lands are acquired through private donations of land or money. Donations are tax deductable. Contact the conservancy's offices for information about preserves the public may visit in Oregon.

Land Conservation and Development Commission

1175 Court St. N.E., Salem, 97310.
Tel: 378-4926
A planning program that continues Oregon's long-standing efforts to protect resources and provide for orderly development. Such efforts began as early as 1899, when beaches in Clatsop County were declared a public highway. In 1913 similar rights of public access were extended to all of Oregon's beaches.

U.S. Forest Service

Pacific Northwest Regional Office, 319 S.W. Pine St., Portland. Mailing address: P.O. Box 3623, Portland, 97208.
Tel: 221-2877
Of the total acreage of Oregon, 49.72% is federally owned, and together the USFS and the BLM manage most of it. The USFS maintains 15,751,338 acres of forest land in Oregon, including 13 national forests, numerous wilderness areas, an experimental watershed area, a grasslands reclamation project; and several national scenic and recreational areas and waterways. Recreation information, including maps, brochures, and books, is available from the Portland office. Specific information about weather, roads, fire conditions, etc., is available from local forest supervisors' offices. See Regional Notes section of this guide for locations of regional offices.

U.S. Bureau of Land Management

825 N.E. Multnomah, 14th Floor, Portland. Mailing address: P.O. Box 2965, Portland, 97208. Tel: 221-2877
Of the total acreage of Oregon, 49.72% is federally owned, and together the USFS and the BLM manage most of it. The BLM manages 15,669,408 acres of land in Oregon. Natural resources managed by the BLM on forest land (west of the Cascades) and rangeland (east of the Cascades) include forest products, livestock forage, minerals, soil, water and air, wildlife habitat, and horses. A wide variety of maps is available from the Portland office. See U.S. Forest Service listing for more information on federally managed lands.

Oregon Department of Fish and Wildlife

506 S.W. Mill, Portland, 97201.
Tel: 229-5403
This department has the important responsibility of speaking up for fish and wildlife resources as other land and water users make plans to modify these essential components of habitat needed by the creatures of the wild, many of whom represent the very essence of Oregon.

Department of Geology and Mineral Industries

1069 State Office Bldg., Portland, 97201.
Tel: 229-5580
The State's information center for geological, mining, oil, gas, geothermal, and geological hazard data. Public information program includes technical library and the publication of investigative research.

Sno-Park Permits

So that the roads can be kept clear in high-use winter recreation areas, Sno-Park permits are required for parking in designated locations between November 15 and April 15. Daily and annual permits are sold at ski areas, Motor Vehicle Division field offices, and many sports and ski stores. The State of Oregon and Washington honor each other's Sno-Park permits.

State Campsite Information Center

Tel: 800-452-5687 (in-state) or 238-7488
Provides current information on campsite availability in Oregon State Parks from the first Monday in March to Labor Day weekend, 8-4:30 Mon-Fri.

Tourism Division

Oregon Economic Development Department, 595 Cottage St. N.E., Salem, 97310. Tel: 373-1200 or 800-233-3306 (in-state) or 800-547-7842 (out-of-state).
Provides travel planning information to prospective visitors to Oregon and travel professionals.

OREGON PUBLIC BROADCASTING

A listener-supported statewide network, OPB strives to provide a useful, intelligent and entertaining radio service to listeners in Oregon and Southern Washington.

Programs are targeted to audiences that OPB considers are underserved by other media. These audiences include classical, jazz, and folk music enthusiasts, ethnic and racial minorities, women, the elderly, confined, and handicapped, and those wanting literate, unbiased news coverage and analysis.

Listeners' favorites include:

NPR's All Things Considered
weekdays 5-7 p.m.,
Sat-Sun 5-6 p.m.

NPR's Morning Edition
weekdays 5-9 a.m.

NPR's Weekend Edition
Sat 8-10 a.m.

Oregon First
weekdays 4:30-5 p.m.

Northwest Week in Review
Mon 7-7:30 p.m.

Portland City Club
Fri 12:30-2 p.m.

Radio Reader
weekdays 7:30-8 p.m.

Northwest Musicians
Sat 12 noon-1 pm

News
weekdays 12 noon, 2 p.m.

Weather
midnight daily

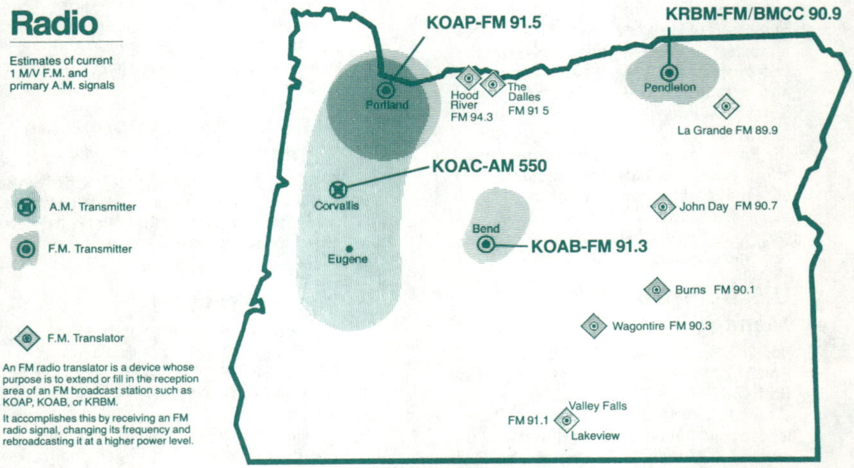

North Coast

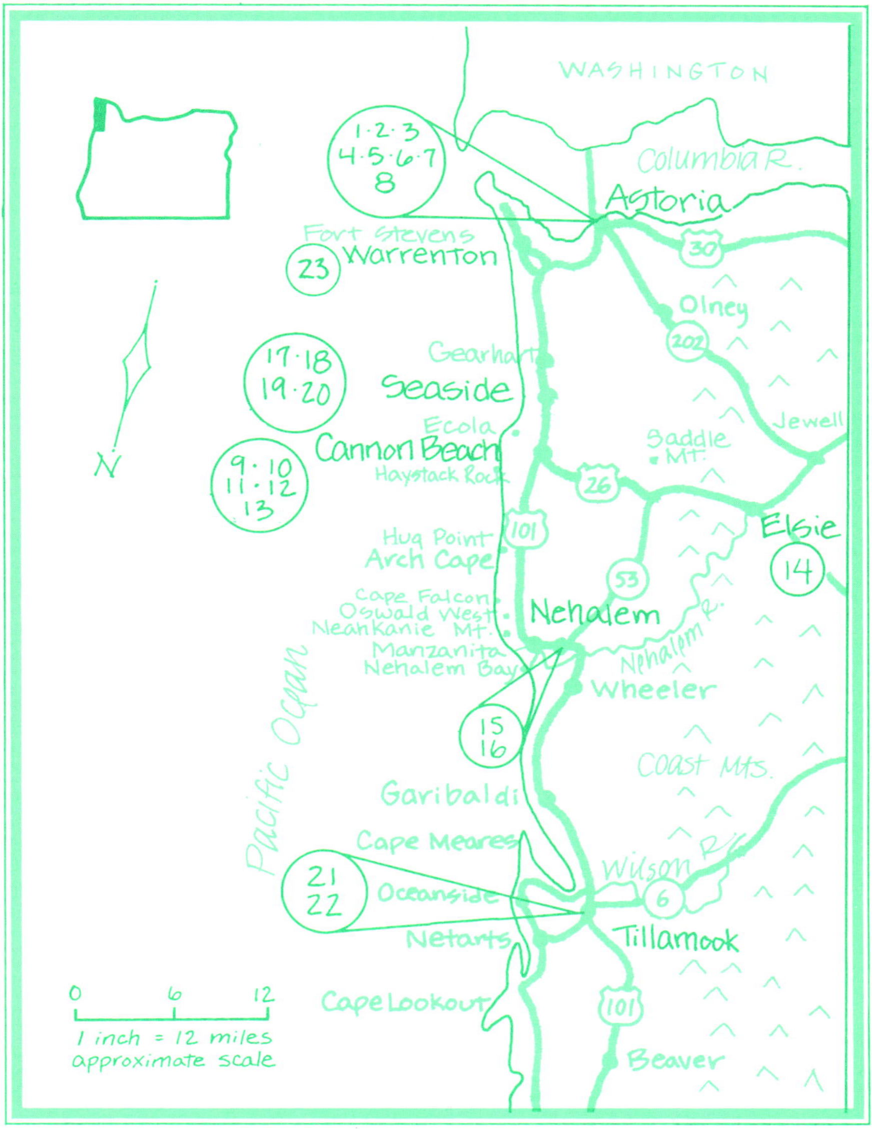
WASHINGTON
Columbia R.
Astoria
30
Olney
202
Jewell
Saddle Mt.
Elsie
14
26
53
1·2·3
4·5·6·7
8
Fort Stevens
Warrenton
23
Gearhart
Seaside
17·18
19·20
Ecola
Cannon Beach
Haystack Rock
9·10
11·12
13
N
101
Hug Point
Arch Cape
Cape Falcon
Oswald West
Neahkanie Mt.
Nehalem
Nehalem R.
Manzanita
Nehalem Bay
Wheeler
15
16
Coast Mts.
Pacific Ocean
Garibaldi
Cape Meares
21
22
Oceanside
Wilson R.
6
Netarts
Tillamook
Cape Lookout
101
Beaver
0
6
12
1 inch = 12 miles
approximate scale

NORTH COAST REGIONAL NOTES

The Coast Range causes many of the moisture-bearing clouds from the Pacific Ocean to deposit seemingly unending amounts of fog, haze, and rain on the North Coast, making it is perpetually mystical and beautiful. The best chance for clear weather is in late summer and early fall; however, the mist is not to be missed.

Fort Stevens *near* **Astoria** *was established to guard the mouth of the Columbia from Confederate attack during the Civil War! The site of the old fort has a memorial rose garden, an interpretive museum, a self-guided history walking tour, numerous old fortification remains, and the rusting skeleton of the Peter Iredale, a four-masted British ship which went aground in 1906.*

Saddle Mountain *contains 2,000 species of flora including the "crucifer," which is believed to grow only there. About two miles east of Highway 101 on the north side of Highway 26 is a 700-year-old* **sitka spruce tree,** *the* **largest in the U.S. Seaside** *and* **Ecola** *mark the end of the trail for the Lewis and Clark expedition; and islands just offshore provide resting places for sea lions and shorebirds. Enormous* **Haystack Rock** *attracts bird watchers, photographers, and watercolorists.* **Oswald West State Park** *is an outstanding coastal headland with a rain forest and massive spruce and cedar trees, under which one can walk to a magic-like beach where the author and her husband once saw two bare-breasted young women in long black skirts under a huge black umbrella, walking in the rain.*

One can now hike to the top of **Neahkanie Mountain,** *the home of the local Indian supreme god called "E-Kah-Ni." The mountain was once an impassable obstacle to Indians and white men alike, about which Don Berry wrote in his book* Trask. *Now, turnouts carved into the lower mountainside afford remarkable views. Roosevelt elk and black-tailed deer are a common sight here, and caution should be taken especially when driving at daybreak or dusk.*

Cape Meares, Cape Lookout, *and* **Cape Kiwanda** *(Central Coast map) can be toured via a* **20-mile scenic drive** *by car, bicycle, or on foot. Follow Scenic Drive signs from Tillamook or Pacific City (Central Coast map). Cape Meares has a large sitka spruce called the Octopus Tree and an 1890 lighthouse which is open to the public during summer months.* **Three Arches National Wildlife Refuge** *is situated offshore from Cape Meares. Cape Lookout is one of Oregon's most primitive ocean shore areas.*

A **46-mile Oregon Coast hiking trail** *extends continuously from Fort Stevens south to near Garibaldi. The trail leads through Ecola, Nehalem Bay, and Oswald West State Parks. Cape Lookout has a three-mile segment of the coast trail, and Cape Meares has a two-mile segment. (The very thoughtfully written* A Hiker's Guide to the Coast Trail: Columbia River to Tillamook Bay, *from which much of the North Coast material is taken, is available from state park offices. See reference page 3.)*

Highway 101 is a favorite **bicycle route.** *Fort Stevens and Nehalem Bay have bicycle paths. There are special camping areas for hikers and bicyclists only at Fort Stevens, Ecola, Hug Point, Nehalem Bay, Cape Meares, and Cape Lookout State Parks.*

There is a boat dock and ramp at Fort Stevens State Park, and boat ramps at Nehalem and Spit State Parks. Nehalem State Park has group horse camp facilities. Club camping and group tent facilities are available at Camp Lookout and Fort Stevens State Parks; club camping at Nehalem Bay State Park; group meeting halls at Cape Lookout State Park and Nehalem Bay State Parks; and group picnic facilities at Fort Stevens.

All beaches in Oregon *below mean high tide, except for a very few miles, are owned by the state and* **are public land.** *Clam digging is popular along the Oregon coast, but check carefully for conditions. The sand beaches are popular spots for rock hounds, beachcombers, and walkers.*

Winter (December to April) is the best time for storms to expose gravel bars that yield **agates, jaspers, petrified wood,** *and a variety of* **fossils.** *Most of the gravel bars tend to be sanded in during the summer. About six miles north of Netarts are large gravel areas containing good* **agates.** *There are also good* **jaspers** *and* **sagenite** *at Netarts Sand Pit and Cape Lookout State Park. The road follows the east side of the sand pit to the state park.*

One of the interesting attractions of the Oregon Coast is the **diversity of ecosystems** *ranging from open sand dunes to old growth forest. All of the ecosystems represent different stages of succession. In the beginning, there is sand. After a few years, one or two hearty pioneer species gain a foothold in the shifting sands. The pioneer plants on the dunes are mostly grasses and a few herbs. These plants modify the environment by* *trapping sand with their extensive root systems to form mounds. Eventually enough sand is held in place to allow more herbs to survive. These herbs are eventually replaced by other herbs and a few shrubs, the shrubs by trees, the trees by other trees, until finally a relatively stable climax forest is reached. (A climax forest, however, is only stable relative to a human lifetime. All living systems are dynamic, constantly changing to meet new conditions.)*

North Coast climax forests consist of **sitka spruce, western hemlock,** *and* **western red cedar.** *The young of these species can all grow in the shade of their parents, eventually replacing them and perpetuating the ecosystem. Douglas fir seedlings cannot grow in the shade of their parents, so this is not a climax species.*

The long bullwhip seaweed found on all Oregon beaches is called the **Bull Kelp.** *It grows under 30 to 40 feet of water, with its blades floating on the surface forming kelp beds. The slippery wide green seaweed is known as* **Sea Lettuce.** *Many of the plants clinging to the rocks of the upper tidal zone have a fork in the tip, with an air bladder in each fork. These are some of the many species of* **Rockweed.** *Bunches of a grasslike plant called* **Surf Grass** *may be found washed up on the beach. It grows at low-tide levels.*

Oregon has an incredible variety of **wildflowers** *throughout the state. Please enjoy them, and please leave them undisturbed for others to enjoy. "A picked wildflower is a thing of beauty, but a joy for only one person for a few minutes." Some wildflowers grow in incredibly delicate environments and can take as long as seven years to bloom again.*

The most obvious feature of the coast is the **shoreline.** *Along much of the Oregon coast, stretches of sandy beach are separated by* **basaltic headlands.** *These headlands appeared when wind and seas ate away the softer earth surrounding a hard volcanic core. The ocean is constantly wearing away headlands and depositing the eroded material in bays and coves, gradually creeping toward a straight coastline. This erosion occurs primarily during heavy winter storms from the southwest.*

Moving inland, a lack of open stream channels is noticeable. This is because precipitation comes in a **steady drizzle** *rather than a hard downpour, allowing the water ample time to soak into the ground where it falls, instead of running off.*

Black sand *is common along the entire length of the Oregon Coast, just enough in the dunes to add an occasional dash of color, but many beaches are broadly splashed with black. The sand contains a variety of minerals, all denser than the quartz and feldspar that comprise most ordinary sand. Magnetite, the magnetic oxide of iron, and ilmenite, a titanium material, are usually the most abundant, but most black sands also contain red garnet, a few glittering grains of zircon, and a brown mineral called monazite, which contains rare-earth elements. Some contain gold. The waves know these heavy minerals by their weight, and neatly sort them into separate deposits. Oregon black sands are more interesting than most, because they generally contain chromite and platinum along with the usual minerals. A few people have made a little bit of money, and a lot of others have gone broke trying to mine the beach sands. (For more detail, see* Roadside Geology of Oregon, *reference page 3.)*

A recent phenomenon of the Oregon coast is the **foredune.** *For some obscure reason, sand dunes seem to offend many people, simply because they move. "Hills should stay firmly rooted in place and not go wandering off." Enormous amounts of taxpayers' money are spent each year to* **"control"** *any number of* **perfectly harmless dunes,** *converting them into characterless heaps of sand. Unfortunately, these efforts at dune control almost always succeed.*

None of the native grasses grow well on sand dunes, so beach grass was introduced from Europe about 1910. Oregon suits it splendidly, and now **European Beach Grass** *grows wild all along the coast, ruining many beautiful tracts of dunes and literally changing the shape of the beachscape. Sand used to blow from the beach back into the dunes; but now, the dense growths of grass immediately behind the beach trap most of it, so a grass-covered ridge is growing just behind the beach, and the dunes are marching inland with their supply lines cut off behind them.*

Closest to land is the **deflation plain,** *where the sand has been removed by the wind down to the groundwater level, and the moist sand cannot be carried off. With plenty of water and protection from sand deposition, many more species of plants can survive here than on the foredune. The high-water mark of a high tide is called the* **high-tide line.** *The low-water mark of the low tide is called the* **low-tide line.** *The area between the high-tide line and the low-tide line is called the* **intertidal zone.** *Areas of organic deposits left by retreating waves marking different tide levels on the beach are called* **swash zones.**

Oregon State University has identified over

34 distinct kinds of driftwood *available on the Oregon Coast. Large reserves of driftwood are always out at sea. What brings them to shore is the right velocity and direction of wind. Some pieces are timber, lost from passing barges and freighters, sometimes exotic woods like mahogany and other Asian hardwoods. Much of our driftwood is the result of storms, floods, snow, rock-slides, and erosion along the shore and along inland streams and rivers. These forces uproot many inland trees and send them downriver; sooner or later, most of them reach the sea.*

Oregon's logging industry accounts for many pieces on our beaches. Logs escape from rafts and storage areas along rivers and in estuaries. Logging near stream banks leaves behind branches and other debris that slowly work their way downhill. Flooding may then carry them downstream to the sea.

Longshore currents paralleling the shore transport driftwood from north to south, and even south to north. For example, redwood is often found on Coos County beaches, although the species grows only in Northern California and the southwest corner of Oregon.

Some coves and beaches act as driftwood reservoirs. They collect it after particularly strong winter storms. On some beaches, driftwood comes and goes. Wave action and seasonal changes cause this fluctuation. At any time, some waves may have enough power to push driftwood specimens relatively high on the shore. This movement can be very dangerous. **Do not ignore the beach safety tips on some of the beaches.** *Strong winter waves alternately thrust whole logs and smaller pieces higher up on the beach and sometimes drag them back down into the sea again. Gentler summer waves return much of the wood that winter action drives out to sea. (See* Identifying Oregon Driftwood, *reference page 3.)*

The Nature Conservancy owns and manages a large system of natural preserves throughout the state of Oreogn. Call 228-9561 or visit the conservancy's offices in Portland (see Statewide Resources section) for information about preserves the public may visit in this region.

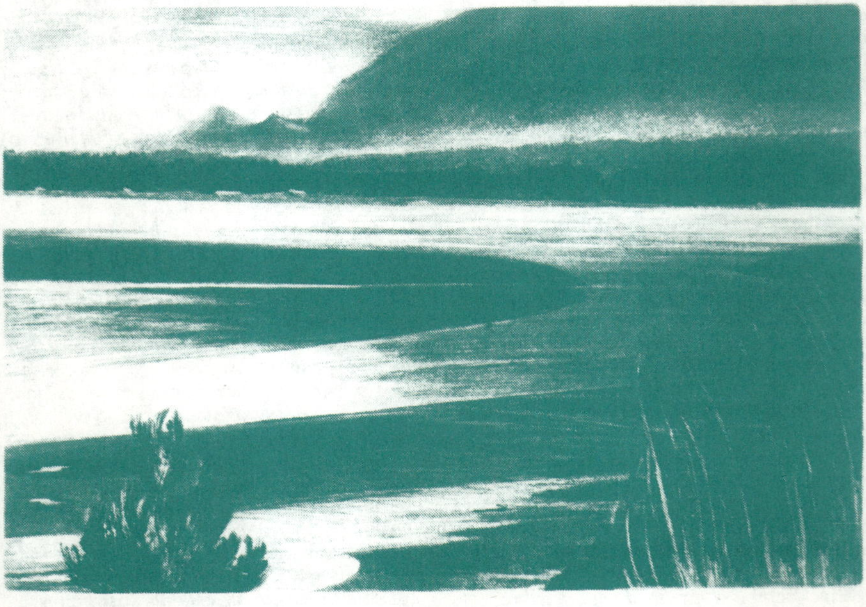

Neahkanie Mountain, © Liza Jones

ASTORIA

1 Greater Astoria Area Chamber of Commerce

111 W. Marine Dr., P.O. Box 176, Astoria, 97103. Tel: 325-6311
Office: 8-8 daily (summer); 8-6 Mon-Fri, 10-6 Sat-Sun (winter)
The oldest American settlement west of the Rockies, Astoria was founded in 1811 and remains a romantic place to explore year around. Rich in historical heritage, the Astoria area offers a variety of experiences: Fort Clatsop National Memorial, Columbia River Maritime Museum, Astoria Column, Flavel House, Heritage Center, Fort Stevens, Battery Russell, and a number of century-old homes, many of which have achieved state and national recognition.

1988 Astoria Area Events include:
April 8-10: Great Astoria Crab Feed & Seafood Festival
April 30: 50's Cruise In, Warrenton
May 14-22: Maritime Week
May 21: Jane Barnes Day
June 17-19: Scandinavian Midsummer Festival
July 4: Warrenton's Old Fashioned Fourth of July Celebration
Aug 1-5: Six Pac Races
Aug 4-7: Clatsop County Fair
Aug 16-21: Astoria Regatta
Aug 20-21: Victorian Homes Tour
Oct 7-9: Oregon Dixieland Jubilee
Oct 15: Great Columbia Crossing Bridge Run

2 Clatsop County Historical Society: Flavel House and Clatsop County Heritage Center and Art Gallery

Flavel House: 441 Eighth St., Astoria, 97103. Heritage Center: 1618 Exchange St., Astoria 97103. Tel: 325-2563 (Flavel House), Tel: 325-8395 (Heritage Center)
Especially notable for its intricate woodwork and sculptured hardware, Flavel House is a splendid Queen Anne-style Victorian mansion built in 1885 by the famous mariner and entrepreneur Captain George Flavel. The house has been restored with lavish period furnishings. Recipient of Oregon Arts Commission tax check-off funds. The Heritage Center and Art Gallery is a general history museum for Clatsop County housed in the 1905 City Hall building. Visa/MC. Both Flavel House and Heritage Center open 10-5 daily (May-Sept), 11-4 daily (Oct-April).

3 Columbia River Maritime Museum

1792 Marine Dr., Astoria, 97103 (at the foot of 17th St. in Astoria, on U.S. Hwy. 30 [Marine Dr.]). Tel: 325-2323.
This museum is a spectacular showcase for the heritage of the Columbia River region and the Northwest. Exhibits include restored fishing and Coast Guard boats, Indian artifacts, operating periscopes, models, figureheads, scrimshaw, the bridge of a WWII destroyer, a Columbia River steamer pilot house, and much more. Moored outside the museum is the lightship "Columbia," the last of its kind active on the West Coast. Visa/MC. 9:30-5 daily (closed Mon, Oct-March).

4 The Edge

120 10th St., Astoria, 97103.
Tel: 325-8151
In 1985 Jerry Schell opened a serious art gallery that shows some of the finest contemporary art in the Northwest including painting, sculpture, ceramics, etchings, and woodcuts. Periodically Jerry also sponsors shows and events of cultural and historical importance such as photographs of local gill netters and performances by special musicians. Visa/MC. 10-5 Tues-Sat. Often open until 7 in the summer.

5 Franklin House Bed and Breakfast

1681 Franklin Ave., Astoria, 97103 (4 blks. from Maritime Museum).
Tel: 325-5044
Karen Nelson's Victorian home has five elegant rooms, all with private baths and queen beds. (The basement has a queen bed plus two twin beds and can accommodate children). Full breakfasts are served. The house can be used for weddings, receptions, and group meetings as well. Visa/MC. Open year around.

6 Franklin Street Station Bed and Breakfast Inn

1140 Franklin St., Astoria, 97103
Tel: 325-4314
James and Renée Caldwell's Inn is in an old Victorian home built by a shipbuilder in the early 1900s. Four richly decorated rooms all have private baths. The Astor Suite can accommodate four people and has a wet bar and deck with a view of the Columbia River. Full breakfasts. Limousine service available. Visa/MC. Open year around.

7 Josephson's Smokehouse and Dock

106 Marine Dr., P.O. Box 412, Astoria, 97103. Tel: 325-2190
Mike and Linda Josephson's smoked salmon (a tradition in the Northwest) is prepared from a 65-year-old family process and available at Josephson's Smokehouse and Seafood Deli and through their mail order service. Available are Scandinavian-style cold-smoked salmon, sturgeon, tuna and cod, pickled salmon, salmon jerky, sturgeon caviar and canned seafoods. 8-6 Mon-Fri, 9-5:30 Sat, 10-4:30 Sun. Longer weekend hours in the summer. Write or call for mail order (wholesale and retail) brochure.

8 Rosebriar Inn Bed and Breakfast

636 Fourteenth St., Astoria, 97103. Tel: 325-7427
Located in a quiet neighborhood, yet convenient to museums, restaurants, and shops, this 1902 Eclectic-Greek Revival home and former convent has nine guest rooms, two with private baths. It is an excellent setting for family reunions, weddings, receptions, and mini-conferences, with a conference room seating 60. Full breakfasts for overnight guests. Ann Leenstra and Judith Papendick are the owners/innkeepers. No smoking. Visa/MC. Open all year.

CANNON BEACH-TOLOVANA PARK

9 Bruce's Candy Kitchen

256 N. Hemlock, P.O. Box 577, Cannon Beach, 97110. Tel: 436-2641
Treva Haskell's handmade chocolates and saltwater taffy have been a tradition with both children and adults in Cannon Beach since 1963. A full view of the cooking of these goodies can be seen from the sidewalk through Mrs. Haskell's front windows. Visa. 10-5 daily.

10 Hannen Stained Glass

987 S. Hemlock, P.O. Box 30, Cannon Beach, 97110. Tel: 436-2761
Established in 1972, Jim Hannen's studio produces originally designed stained glass windows and lamps by commission. A large selection of finished works is also available. Visa/MC/AmEx. 9-5:30 Thurs-Mon or by appointment.

11 Sea Sprite

280 Nebesna St., P.O. Box 66, Tolovana Park, 97145. Tel: 436-2266
One of the last small family-style guest lodgings left on the north Oregon coast, Sea Sprite is right on the beachfront with views of Haystack Rock and Ecola State Park. Reminiscent of old-fashioned beach cabins where friends and family gather, there are five units in one building and a separate cottage, all with kitchens, most with fireplaces. Dishes, firewood, towels, linens provided. No pets. Visa/MC. Open year around. Reservations advised.

12 White Bird Gallery

North end of Hemlock St., P.O. Box 502, Cannon Beach, 97110. Tel: 436-2681 (If no answer call Portland: 292-4347)
This fine art, crafts and fibers gallery features paintings, sculpture, prints, glass, clay, weavings, wearable art, handmade paper and soft sculpture. While much of the work is from Oregon, the gallery's reputation has attracted work by other nationally known artists and craftspeople —many of whom have received awards from the National Endowment for the Arts and the Oregon Arts Commission. Evelyn Georges and her assistant director host openings for changing exhibits, March through Dec. Visa/MC/AmEx. 11-5 daily (summer), 11-5 Fri-Mon (other seasons and holidays).

13 Worcester Glassworks

116 E. Gower St., Cannon Beach, 97110 (corner of Hemlock and Gower St., near Haystack Rock). Tel: 436-2359.
Sally and William Worcester have produced high-quality, one-of-a-kind blown and etched glass vases, bowls, paperweights, and sculpture at their glassblowing studio since 1972. Their work can often be seen in *American Craft Magazine* and at A.C.E. fairs. Visitors are invited to their studio to watch the fascinating process of handblown glass being made. Visa/MC/AmEx. 12-5 daily (June-Oct).

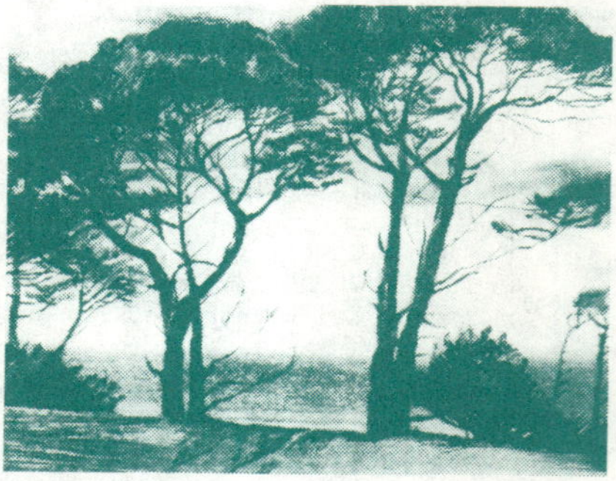

Manzanita Pines, © *Liza Jones*

ELSIE

14 Camp 18 Logging Museum

On Sunset Hwy., 1 mi. west of Elsie. Mailing address: Elsie Rt. Box 195, Seaside, 97138. Tel: 755-2476 (gift shop), 755-0113 (restaurant)
Visitors are welcome anytime to view this incredible collection of old-time logging equipment, including "steam donkeys." An adjacent authentic log building houses a gift shop and restaurant. Meals are served daily by Morris' at Camp 18, famous for its "Logger's Breakfast." Family-style dining after 5 PM. Banquet and meeting facilities also available. Visa/MC/AmEx/Diners/CB/Discover. Gift shop: 10-6 Mon-Thurs, 10-8 Fri-Sun. Restaurant: 7 AM-9 PM Mon-Thurs, 7 AM-10 PM Fri-Sun.

NEHALEM

15 Nehalem Bay Winery

34965 Hwy. 53, Nehalem, 97131 (1 mi. east of Hwy. 101 on Hwy. 53).
Tel: 368-5300
Established in 1973 by Pat McCoy, the Nehalem Bay Winery produces varietal wines and fruit and berry wines. Cellarmaster Jeff Daniels invites visitors to the winery's tasting room and picnic facilities. Tours of the winery are also available. The winery anchors the Tillamook County Cheese food and winery tour. Visa/MC. 10-5 daily.

16 The Peacock Gallery

Center of Nehalem on Hwy. 101, P.O. Box 67, Nehalem, 97131. Tel: 368-6924
Patricia Rinehart brought art to Nehalem with the opening of her gallery in 1984. Complementing other galleries up and down the coast, she supports north Oregon coast artists by featuring prints and pastels by Liza Jones, spirit masks and pins by Lillian Pitt, and Native American sculpture by James Jackson. Also available are Oregon specialty foods, myrtlewood, and pottery. Some of the artists represented have received awards from the National Endowment for the Arts and the Oregon Arts Commission. Visa/MC/AmEx. 11-5 daily (summer), 11-5 Fri-Mon (winter).

SEASIDE

17 Seaside Chamber of Commerce and Visitors Bureau

7 North Roosevelt, P.O. Box 7, Seaside, 97138. Tel: 738-6391 or 800-444-6740 (nationwide)
Office: 9-5 Mon-Fri, 10-4 Sat, 12-4 Sun.
Seaside's wide sandy beaches allow for plenty of fun, including beach volleyball, kite flying, swimming, sandcastle building, and much more. A two and one-half mile promenade parallels the beach and provides views of charming old beach homes. Splitting the promenade is Broadway Street, Seaside's newly renovated main street with an assortment of small gift shops, restaurants, food stands, and family entertainment centers. An automobile turnaround marks the end of the Lewis and Clark Trail and allows visitors the same panoramic view of the ocean the explorers had. Accommodations ranging from bed and breakfast inns and cozy motels to ocean-front hotels help support Seaside's growing reputation as a coastal convention center.

1988-89 Seaside Area Events include:

1988

May 21: Cannon Beach Sandcastle Contest
July 4: Fireworks Display
July 7-10: Miss Oregon Pageant
Aug 12-14: Volleyball Tournament on the Beach
TBA: Cruisin' the Turnaround
Sept 23-25: Oktoberfest
Oct 7-9: Oregon Dixieland Jubilee
Nov 25-27: Christmas Gift Fair
Nov-Dec: Yuletide at Seaside

1989

Jan 20-21: Barbershop Quartet Cabaret
Feb 25: Trail's End Marathon
March 17-19: North Coast Home & Garden Show

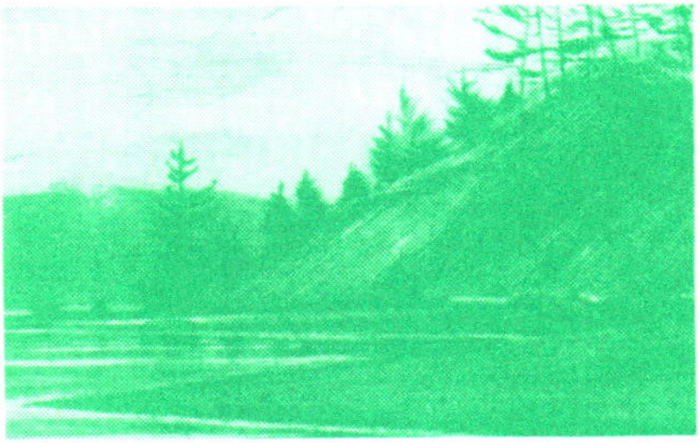

Nehalem June, © Liza Jones

18 The Boarding House Bed and Breakfast

208 N. Holladay Dr., Seaside, 97138 (2 blks. from downtown). Tel: 738-9055
Each of the six intimate sleeping rooms at this 1898 Victorian "boarding house" on the banks of the Necanicum River has a private bath, color TV, down quilt, and wicker and wood mingled with country charm. Continental breakfasts are served in the dining room or on the wrap-around porch. No smoking. No pets. Major credit cards accepted. Open all year.

19 The Gilbert Inn

341 Beach Dr., Seaside, 97138 (1 blk. south of Broadway, 1 blk. from ocean). Tel: 738-9770
This 1894 Queen Anne-style home has been reopened recently by Carole and Dick Rees, and Carole says it's "absolutely elegant." There's the "1800s suite," where Mr. Gilbert lived while the rest of the house was being built, a garret room, and three smaller guest rooms. All have private baths, TVs, and are furnished with tall four-poster or brass beds and lots of wicker. The home has its original, never-painted fir woodwork, a large living room, and wonderful, new dining area. Full breakfasts. Available for weddings, anniversaries, parties. No smoking. Visa/MC/AmEx. Open all year.

20 Riverside Inn Bed and Breakfast

430 S. Holladay Dr., Seaside, 97138. Tel: 738-8254
This charming 11-unit inn on the Necanicum River offers the enchantment of Grandmother's house, yet private baths and separate entrances give each unit the seclusion of a quaint hotel. Country-flavor with quilts, plants, library, equipped kitchens, color TVs, skylights, views, and spectacular river-front deck. Complimentary homemade breakfast. Just 3½ blocks to beach or downtown. Visa/MC. Open year around.

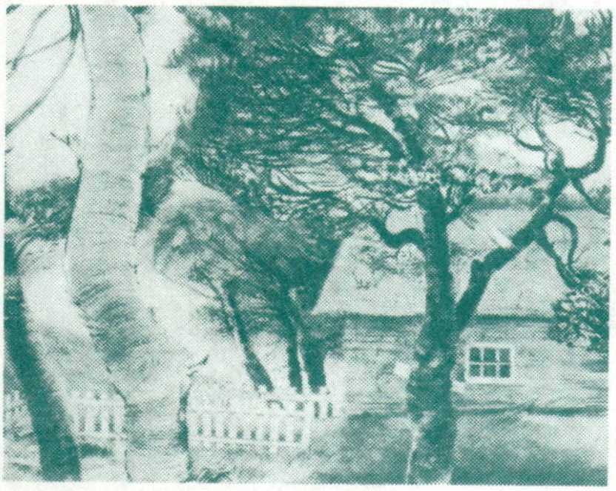

TILLAMOOK

21 Tillamook County Creamery Association

4175 Hwy. 101 N., P.O. Box 313, Tillamook, 97141. Tel: 842-4481
Home of world-famous Tillamook cheese, now a consolidation of local Tillamook dairies. Observation room affords view of cheese being made. Ongoing video show describes history of the company and the area. Cheese and gift shop features ice cream bar, deli and some other Northwest products. 8-6 daily Labor Day to June 15 except Christmas and Thanksgiving; 8-8 June 15 to Labor Day.

22 Whiskey Creek Bed and Breakfast

7500 Whiskey Creek Rd., Tillamook, 97141 (2 mi. north of Cape Lookout State Park). Tel: 842-2408
Whiskey Creek is Allison Asbjornsen's 1900-vintage home snuggled into the woods on the shores of Netarts Bay. Located on three secluded acres, it offers guests great bird watching, canoeing, hiking, or just plain sitting. Cozy bedrooms with a shared bath have queen-sized beds. There is also a two-bedroom suite with private entry, bath, kitchen, and living room. Children welcome. No pets or smoking. Open year around. Reservations recommended.

TOLOVANA PARK

See CANNON BEACH-TOLOVANA PARK

WARRENTON

23 Fisherman's Choice

P.O. Box 818, Warrenton, 97146. Tel: 861-3511
"For three generations we've been a fishing family and are proud of our heritage and the seafood Oregon is famous for," says Stephanie Miller of Fisherman's Choice. Their seafood gift packs feature assortments of custom smoked or canned coho, Chinook, or sockeye salmon, albacore tuna, sturgeon, and Pacific shrimp. The packs come with recipes and can be shipped anywhere. Available wholesale or retail. Call or write for brochure. Visa/MC.

Portland Avenue (Artists' studio, Manzanita),
© Liza Jones

Central Coast

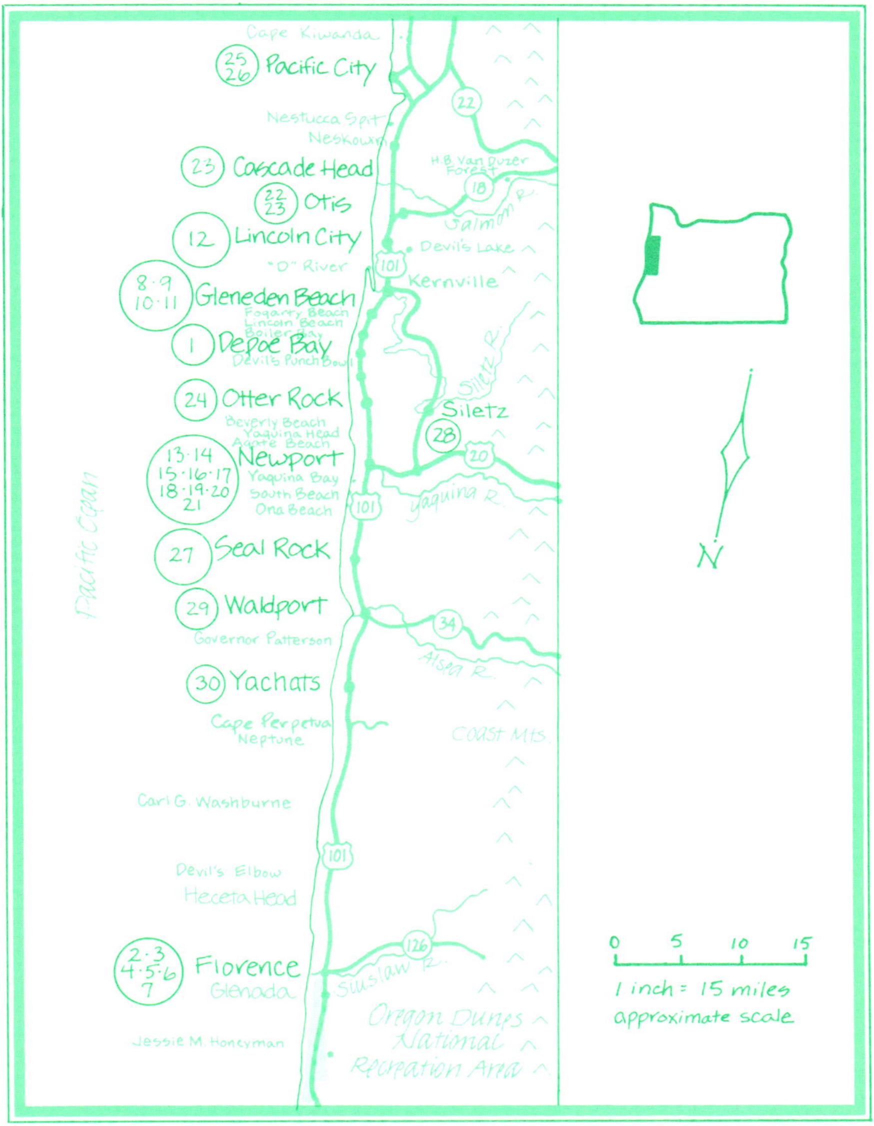

CENTRAL COAST REGIONAL NOTES

The colorful sandstone headland, **Cape Kiwanda,** *with sand dunes nearby, is where* **silver salmon** *fishermen still fish with* **flat-bottom dories** *that are launched from the beach.* **Cascade Head** *is a several-hundred-acre Nature Conservancy-***wildlife refuge** *and experimental forest where research is conducted on the management of Oregon's forest reserves. Some areas are open for public enjoyment. The Nature Conservancy owns and manages a large system of natural preserves throughout the state of Oregon. Call 228-9561 or visit the conservancy's offices in Portland (see Statewide Resources section) for information about preserves the public may visit in this region. The Salmon River offers multiple opportunities for estuary studies.*

The **"D" River** *is the* **shortest river in the world,** *and it is up the* **Siletz River** *where Ken Kesey located* Sometimes a Great Notion. **Devil's Elbow** *and* **Otter Crest** *provide picturesque views of a lighthouse and the rugged Oregon coastline. The* **Devil's Punchbowl** *and* **Boiler Bay Waysides** *have* **extensive marine gardens** *and ocean-carved caverns where sea life can be observed. Yaquina Bay is the home of the 1871* **Yaquina Bay Lighthouse** *(Newport's oldest surviving building, which some people say is haunted), now authentically refurbished and open to the public during summer months.* **Neptune** *has a primitive, scenic, rocky shoreline.* **Carl G. Washburne** *is a favorite spot for elk, which can be viewed in campgrounds and nearby meadows.* **Darlingtonia** *features unusual* **carnivorous plants** *that consume insects, and* **Jessie M. Honeyman** *is famous for its sand dunes, lakes, and wild rhododendron.*

Signs on the way up to **Cape Perpetua** *read: "Wind: is the greatest continual force shaping the coastal environment. On Columbus Day, October 12, 1962, a raging storm with 150 m.p.h. winds attacked the Pacific Northwest. Trees on this slope were among the millions to topple. The wind falls were salvaged and the young trees you see were planted in 1964 to replace them. Rain: The forest floor, like a sponge, absorbs moisture; however, a week of torrential rains during the winter of 1964-65 saturated the forest soils beyond their capacity. A flood of water swept down this ravine carrying rocks, trees, and soil with it. Now alders are beginning to grow on the scarred slopes."*

At the top of the drive is the short "Trail of the Whispering Spruce" which "leads through the forest to grassy cliffs overlooking the Pacific Ocean. Signs identify natural features, wildflowers, and big game animals. There are exceptional views of the ocean and coastline extending from Cape Foulweather to Cape Blanco, a distance of over 150 miles."

Several state parks have hiking trails, including Beverly Beach, Neptune, Carl G. Washburne, and Jessie M. Honeyman. Highway 101 is a favorite **bicycle route.** *There are special camping areas for hikers and bicyclists only at H. B. Van Duzer, Devil's Lake, Beverly Beach, South Beach, and Jessie M. Honeyman State Parks.*

There are boat docks and ramps at the Nestucca Spit and on lakes at East Devil's Lake and Jessie M. Honeyman State Parks, and a boat ramp to creek at Ona Beach State Park. Beverly Beach and Jessie M. Honeyman State Parks have group tent facilities. Club camping is available at Devil's Lake, South Beach, Beverly Beach, and Jessie M. Honeyman State Parks.

All beaches in Oregon *below mean high tide, except for a very few miles, are owned by the state and* **are public land.** *Clam digging is popular along the Oregon coast, but check carefully for conditions. The sand beaches are popular spots for rock hounds, beachcombers, and walkers. Winter (December to April) is the best time for storms to expose gravel bars that yield* **agates, jaspers, petrified wood,** *and a variety of* **fossils.** *Most of the gravel bars tend to be sanded in during the summer.*

The beaches just west of the post office in Lincoln City produce "cloud agates," jasper, and fossilized coral. Pools at low tide in rocky reefs produce agates, shells, etc. DANGEROUS! BE CAREFUL! There are good beaches from Otter Rock south to Yaquina Head. Cliffs just north and south of Spencer Creek at Beverly Beach State Park are full of fossilized clams and other shells. On Moodlock Beach from the mouth of Moodlock Creek south to Yaquina Bay is a good beach to hunt fossils. Agate Beach is good for agate hunting when gravel beds are exposed; however, it is often sanded in. At the north jetty in Newport, proceed to Yaquina Bay State Park by turning west at the north edge of the bay bridge when on U.S. 101. Walk down the steps to the beach and look for exposed gravel bars (wintertime is best). Sagenite, blue-banded green and multicolored agate, jasper, fossilized wood and clams are common. When the gravel bars are exposed at Ona Beach, one can find lots of agates, jaspers, carnelian, sagenite, teredo wood, fossils, etc. Starting at Yachats, south to Heceta Head are many creeks (Cummins, Bob, Agate, Tenmile, Rock, Big, China, etc.) which near the mouth produce sagenite, bloodstone, jasper, and agate. Big Creek has large cutting agate in the winter. There is a great variety of agates during the winter on the north side of Alsea Bay near Waldport and Seal Rock. There are agates, sagenite and jasper on the north beach of Yachats and at Agate Point just south of Yachats. Beaches in the general area between Yachats and Heceta Head often provide rounded agates about the size of golf balls after each major storm. There is also an **old volcanic flow** *at Agate Point. The long, wide beach at Carl G. Washburne State Park is unpredictable, although good when the gravel bars show. There are few agate-producing beaches from Florence to Coos Bay.*

One of the interesting attractions of the Oregon Coast is the **diversity of ecosystems** *ranging from open sand dunes to old growth forest. All of the ecosystems represent different stages of succession. In the beginning, there is sand. After a few years, one or two hearty pioneer species gain a foothold in the shifting sands. The pioneer plants on the dunes are mostly grasses and a few herbs. These plants modify the environment by trapping sand with their extensive root systems to form mounds. Eventually enough sand is held in place to allow more herbs to survive. These herbs are eventually replaced by other herbs and a few shrubs, the shrubs by trees, the trees by other trees, until finally a relatively stable climax forest is reached. (A climax forest, however, is only stable relative to a human lifetime. All living systems are dynamic, constantly changing to meet new conditions.)*

The long bullwhip seaweed found on all Oregon beaches is called the **Bull Kelp.** *It grows under 30 to 40 feet of water, with its blades floating on the surface forming kelp beds.*

Oregon has an incredible variety of **wildflowers** *throughout the state. Please enjoy them, and please leave them undisturbed for others to enjoy. "A picked wildflower is a thing of beauty, but a joy for only one person for a few minutes." Some wildflowers grow in incredibly delicate environments and can take as long as seven years to bloom again.*

The most obvious feature of the coast is the **shoreline.** *Along our coast, stretches of sandy beach are separated by* **basaltic headlands.** *These headlands appeared when wind and seas ate away the softer earth surrounding a hard volcanic core. The ocean is constantly wearing away headlands and depositing the eroded material in bays and coves, gradually creeping toward a straight coastline. This erosion occurs primarily during heavy winter storms from the southwest. Moving inland, a lack of open stream channels is noticeable. This is because precipitation comes in a* **steady drizzle** *rather than a hard downpour, allowing the water ample time to soak into the ground where it falls, instead of running off.*

Black sand *is common along the entire length of the Oregon Coast, just enough in the dunes to add an occasional dash of color, but many beaches are broadly splashed with black. The sand contains a variety of minerals, all denser than the quartz and feldspar that comprise most ordinary sand. Magnetite, the magnetic oxide of iron, and ilmenite, a titanium material, are usually the most abundant, but most black sands also contain red garnet, a few glittering grains of zircon, and a brown mineral called monazite, which contains rare-earth elements. Some contain gold. The waves know these heavy minerals* **by their weight**, *and neatly sort them into separate deposits. Oregon black sands are more interesting than most, because they generally contain chromite and platinum along with the usual minerals. A few people have made a little bit of money, and a lot of others have gone broke trying to mine the beach sands. (For more detail, see* Roadside Geology of Oregon, *reference page 3.)*

A recent phenomenon of the Oregon coast is the **foredune.** *For some obscure reason, sand dunes seem to offend many people, simply because they move. "Hills should stay firmly rooted in place and not go wandering off." Enormous amounts of taxpayers' money are spent each year to* **"control"** *any number of* **perfectly harmless dunes,** *converting them into characterless heaps of sand. Unfortunately, these efforts at dune control almost always succeed.*

None of the native grasses grow well on sand dunes, so beach grass was introduced from Europe about 1910. Oregon suits it splendidly, and now **European Beach Grass** *grows wild all along the coast, ruining many beautiful tracts of dunes and literally changing the shape of the beachscape. Sand used to blow from the beach back into the dunes; but* *now, the dense growths of grass immediately behind the beach trap most of it, so a grass-covered ridge is growing just behind the beach, and the dunes are marching inland with their supply lines cut off behind them.*

Closest to land is the **deflation plain,** *where the sand has been removed by the wind down to the groundwater level, and the moist sand cannot be carried off. With plenty of water and protection from sand deposition, many more species of plants can survive here than on the foredune. The high-water mark of a high tide is called the* **high-tide line.** *The low-water mark of the low tide is called the* **low-tide line.** *The area between the high-tide line and the low-tide line is called the* **intertidal zone.** *Areas of organic deposits left by retreating waves marking different tide levels on the beach are called* **swash zones.**

Going south, about 8 miles north of Florence the basalt ends and a long stretch of smooth and sandy coast begins, because the waves are eroding soft, sedimentary rocks which contain a lot of sand. Sutton Lake and Mercer Lake, just north of Florence, both exist because sand dunes migrating inland from the beach have dammed the drainage of small streams. The outlets of both lakes are by seepage through the sand.

Just south of Florence at Honeyman State Park, **active sand dunes,** *overtaking and burying forest, are also moving northeastward into Cleawox Lake at about 17 feet a year.*

Oregon State University has identified over **34 distinct kinds of driftwood** *available on the Oregon Coast. Large reserves of driftwood are always out at sea. What brings them to shore is the right velocity and direction of wind. Some pieces are timber, lost from passing barges and freighters, sometimes exotic woods like mahogany and other Asian hardwoods.*

Much of our driftwood is the result of storms, floods, snow, rock-slides, and erosion along the shore and along inland streams and rivers. These forces uproot many inland trees and send them downriver; sooner or later, most of them reach the sea.

Oregon's logging industry accounts for many pieces on our beaches. Logs escape from rafts and storage areas along rivers and in estuaries. Logging near stream banks leaves behind branches and other debris that slowly work their way downhill. Flooding may then carry them downstream to the sea.

Longshore currents paralleling the shore transport driftwood from north to south, and even south to north. For example, redwood is often found on Coos County beaches, although the species grows only in Northern California and the southwest corner of Oregon.

Some coves and beaches act as driftwood reservoirs. They collect it after particularly strong winter storms. On some beaches, driftwood comes and goes. Wave action and seasonal changes cause this fluctuation. At any time, some waves may have enough power to push driftwood specimens relatively high on the shore. This movement can be very dangerous. **Do not ignore the beach safety tips on some of the beaches.**

Strong winter waves alternately thrust whole logs and smaller pieces higher up on the beach and drag them back down into the sea again. Gentler summer waves return much of the wood that winter action drives out to sea. (See Identifying Oregon Driftwood, *reference page 3.)*

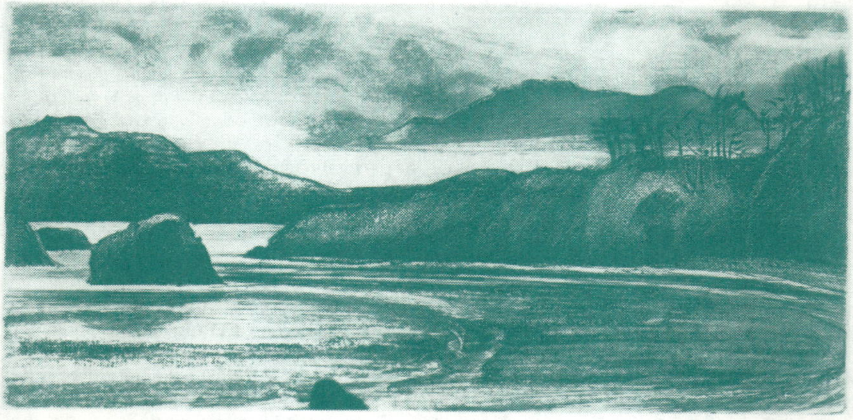

Pine Cove (North Coast), © Liza Jones

CASCADE HEAD

○ **Sitka Center for Art and Ecology**

See OTIS for listing.

DEPOE BAY

1 Channel House Bed and Breakfast Inn

Foot of Ellingson St. on south side of Depoe Bay Channel, P.O. Box 56, Depoe Bay, 97341. Tel: 765-2140

Paul Schwabe's bed and breakfast inn is set high on the rocks overlooking the coast and entrance to Depoe Bay. Six of the eleven rooms have their own fireplace and private hot tub with view of the ocean, where whales are often spotted feeding offshore. Outside decks, breakfast room, and library add to guests' enjoyment. Limited smoking. Vi Stavatis is the resident innkeeper. Visa/MC. Open year around.

FLORENCE

2 B.J.'s Ice Cream Parlors—48 Flavors

Two locations: 2930 Hwy. 101N, Florence, 97439 (just north of Florence on east side of Hwy. 101) and 1441 Bay St., Florence, 97439 (in Florence's Old Town). Tel: 997-7286

Brian and Jodie Cole have been making homemade ice cream since 1978, and it's famous all over the state. They have full fountain service and make their own ice cream cakes, cheesecakes, pies, waffle cones, and a large variety of all-natural yogurts. Oregon-made salt water taffy also available. B.J.'s wholesales ice cream too. Main store: 11-11 Mon-Sat, 11-10 Sun (summer), 11-10 Mon-Sat, 12-9 Sun (winter). Bay St. store: 10-9 daily (summer), 10-6 daily (winter).

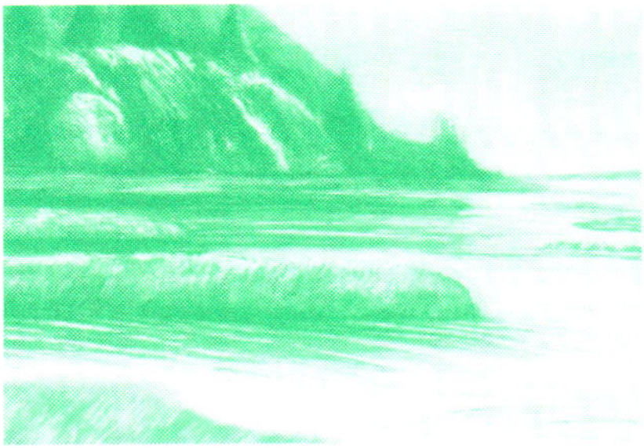

Netarts (North Coast), © Liza Jones

3 Coast House

P.O. Box 1892, Florence, 97439. Tel: 997-8000

Coast House is a split-level cedar cabin on a secluded wooded cliffside ten miles north of Florence. Bay windows overlook the ocean and two sleeping lofts rest beneath skylights. There's a tubroom with a view of the woods and sea, spacious deck, and deckside shower sheltered by a large evergreen. The cabin has both electrical heat and a woodburning stove and comes furnished with bedding, towels, cookware, and dishes. Visa/MC. For reservations contact Jayne Fraese at above address.

4 Johnson House Bed and Breakfast Inn

216 Maple St. (1 blk. north of riverfront in Old Town Florence and 1½ blks. east of Hwy. 101), P.O. Box 1892, Florence, 97439. Tel: 997-8000

The Johnson House, built in 1892, has been perfectly restored into a bed and breakfast inn by Jayne and Ron Fraese. Gourmet breakfasts and antique furnishings (including feather beds) in every room delight guests and evoke the atmosphere of warm, plain living on the Oregon coast nearly a century ago. Jayne and Ron serve and sell their Johnson House local wild berry conserves: blackberry, elderberry, blueberry, and huckleberry. Visa/MC. Open year around.

5 Moonset

P.O. Box 1892, Florence, 97439. Tel: 997-8000

Moonset is a landmark seaview retreat for two, nine miles north of Florence. Sited high on a one-acre meadow, it has a breathtaking panoramic view of woods, lake, and sea from sunrise to sunset, season to season. The architecturally stunning cabin has a king-sized sleeping loft with goosedown pillows and comforter, and is provided with linens, cookware, dishes, and plenty of firewood. Visa/MC. For reservations contact Jayne Fraese at above address.

6 Sea Lion Caves

91560 Hwy. 101, Florence, 97439 (11 mi. north of Florence and 38 mi. south of Newport on Hwy. 101). Tel: 547-3111

America's largest sea cave and nature's home for wild sea lions and a variety of sea birds. A 215-foot long elevator ride takes visitors to a viewing area just above sea level. Passing whales, a gift shop and a full-size bronze sculpture of a Steller sea lion family are added attractions. Visa/MC. 9 AM to dusk, daily except Christmas.

7 Windward Inn Restaurant

3757 Hwy. 101 N., Florence, 97439 (north of Florence on westside of Hwy. 101). Tel: 997-8243
Famous for their fresh mussels broiled on the half shell, Dave Haskell and Lynnette Wickstrom specialize in carefully prepared fresh Oregon seafood. The Windward Inn also makes all its own pastries and bread and has one of the finest selections of Oregon wines. Gift shop. Visa/MC/AmEx/ Diners. 8 AM-9 PM daily (breakfast served from 8-11:30 AM).

GLENEDEN BEACH

8 Alder House Glassblowing Studio

Halfway between Kernville and Salishan Lodge on Hwy. 101; go east on Immonen Rd. 3/4 mi. (1/4 mi. past Mossy Creek Pottery). Mailing address: 611 Immonen Rd., Lincoln City, 97367. Tel: 996-2483
Buzz and Annie Williams' glassblowing studio, housed in a geodesic dome in an old grove of alder, produces handblown goblets, vases, bowls and other objects using a 2,000-year-old process. Molten glass can be seen transformed into a myriad of shapes by experienced craftsmen. Visa/MC. 10-5 daily (March 15-Nov 30).

9 Mossy Creek Pottery

Halfway between Kernville and Salishan Lodge on Hwy. 101; go east on Immonen Rd. 1/2 mi. towards Alder House Glass Studio. Box 368, Immonen Rd., Gleneden Beach, 97388. Tel: 996-2415
The work of resident potters Tom and Joanne Davis, whose stoneware and porcelain is noted for its blend of traditional and contemporary concepts, is featured along with that of several other local Oregon potters at Mossy Creek, established in 1973. Visa/MC. 9-5 daily.

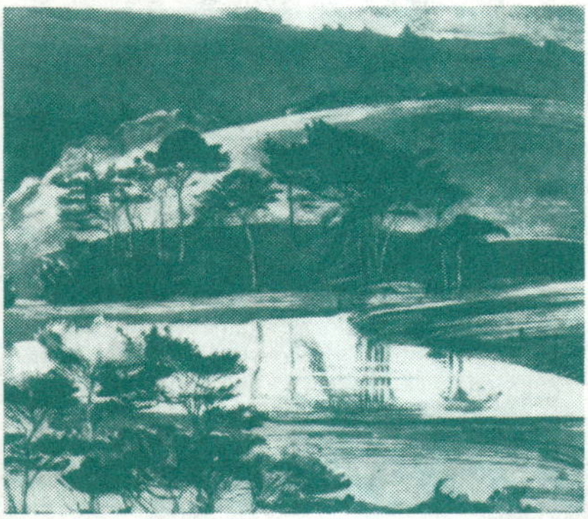

10 The Gallery and "Out of the Woods" Gift Shop at Salishan Lodge

P.O. Box 118, Gleneden Beach, 97388. Tel: 764-2371
When John and Betty Gray created Salishan in 1965 they incorporated Oregon art into the buildings (each guest room has its own original print). The gallery continues to exhibit the work of Northwest artists and craftsmen, many of whom have received awards from the Oregon Arts Commission and the National Endowment for the Arts. Recently the gift shop has assembled a collection of wood toys, clocks, furniture, decoys, and even gift boxes for wine which can be purchased from the lodge's wine cellar. Personal checks for artwork, all major credit cards for food, lodging, etc. 8 AM-10 PM daily.

11 Lawrence Gallery

Marketplace at Salishan (3 mi. south of Lincoln City, across from Salishan Lodge), Gleneden Beach, 97388. Tel: 764-2318
Monthly exhibits highlight important new works of the region, including paintings, ceramics, glass, jewelry, prints, and sculpture by Northwest artists and craftsmen, many of whom have received awards from the Oregon Arts Commission and the National Endowment for the Arts. The Lawrence Gallery offers art consulting, delivery, installation, packing and shipping services. Visa/MC/AmEx/ Discover. 10-6 Mon-Sat, 10-5 Sun.

LINCOLN CITY

12 Shipwreck Cellars—Oak Knoll Wine Tasting Room

3521 S.W. Hwy. 101 (in the Nelscott area), Lincoln City, 97367 Tel: 996-3221
This wine-tasting room features sampling and sales of award-winning Oregon wines from Oak Knoll Winery and other premium Oregon vintners. Hosts Harry and Mary Lockwood invite visitors to come in and learn about the growing acclaim of Oregon wines. No charge for tasting. Visa/MC. 11-5 Mon-Sat, 12-5 Sun. (See Hillsboro, Northern Willamette Valley, for Oak Knoll Winery listing.)

After Rain (Neskowin), © Liza Jones

NEWPORT

13 Canyon Way Restaurant and Bookstore

1216 S.W. Canyon Way, Newport, 97365 (½ blk. up from the bay front).
Tel: 265-8319
Established in 1971, and specializing in fresh everything! They use local seafood and make breads, pasta, croissants, and decadent desserts daily. Carry-out shop features homemade sauces, sticky buns, cinnamon rolls, chocolate chip cookies, pasta salads, and filled croissants. Variety of beers, Oregon wines, and espresso coffee drinks. Outdoor patio dining in summer. Local artists display works in watercolor, oils, and stained glass in restaurant. Bookstore features the usual and unusual in cards and books, including children's books. Visa/MC/AmEx. Restaurant: 11-3 Mon-Sat (lunch), 5-9 daily (dinner). Reservations suggested. Bookstore: 10-9 daily.

14 Oar House Bed and Breakfast

520 S.W. Second St., Newport, 97365 (turn off Hwy. 101 towards ocean on Hurbert, go to second stop sign).
Tel: 265-9571
Built at the turn of the century and now completely remodeled, this three-story house has an ocean view from every floor and a lookout tower with a 360° view. The Oar House is "nautical . . . but nice" and innkeeper Carol Sutherland waits on guests hand and foot. Indoor spa, sauna, and two guest rooms with private baths. The "Captain's Quarters" has a queen-sized bed, shower, bidet, dressing room, and sitting room. The "Port of Call" has a king-sized bed and claw-foot tub. Full breakfasts and hors d'oeuvres. No children or pets. Smoking outdoors on covered decks only. Open from mid-Feb through Dec.

15 Ocean House Bed and Breakfast

4920 N.W. Woody Way, Newport, 97365 (north edge of Newport, off Hwy. 101).
Tel: 265-6158 or 265-7779
Ocean House overlooks both gardens and the surf at Agate Beach, near the center of year-around coastal activities. A short private trail leads to the beach and tide pools. Cozy upstairs bedrooms with private baths open toward the sea. Full breakfast is served in the spacious living room or on the porch or decks. Owner/hosts Bette and Bob Garrard say relaxing and storm-watching by an open fire is unforgettable. No smoking. Visa/MC. Open year around except Dec 15 to Jan 1.

16 Oceanic Arts

444 S.W. Bay Blvd., Newport, 97365 (on Newport's bay front). Tel: 265-5963
Representing over 100 Northwest artists, the gallery offers contemporary crafts and jewelry, watercolors, oils, and prints. Custom framing, designed by owner Stan Pickens, also available. Wide selection of reproductions by nationally known artists Rie Muñoz, Yvonne Davis, Bev Doolittle, and Charles Wysocki. Visa/MC/AmEx/Discover. 10-6 daily.

17 Oregon Coast Council for the Arts

Naterlin Community Center, 609 N.E. Coast Hwy., P.O. Box 1315, Newport, 97365. Tel: 265-9231
Maintains information for all coastal arts activities and sponsors events, competitions, exhibitions, and performances. Hosts annual Performance Series at Salishan Lodge in November, January, and February; an Exhibition Series December through March at the Newport Visual Arts Center; and a Literary Series. Sponsors classes and children's events throughout the summer. Will open and manage Newport Performing Arts Center in 1988. Call or write for monthly newsletter. OCCA projects are often supported by grants from the Oregon Arts Commission and the National Endowment for the Arts. 9-5 Mon-Fri.

18 Oregon Oyster Company

6878 Yaquina Bay Rd., Newport, 97365 (on Bay Rd. about 8 mi. up Yaquina Bay).
Tel: 265-5078
Established in 1907 and still owned by the Wachsmuth family, the Oregon Oyster Company farms and harvests three types of oysters. Visitors are welcome to watch the process and buy fresh oysters daily. Wholesale and retail available. 9-4 daily.

19 Sylvia Beach Hotel and "Tables of Content" Restaurant

267 N.W. Cliff, Newport, 97365.
Tel: 265-5428
Sally Ford and Goody Cable recently remodeled this 1910 historic oceanfront hotel into a bed and breakfast for book lovers. There are 20 guest rooms, all with private baths, and each furnished in the style of a different author. A large library overlooks the ocean. The restaurant offers not only breakfasts but also serves family-style dinners. Reservations are required for dinner. Ken Peyton is the innkeeper. No smoking or pets. Visa/MC. Open year around.

20 The Whale's Tale

452 S.W. Bay Blvd., Newport, 97365 (on Newport's historic bay front). Tel: 265-8660

Begun as a small delicatessen in 1976 by Dick Schwartz and Kate Kelly, The Whale's Tale has evolved into a full-service restaurant and is now an important part of the Newport community. Specialties include Eggs Newport made with local Oregon shrimp, fresh seafood poached or sauteed, poppyseed pancakes, and vegetarian fare. All breads are baked on the premises and Oregon wines and beer are featured. Folk music by local musicians. Children welcome. All major credit cards. 7 AM-9 PM Mon-Thurs, 7 AM-10 PM Fri, 9 AM-10 PM Sat-Sun. Closed Wed in winter.

21 The Wood Gallery

818 S.W. Bay Blvd., Newport, 97365 (on Newport's bay front). Tel: 265-6843

Kelly Barker represents 250 different woodworkers, painters, potters, ivory workers, jewelers, metalsmiths, sculptors and fiber artists. A 6 cyl Porsche engine made completely of wood that works just like a regular engine with everything moving, all-wooden clocks that keep accurate time and full-size ceramic furniture are available here. Alpine Vineyards Tasting Room. Visa/MC/AmEx/Diners/CB. 10-6 daily.

OTIS

22 Otis Cafe

At Otis Jct. on Hwy. 18, 5 mi. northeast of Lincoln City, P.O. Box 114, Otis, 97368. Tel: 994-2813

Otis Daily Bread and Hot Sweet Mustard are some of the things "fresh made" from family recipes here. Owner Virginia Morgan provides wholesome food at her old-fashioned, unpretentious cafe along with information about which hiking trails are best on Cascade Head, and when and where the next chamber music or jazz concert will take place. 7 AM-3 PM Mon-Wed, 7 AM-9 PM Thurs-Sat, 8 AM-9 PM Sun.

23 Sitka Center for Art and Ecology

On Cascade Head Ranch (north of Lincoln City on Hwy. 101, turn west on Three Rocks Rd. and follow signs to Sitka). P.O. Box 65, Otis, 97368. Tel: 994-5485

Situated on the slopes of Cascade Head, near a Nature Conservancy area and the Salmon River Estuary, and dedicated to the expression of the strong relationship between art and nature, Sitka offers summer sessions of learning and experiencing through a combination of classroom techniques and out-of-doors activities. Program partially sponsored by grants from the Oregon Arts Commission and the National Endowment for the Arts. Classes run June-August. Write or call for complete brochure and schedule of activities. Office: 10-5 almost daily (summer), 12-4 (winter).

OTTER ROCK

24 Pottery West

Next to state park, P.O. Box 19, Otter Rock, 97369. Tel: 765-2528

Established in 1976, Pottery West features hand-thrown stoneware made by Dan Hagstrom in his own studio plus the work of several leading Oregon potters who began their careers as apprentices at Pottery West. Visa/MC. 10-4 daily (summer), weekends only (winter).

PACIFIC CITY

25 Pacific View Bed and Breakfast

34930 Hillcrest, P.O. Box 28, Pacific City, 97135. Tel: 965-6498

Aptly named, this sea captain's home built in the late 1930s is on the first hill in from the ocean. The three-bedroom home, owned by hosts Jim and Maxine Wright, affords panoramic views of Cape Kiwanda, Haystack Rock, Nestucca River, and coast range. There's a glassed-in "widow's walk," picture windows, and gardens for watching whale migrations, spectacular sunsets, or powerful storms. Private or shared bath. Full breakfast. Limited smoking, no pets. Visa/MC/AmEx. Open daily May-Jan.

26 The Riverhouse Restaurant

34450 Brooten Rd., P.O. Box 223, Pacific City, 97135. Tel: 965-6722
Steven Neufeld offers pleasant dining overlooking the Nestucca River, featuring fresh coastal seafood dinners, mouth-watering sandwiches, home-baked desserts and Saturday night concert series of Oregon musicians in a variety of musical traditions. Cocktails available. Visa/MC. 11-9 daily, Sat and Sun open until 10 (summer); 11-8 Tues-Sun, Fri and Sat open until 9 (winter). 10-2 Sun brunch.

SEAL ROCK

27 Seal Rock Art Gallery

10 mi. south of Newport on Hwy. 101 at Grebe St. in center of downtown Seal Rock. P.O. Box 89, Seal Rock, 97376. Tel: 563-2576 or 563-2016 for appointment
Martin and Ruth Kallman invite you to view some of the most outstanding art exhibits on the Oregon coast. New shows monthly feature painting, drawing, ceramics, jewelry, and art glass by Oregon artists exclusively. Art supplies also available. Many workshops and live concerts of music and dance are featured during a changing calendar of events. Visa/MC. 11-5 daily (June-Dec), 11-5 Fri-Mon (Jan-May).

SILETZ

28 The Confederated Tribes of the Siletz

P.O. Box 549, Siletz, 97380.
Tel: 444-2532
The People and the Land: The people of the Confederated Tribes of the Siletz number 1800 strong and all share roots that connect them to the Oregon and Northern California coasts where for thousands of years their forebears lived in peace and prosperity.

In the 1850s their ancestors were forced from their lands by soldiers onto the Coast Reserve, later called the Siletz Reservation. Many of them live in the town of Siletz, named after its river, the Siletz, meaning "twisted as a snake or rope."

For the many who live outside the Siletz area, Government Hill in the town of Siletz is the place they come each August to visit family and friends at the annual Nesika Illahee PowWow (August 12, 13, and 14 in 1988). This is very much a public event, with Indian arts and crafts and lots of food, including Indian fry bread and Indian tacos. While people come from many states, most are from the Northwest.

Aug 12: Friday evening starts with a very formal Grand Entry with drumming and singing followed by intertribal dancing where people not dressed in regalia or for dancing may participate informally.

Aug 13-14: On Saturday and Sunday, beginning at noon and in the evening there is Competition Dancing between people from various Indian tribes.

Exhibition Dancing takes place throughout the weekend.

Indian Cove (North Coast), © Liza Jones

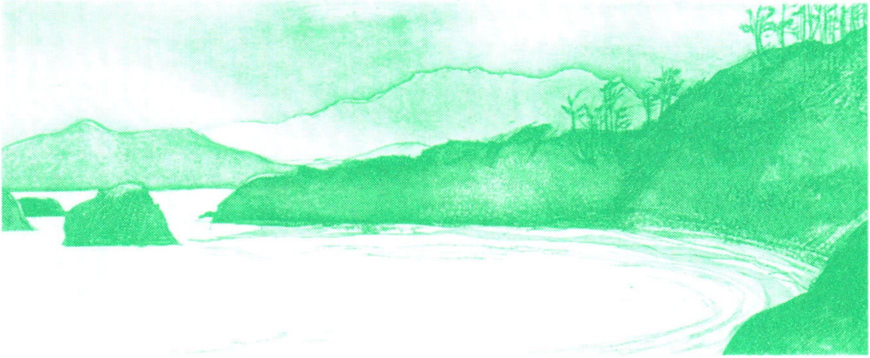

WALDPORT

29 Gale Gallery, Glashaus Pottery, and Heather Cottage

Yaquina John Point (½ mi. south of Waldport on ocean side of Hwy. 101 at Adahi Ave.), P.O. Box 528, Waldport, 97394. Tel: 563-3620

The gallery features Oregon artists and specializes in stoneware made on the premises, watercolor exhibits, carved carousel horses, other American folk art. Also fabric inlay designer kites, handcrafted walking sticks, ornaments, candles, soap, notes, toys, and more. Heather Cottage is a cozy, one-bedroom, fully furnished vacation rental a few minutes walk from the ocean beach and mouth of the Alsea River. A non-smokers' delight available by day, week, or month, year around. Visa/MC. Gallery: 11-5 daily (summer), 12-5 Fri-Mon (winter), or by appointment.

YACHATS

30 Ziggurat Bed and Breakfast

95330 Hwy. 101, Yachats, 97498 (6½ mi. south of Yachats). Tel: 547-3925

"Ziggurat" means "terraced pyramid," explain owner/hosts Mary Lou Cavendish and Irv Tebor, and this one is a spectacular four stories tall. It has been called a sculpture-by-the-sea. Guests have the privacy of the entire first floor with two bedrooms, queen-sized beds, bath, sauna, and library/living room. There's ocean viewing from the surrounding tiled solarium, from the open-air decks, or from the second floor, where a full breakfast is served. No children under 14 or pets. Open year around.

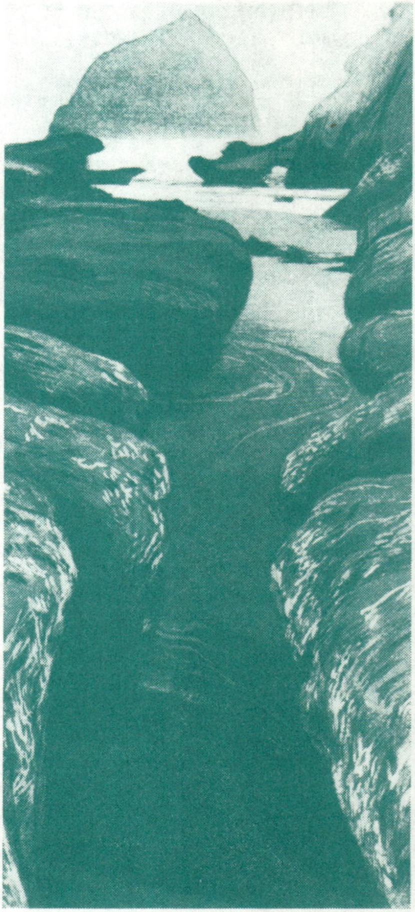

Pathway (Cape Kiwanda), © Liza Jones

BEACH SAFETY TIPS

1. **Never turn your back on the sea.**
2. **Waves are unpredictable.** *Forget anything you ever heard about "that 7th or 11th wave" that is supposed to be the bad one. The larger, more dangerous waves cannot be predicted by any system.*
3. *Even* **a small wave** *(a 3-footer)* **can knock down an adult.**
4. **"Sneaker waves"** *are just that—completely unpredictable, even on outgoing tides.*
5. **Check tide table** *before setting out for the beach. Incoming tides can be the most dangerous for unwary explorers, but watch outgoing tides too—they can tumble huge logs along with them.*
6. **Never, ever, stand on—or get near—a log that is in the surf or on the wet portion of the beach.** *Unpredictable waves can toss or roll it—and injure a person seriously if he happens to be in the way.*
7. *When beachcombing, be sure to* **leave word** *with someone about where you plan to go on the beach and how long you will be there.*

South Coast

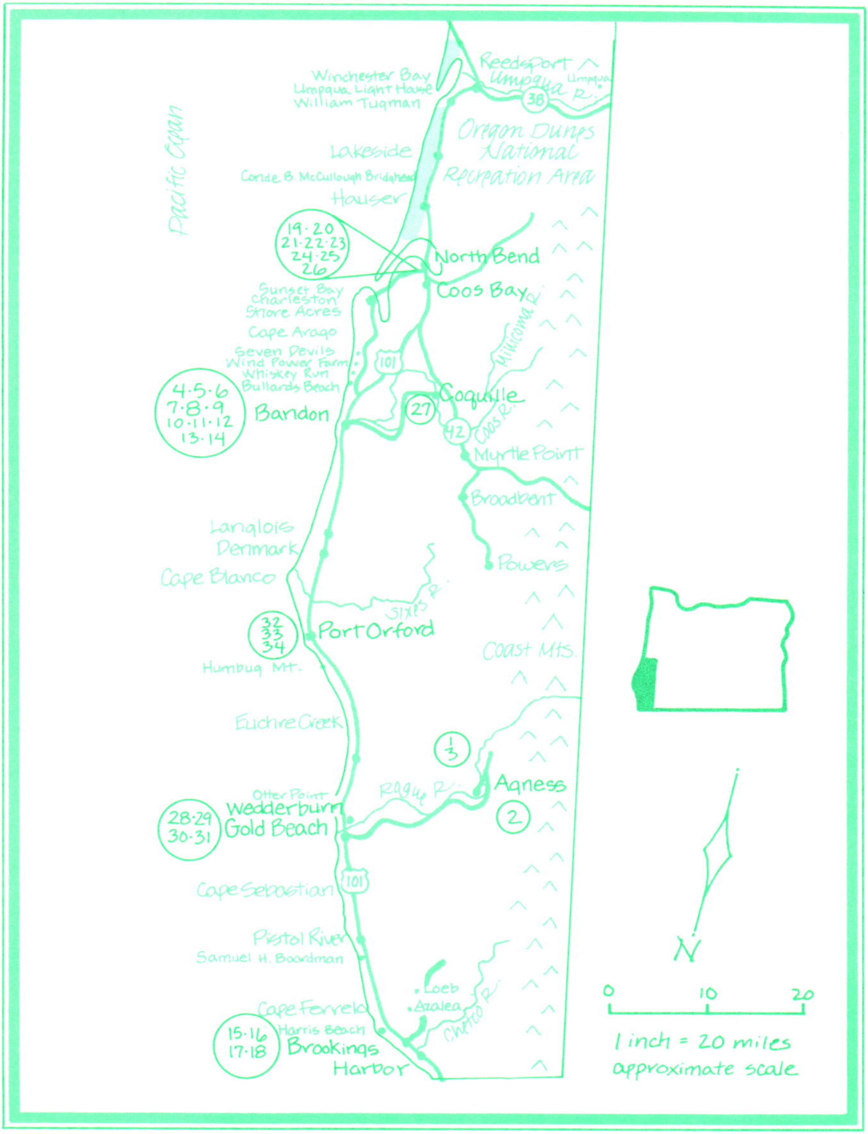

Reedsport
Umpqua
Umpqua R.
38
Winchester Bay
Umpqua Light House
William Tugman
Oregon Dunes National Recreation Area
Pacific Ocean
Lakeside
Conde B. McCullough Bridgehead
Hauser
19·20 21·22·23 24·25 26
North Bend
Coos Bay
Sunset Bay
Charleston
Shore Acres
Cape Arago
Millicoma R.
Seven Devils
Wind Power Farm
Whiskey Run
Bullards Beach
101
4·5·6 7·8·9 10·11·12 13·14
Bandon
27
Coquille
42
Coos R.
Myrtle Point
Broadbent
Langlois
Denmark
Cape Blanco
Powers
Sixes R.
32 33 34
Port Orford
Humbug Mt.
Coast Mts.
Euchre Creek
1 3
Rogue R.
Agness
Otter Point
Wedderburn
2
28·29 30·31
Gold Beach
101
Cape Sebastian
Pistol River
Samuel H. Boardman
N
0 10 20
1 inch = 20 miles
approximate scale
Loeb
Azalea
Chetco R.
Cape Ferrelo
Harris Beach
15·16 17·18
Brookings
Harbor

SOUTH COAST REGIONAL NOTES

In sharp contrast with the lush greenery elsewhere along the Oregon coast, miles of sand dunes rise abruptly from sea level. The highlight of Oregon's dune country is a 40-mile stretch along the coast from Coos Bay north to the Siuslaw River. This probably has the **most spectacular tract of coastal sand dunes in the country.** *Rivers carried some of the sand to the sea, and waves battering the sandstones exposed in the sea cliff supplied the rest. Every time the tide comes in, waves carry new high sand onto the beach. They leave it there, where it dries as the tide goes out, and then the wind blows it inland into the dunes.*

Prevailing winds blow onto the Oregon Coast from the southwest in winter and northwest in summer, so the waves tend to drive sand northward along the beach all winter and then back south again in the summer. Along some sections of the coast the winter waves prevail, and sand pits grow from south to north; in others, the summer waves hold upper hand and sand pits build southward. The mouth of the Siuslaw River at Florence (see Central Coast Regional Notes), for example, has been diverted about three miles north by growth of a sand pit; whereas those of the Umpqua River at Reedsport and the Millicoma River at Coos Bay have been diverted several miles to the south.

Coastal sand dunes also show the influence of the changing seasonal pattern of prevailing winds. Heavy winter storms bring strong onshore gales out of the southwest, shaping the major outlines of the dunes. Then the gentler winds of summer form cross-ridges which are quite conspicuous by fall but disappear entirely before the next spring. So the dunes change in character with the passing of the seasons as well as from day to day, with every change in the weather.

Most of this region is protected by the **Oregon Dunes National Recreation Area.** *Off-road vehicles are restricted to a few areas. Backpacking is popular between the Siltcoos and Umpqua Rivers. Beaches can also be walked or just visited for a picnic. The ''islands'' of pine and spruce in the basins surrounded by parabolic dunes are one interesting aspect of the Oregon dunes. The dunes reach a width of more than two miles between the Umpqua Lighthouse and Tenmile Creek. This is an easy place to get lost, if compass readings are not frequently taken. Carry a windbreaker.*

Umpqua Lighthouse State Park *has massive open sand dunes. Nearby on Lighthouse Road is the Umpqua River Lighthouse, a former U.S. Coast Guard station now converted into an historical display and information center.* **Sunset Beach** *is a charming horseshoe-shaped beach that often has warmer than usual waters.* **Shore Acres Arboretum and State Park,** *once the estate of a wealthy Coos Bay lumberman, now maintains formal floral gardens and interpretive displays. Just south of* **Seven Devils' Wayside** *there is a* **wind-power farm,** *where over 40 windmills generate electricity from the wind blowing off the Pacific Ocean. It is an astonishing sight. The Coquille Lighthouse at* **Bullards Beach State Park** *was built in 1896 and is open during the summer months.*

All around this area grows a very thorny shrub called gorse or Irish furze that blooms twice a year and was imported by Bandon's early settlers as a remembrance of the British Isles where it is trimmed into impenetrable hedgerows. On the South Oregon Coast, however, it has become a rapidly spreading pest that is especially susceptible to fire and was once responsible for a fire that burnt Bandon to the ground.

The **South Slough National Estuarine Sanctuary,** *established in 1972, is the first estuarine sanctuary in the nation. It contains 4,000 acres of land and 600 acres of tidelands at the southern part of the South Slough of Coos Bay. The purposes of the sanctuary are to serve as a source of scientific information to provide some of the information essential to coastal zone management decision making and to serve as an educational facility to bring to students, teachers, and the public an appreciation of estaries and their complexity. One can canoe, bird-watch, and hike on three self-guided trails.*

The beach loop at **Bandon** *affords views of Face Rock and other large remnants of the shoreline now stranded in the ocean. Note the cranberry bogs in this area that supply Bandon's famous cranberry industry.* **Cape Blanco** *has an unusual black sand beach.* **Port Orford Head** *is good for whale watching (in season) . . . as are many places along the entire Oregon Coast.*

Azalea State Park *is named after the large native azaleas that grow in the area, often referred to as the banana belt of the Oregon Coast. The mildness of the weather allows hummingbirds to winter over on the southern Oregon coast, and most of the Easter lilies sold in America are raised in this area.*

A portion of the **Oregon Coast Trail** *is located on Cape Arago, Sunset Bay, and Shore Acre State Parks. Other segments are located in Cape Sebastian, Humbug Mountain, and Samuel H. Boardman State Parks.*

Highway 101 is a favorite **bicycle route.** *There are special camping areas for hikers and bicyclists and Umpqua Lighthouse, William T. Tugman, Cape Arago, Bullards Beach, Cape Blanco, Humbug Mountain, Samuel H. Boardman, Loeb, and Harris Beach State Parks.*

There are boat docks and ramps at Bullards Beach and William M. Tugman State Parks, and a boat ramp to the bay at Conde B. McCullough Bridgehead State Park, and to the river at Umpqua State Park. Club camping is available at Bullards Beach, Harris Beach, and Sunset State Parks. The garden and garden house are available for special occasions at Shore Acres State Park.

All beaches in Oregon *below mean high tide, except for a very few miles, are owned by the state and* **are public land.** *Clam digging is popular along the Oregon coast, but check carefully for conditions. The sand beaches are popular spots for rock hounds, beachcombers, and walkers. Winter (December to April) is the best time for storms to expose gravel bars that yield* **agates, jaspers, petrified wood,** *and a variety of* **fossils.** *Most of the gravel bars tend to be sanded in during the summer.*

Cape Arago (follow signs from North Bend) is a fairly good place to hunt agates, marine shells, flower jasper, and petrified wood. Merchants, Whiskey Run, and Bullard Beaches on Seven Devils Road are all good producers of agates, agatized myrtlewood, jasper, chert, quartz, etc. Marine fossils are in the cliffs, and traces of gold can be found in panned beach sand. The beaches from the mouth of the Sixes River to Cape Blanco and on south to Port Orford produce good agates. Chert Cove, between Sixes Rock (old port) and Euchre Creek (near Orphir) have cutting-size picture chert. The cove is reachable only when the tide is out or going out. The beach south of Euchre Creek has fine multicolored gravel. Agates can be found south of Hubbard Mound (near Nesika Beach) to Gold Beach. Blue-green serpentine has been found on the north side of the Rogue River, just back of the bridge, and talc and nephrite jade on the beaches north and south of the Rogue River. Milky quartz, agates, chert, and jade are found on the beaches north and south of Pistol River. Lone Ranch is the site of a boran mine. The beaches from Cape Farrago to Brookings have a lot of metamorphic rocks, including serpentine and grossularite garnet (a pseudo-jade that comes in pink, white, yellow, and green). Rainbow Cove (1 mile south of Lone Creek Ranch State Park) does not sand in, and has good agate chert. It is windy, however, and can only be entered at low tide. (See Rockhound's Map of Oregon, *reference page 3.)*

One of the interesting attractions of the Oregon Coast is the **diversity of ecosystems** *ranging from open sand dunes to old growth forest. All of the ecosystems represent different stages of succession. In the beginning, there is sand. After a few years, one or two hearty pioneer species gain a foothold in the shifting sands. The pioneer plants on the dunes are mostly grasses and a few herbs. These plants modify the environment by trapping sand with their extensive root systems to form mounds. Eventually enough sand is held in place to allow more herbs to survive. These herbs are eventually replaced by other herbs and a few shrubs, the shrubs by trees, the trees by other trees, until finally a relatively stable climax forest is reached. A climax forest is only stable relative to a human lifetime. All living systems are dynamic, constantly changing to meet new conditions.*

The long bullwhip seaweed found on all Oregon beaches is called the **Bull Kelp.** *Growing under 30 to 40 feet of water, its blades float on the surface forming kelp beds.*

Oregon has an incredible variety of **wildflowers** *throughout the state. Please enjoy them, and please leave them undisturbed for others to enjoy. "A picked wildflower is a thing of beauty, but a joy for only one person for a few minutes." Some wildflowers grow in incredibly delicate environments and can take as long as seven years to bloom again.*

Myrtlewood *and the objects made from it are rapidly becoming a thing of the past as the older craftsmen are dying and the trees are being cut as slash. Northern California and Southern Oregon are the only places in the Americas where myrtlewood is grown. It takes one hundred years to "get the right grain," yet no one is planting myrtlewood for future generations.*

The most obvious feature of the coast is the **shoreline.** *Along our coast, stretches of sandy beach are separated by* **basaltic headlands.** *These headlands appeared when wind and seas ate away the softer earth surrounding the hard volcanic core. The ocean is constantly wearing away headlands and depositing the eroded material in bays and coves, gradually creeping toward a straight coastline.*

This erosion occurs primarily during heavy winter storms from the southwest.

Moving inland, a lack of open stream channels is noticeable. This is because precipitation comes in a **steady drizzle** *rather than a hard downpour, allowing the water ample time to soak into the ground where it falls, instead of running off.*

Black sand *is common along the entire length of the Oregon Coast, just enough in the dunes to add an occasional dash of color, but many beaches are broadly splashed with black. The sand contains a variety of minerals, all denser than the quartz and feldspar that comprise most ordinary sand. Magnetite, the magnetic oxide of iron, and ilmenite, a titanium material, are usually the most abundant, but most black sands also contain red garnet, a few glittering grains of zircon, and a brown mineral called monazite, which contains rare-earth elements. Some contain gold. The waves know these heavy minerals by their weight, and neatly sort them into separate deposits. Oregon black sands are more interesting than most, because they generally contain chromite and platinum along with the usual minerals. A few people have made a little bit of money, and a lot of others have gone broke trying to mine the beach sands. Rising prices of many mineral commodities may yet make it worthwhile.*

A recent phenomenon of the Oregon coast is the **foredune.** *For some obscure reason, sand dunes seem to offend many people, simply because they move. "Hills should stay firmly rooted in place and not go wandering off." Enormous amounts of taxpayers' money are spent each year to* **"control"** *any number of* **perfectly harmless dunes,** *converting them into characterless heaps of sand. Unfortunately, these efforts usually succeed.*

None of the native grasses grow well on sand dunes, so beach grass was introduced from Europe about 1910. Oregon suits it splendidly, and now **European Beach Grass** *grows wild all along the coast, ruining many beautiful tracts of dunes and literally changing the shape of the beachscape. Sand used to blow from the beach back into the dunes; but now, the dense growths of grass immediately behind the beach trap most of it, so a grass-covered ridge is growing just behind the beach, and the dunes are marching inland with their supply lines cut off behind them.*

Closest to land is the **deflation plain,** *where the sand has been removed by the wind down to the groundwater level, and the moist sand cannot be carried off. With plenty of water and protection from sand deposition, many more species of plants can survive here than on the foredune. The high-water mark of a high tide is called the* **high-tide line.** *The low-water mark of the low tide is called the* **low-tide line.** *The area between the high-tide line and the low-tide line is called the* **intertidal zone.** *Areas of organic deposits left by retreating waves marking different tide levels on the beach are called* **swash zones.**

Oregon State University has identified over **34 distinct kinds of driftwood** *available on the Oregon Coast. Large reserves of driftwood are always out at sea. What brings them to shore is the right velocity and direction of wind. Some pieces are timber, lost from passing barges and freighters, and are sometimes exotic woods like mahogany and other Asian hardwoods. Much of our driftwood is the result of storms, floods, snow, rock-slides, and erosion along the shore and inland streams and rivers. These forces uproot many inland trees and send them downriver; sooner or later, most of them reach the sea.*

Oregon's logging industry accounts for many pieces on our beaches. Logs escape from rafts and storage areas along rivers and in estuaries. Logging near stream banks leaves behind branches and other debris that slowly work their way downhill. Flooding may then carry them downstream to the sea.

Longshore currents paralleling the shore transport driftwood from north to south, and even south to north. For example, redwood is often found on Coos County beaches, although the species grows only in Northern California and Southwestern Oregon.

Some coves and beaches act as driftwood reservoirs. They collect it after particularly strong winter storms. On some beaches, driftwood comes and goes. Wave action and seasonal changes cause this fluctuation. At any time, some waves may have enough power to push driftwood specimens relatively high on the shore. This movement can be very dangerous. **Do not ignore the beach safety tips on some of the beaches.**

Strong winter waves alternately thrust whole logs and smaller pieces higher up on the beach and drag them back down into the sea again. Gentler summer waves return much of the wood that winter action drives out to sea. *(See* Identifying Oregon Driftwood, *reference page 3.)*

The Nature Conservancy owns and manages a large system of natural preserves throughout the state of Oregon. Call 223-9561 or visit the conservancy's offices in Portland (see Statewide Resources section) for information about preserves the public may visit in this region.

AGNESS AND BEYOND

1 Clay Hill Lodge

45 mi. up the Rogue River from Gold Beach, accessible only by 6 mi. hike, float trip, or jet boat tour from Gold Beach, P.O. Box 18, Agness, 97406.
Tel: 247-6215
This small lodge in the Wild Section of the Rogue River, surrounded by national forest, is operated by Larry and Clare Bowen. Private rooms and home-cooked meals offer the atmosphere and comfort of a bed and breakfast in the midst of the pristine wilderness. Beautiful scenery, panoramic views, and abundant wildlife encourage hiking, fishing, swimming, boating, or just relaxing. Visa/MC. Open daily April-Nov. Reservations required.

2 Lucas Pioneer Ranch and Lodge

3904 Cougar Lane, Agness, 97406 (from Hwy. 101 take Jerry's Flat Rd. at the south end of Gold Beach Bridge 35 mi. to Agness, or come I-5 to Merlin Exit, 3 mi. north of Grants Pass, and drive to Agness on scenic, partially-paved Forest Service road over mountain range—about 2 hours—or come via daily boats from Gold Beach or on pre-arranged float trips from Grants Pass). Tel: 247-7443
This historic country inn has been in the Lucas family since the early 1900s. In a peaceful setting at the junction of the Rogue and Illinois rivers, it serves family-style, home-cooked meals with ranch-grown fresh vegetables and sweet corn in season. Comfortable, rustic cabins. Country-fried chicken noon meals served to the public at 11:30 AM from Mother's Day to Oct 31. Reservations required. The Agness Store, featuring a gift shop with all items made or grown in Oregon, is located on the ranch.

3 Paradise Bar Lodge

52 mi. up the Rogue River from Gold Beach, accessible only by boat, trail, or private plane, P.O. Box 456, Gold Beach, 97444. Tel: 247-6022 (Reservations: P.O. Box 548, Gold Beach, 97444. Tel. 247-6504)
This rustic lodge in the Rogue "Wild River" section with ranch-style meals, fresh-baked bread, home-grown fruits and vegetables, cold beverages and cocktails, and comfortable, rustic rooms and cabins has been offering hospitality for over 30 years in its hideaway location. Manager Allen Boice has many tall tales to tell about the Rogue River. Fishing, hiking, swimming and gold panning available. Visa/MC. Lodge: 6 AM-10 PM daily. Reservation service: 9-6 Mon-Sat. Reservations necessary.

BANDON

4 Bandon Storm Watchers

P.O. Box 1693, Bandon, 97411.
Tel: 347-2779 or 347-3983
Bandon, the "Winter Storm Capital of the Coast," is promoted by this award-winning community organization. With coastal temperatures invariably warmer than inland, the Storm Watchers say Bandon is a great place to spend a few days in the wintertime . . . and that the thrill of standing on the shore and watching one of the wintertime "timber-rattlers" defies description. The all-volunteer group sponsors a variety of lectures and programs, highlighted by a city-wide Wine and Seafood Festival, the season's-end finale, on Memorial Day weekend.

1988-89 Bandon Area Annual Events include:

Every Sat, Jan-April: Informative public lectures on coastal environment, happenings, and history, 3 PM, Community Center in Bandon City Park. No charge. (Sample lecture titles listed below.)

1988

April 2: "Introduced Species into the Ocean" by James Carlton

April 9: "Marine Artifacts" by James White

April 16: "Field Trip on Coastal Plants" by Gwen Llewellyn (meeting place TBA)

Memorial Day Weekend, May 28-29: Wine and Seafood Festival and Arts and Crafts Exhibit, 11 AM-5 PM, Community Center in Bandon City Park with Oregon wine-tasting booths, Bandon restaurants featuring seafood delicacies

5 Andrea's Old Town Cafe

160 Baltimore, Bandon, 97411 (in Oldtown Bandon between 1st and 2nd streets). Tel: 347-3022
Since 1977, Andrea Gatov has specialized in homemade gourmet foods: fresh, local seafood, wild berries and mushrooms, home-raised lamb and her own famous cheese cakes. She is well known for her exceptional recipes and reasonable prices. Live piano music often entertains local residents and returning visitors. 8 AM–9 PM Mon-Sat, 10 AM–9 PM Sun (summer); 9 AM–3:30 PM Mon-Thurs, 9 AM–9 PM Fri, Sat; 10:30 AM–3 PM Sun (winter).

6 Bandon Tasting Room

350 Second St., Bandon, 97411 (two doors east of Bandon's Information Center). Tel: 347-9129
The home of Jon Marker's Cabernet Rose, "Oregon's Breakfast Wine," this is Jonicole Vineyard's satellite tasting room as well as a generic Oregon wine-tasting room where Bill and Nancy educate people about Oregon wines. Nancy also organizes tours of Umpqua Valley wineries from here. The Tasting Room is usually open 12-5 daily but always on weekends, year around. Visa/MC. (See Roseburg, Southern Oregon, for Jonicole Vineyards listing.)

7 Cliff Harbor Bed and Breakfast Inn

9th St. and Beach Loop Rd., P.O. Box 769, Bandon, 97411. Tel: 347-3956
This spacious, modern home is dramatically sited at cliff's edge overlooking wide, sandy beaches and an expanse of ocean and coastline. The Inn's interior features the woodworking, cabinetry, and fine furniture of Eugene craftsman, Douglas Haines. There are two suites, both with private baths and entrances, one with kitchen and fireplace. Smoking restricted. No pets. Open year around.

8 Cranberry Sweets Company

Corner 1st & Chicago streets (in Oldtown Bandon on the waterfront), P.O. Box 501, Bandon, 97411. Tel: 347-9475
Cliff and Margaret Shaw's remarkable, all-natural, cranberry candies are handmade from a 25-year-old recipe and have no salt, artificial flavorings, starch, gelatin or preservatives. Some are dipped in chocolate, others in sugar. There are even lemon meringue and apple pie varieties tasting just like their namesakes! Call or write for brochure, price list or telephone ordering. Visa/MC. 9-5:30 daily.

9 Exhibit Hall

210 Second St., Bandon, 97411 (in Oldtown Bandon). Tel: 347-9712
It is anticipated that the Continuum exhibit will be coming back to Bandon to be permanently displayed at the Bandon Exhibit Hall. The nationally acclaimed Continuum exhibit presents man's thoughts about his own consciousness with fascinating and thought-provoking information from the fields of science, technology, parapsychology, philosophy, religion, medicine, and the arts.

10 Harbor Hall

325 Second St., Bandon, 97411 (in Oldtown Bandon). Tel: 347-4404
This new 350-seat, accoustically treated auditorium with state-of-the-art lighting and sound capabilities is rapidly becoming *the* entertainment spot on the south coast. Some of its offerings in 1988 include "Little Mary Sunshine" (May 27–June 25), "The Rainmaker" (Sept 16–Oct 1), "Barefoot in the Park" (Dec 2-17), and "Gypsy" in February, 1989. Besides its usual repertoire of fine concert entertainment, Harbor Hall will also be presenting "Insomni ACTS" (an after-dinner late-night theater for insomniacs with mime, black-out skits, reader theater, dance, etc.) through much of the summer and fall.

11 Northwest Collectors Gallery

In Laurel Grove, approximately 7 mi. south of Bandon on Hwy. 101. Rt. 1, Box 1310, Bandon, 97411. Tel: 347-9332
Kirk and Elizabeth Day have created one of Southern Oregon's most contemporary collections of modern art glass, hand-crafted furniture, ceramics, sculpted metal, paintings, and jewelry. Amidst massive beams and skylights, the gallery currently features the recent work of John Richen, Philip Clausen, Michael Schlicting, Hawthorne and Nowak, Richard LaLonde, Etsuko Sakamura, Kevin Kadar, Don McMichael, Dennis Jones, Ruth Brockman, and K. Arnot Day. Visa/MC. 10-5:30 daily (March 15–Dec 31).

12 Spindrift Bed and Breakfast

2990 Beach Loop Rd., Bandon, 97411. Tel: 347-2275
Guests can enjoy a panoramic 180° ocean view from the Common Room where hostess Robbie Smith serves luxurious, filling breakfasts. (Wine and cheese available to those arriving before 5 PM.) The Seaview room has its own fireplace and private entrance and bath. The Surfsand room has a shared bath. No small children, pets or smoking. Visa/MC. Open year around.

13 230 Second Street Gallery

In Oldtown Bandon, P.O. Box 1736, Bandon, 97411. Tel: 347-4133
Ruth and Hugh Harrison invite visitors to discover regional fine art and quality crafts by more than 80 dedicated artists and craftsmen whose mediums include glass, bronze, wood and steel sculpture, fiber, ceramics, oil, watercolor and acrylic paintings, mezzotints, silk screens, lithographs, and etchings. Housed in one of Bandon's restored historical buildings, the gallery is staffed by practicing professional artists. A number of the artists and craftsmen represented have received awards from the Oregon Arts Commission and the National Endowment for the Arts. Visa/MC. 10-5:30 daily.

14 The Wool Company

990 Second St., Bandon, 97411.
Tel: 347-3912
"Wools from start to finish" is their motto. Local wools are washed, dyed, carded, spun, knitted and woven—some blended with silk, linen, llama, dog hair, with over 200 colors in stock. Custom yarns, sweaters, blankets, rugs, and felt as well as spinning wheels, lessons and quick, quality carding service also available. 10-5:30 Mon-Sat.

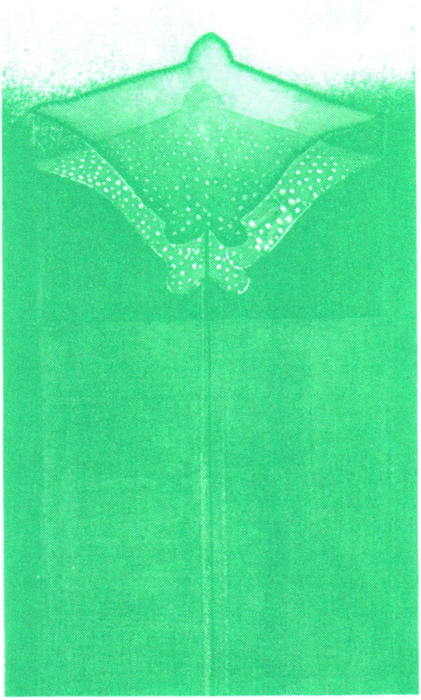

Two Skates, © *Liza Jones*

BROOKINGS-HARBOR

15 Brookings-Harbor Chamber of Commerce

97949 Shopping Center Ave.,
P.O. Box 940, Brookings, 97415.
Tel: 469-3181.
Office: 9-5 daily.
"Majestic" and "spectacular" are often used to describe the Southern Oregon coastline. The community of Brookings-Harbor is located just six miles from the California border. In addition to beautiful scenery and incredible fishing (both ocean and river), the area boasts the mildest winter climate in all of Oregon. So mild in fact that the area is nicknamed the "Banana Belt." There are many motels, bed and breakfast homes, RV parks, restaurants, and plenty of recreational opportunities. Ocean charters are available at the Port of Brookings, which has the safest bar crossing on the Oregon Coast. River fishing guides are also available to the fishing enthusiast.

1988 Brookings-Harbor Area Events include:
March 26-27: Beachcombers Festival
May 27-30: Azalea Festival
Sept 16-17: Oregon Bike Rally Celebration

16 Chetco Inn

417 Fern, P.O. Box 1386, Brookings, 97415 (on the hill above the Shell station). Tel: 469-9984
The current face lift of the historic Chetco Inn, built in 1915, is a labor of love by innkeepers Bill and Victoria Roberts and family. Thirty-two rooms, 20 with private baths, have been restored to their original use. The parlor is large enough for reunions and meetings. A delightful change from the ordinary. Children and pets welcome. Visa/MC. Always open.

17 Holmes Sea Cove Bed and Breakfast

17350 Holmes Dr., Brookings, 97415 (2 mi. north of Brookings, turn onto Dawson Rd. from Hwy. 101). Tel: 469-3025
Jack and Lorene Holmes have a separate guest cottage and two bedrooms on the lower level in their home just up a winding trail from a private park with picnic tables and creek and the beach. All rooms have private baths and entrances. Continental breakfasts are brought to guests' rooms. No pets and no smoking in rooms. Visa/MC. Open year around.

18 Ward House Bed and Breakfast

516 Redwood St., P.O. Box 86, Brookings, 97415 (1 blk. off Hwy. 101).
Tel: 469-5557
Shell and Gro Lent have restored the classic 1917 home of former mill manager William Ward to capture the flavor of that time. Overlooking downtown Brookings, the home has an ocean view and warm, friendly atmosphere. A hot tub and sauna are available to guests. Gro's Norwegian hospitality highlights the gourmet breakfast. Visa/MC. Open all year. Reservations required.

COOS BAY-NORTH BEND

19 Coos Art Museum

235 Anderson Ave., Coos Bay, 97420 (in Old Post Office Building in downtown Coos Bay). Tel: 267-3901
The only coastal art museum between San Francisco and the Canadian border and the cultural center for the area's 75,000 residents, Coos Art Museum attracts thousands of visitors who annually travel Hwy. 101. Mounting six to eight exhibitions each year, the museum focuses its programming on the successful integration of art, education, and participation. Its programs are often supported by grants from the Oregon Arts Commission and the National Endowment for the Arts. Visa/MC. 11-5 Tues-Fri, 12-4 Sat-Sun.

20 Cozette's Gourmet Foods

1149 Juniper St., Coos Bay, 97420.
Tel: 267-4547
"Gourmet" cranberries are Cozette's specialty . . . brandied cranberries, cranberries in port wine, cranberry marmalade, and cranberry hazelnut compote with rum. Other "Indecently Delicious" products include pear condiments, chutneys, savory sauces, and natural macadamia nuts with no added salt or oil. Available in myrtlewood gift packs. A Neiman-Marcus selection, Cozette's products are also carried in specialty stores throughout Oregon and in Coos County at the House of Myrtlewood, Cone-9, Greater Things, Cranberry Sweets Co., and Bandon Berries. Write for wholesale or retail price list.

21 The Highlands Bed and Breakfast

608 Ridge Rd., North Bend, 97459.
Tel: 756-0300
This contemporary cedar home is located on six acres that have been left purposely hospitable to wildlife. The family homestead includes resident chickens that supply fresh eggs for thoughtfully prepared breakfasts which are served on the wrap-around deck (weather permitting). One large guest room with double bed and adjoining private bath and one smaller guest room with double bed and adjoining whirlpool bath. Cozy quilts, soapstone woodburning stove, and spectacular views of the coast range. Smoking on deck only. No children or pets.

22 The House of Myrtlewood

1125 S. First (south end of Coos Bay, visible from Hwy. 101), P.O. Box 457, Coos Bay, 97420. Tel: 267-7804
A small area on the Pacific coast contains the world's primary supply of the rare hardwood—myrtlewood. Founded in 1929, The House of Myrtlewood gives complimentary factory tours daily to watch the production process from log to finished product, and then invites visitors to browse through its gift shop and Oregon gourmet food room. Visa/MC. 8:30-5:30 daily.

23 Hurry Back! Cafe

100 Commercial, Coos Bay, 97420 (on Hwy. 101 S. at turn-off to Charleston).
Tel: 267-3933
Wim de Vriend serves wholesome, homemade, hearty food in a sidewalk cafe atmosphere. The part-seafood, all-natural menu includes homemade croissants, fancy pastries, fresh-baked breads, including the only 100% rye sourdough on the West Coast, fresh pasta, freshly squeezed juices, espresso, and a variety of wines and beers. Live music Friday and Saturday evenings. Visa/MC. Opens 8 AM Mon-Sat and closes between 9 and 11 PM, depending on crowd. 9 AM-3 PM Sun.

24 **Oregon Coast Music Festival**
P.O. Box 663, Coos Bay, 97420.
Tel: 269-4150
(Daytime & evening concerts in Coos Bay, Charleston and North Bend)
Lovely combination of great music and scenic beauty of the Oregon coast featuring chamber, symphonic, folk, jazz, concert band and dance music at various locations. Generally held the third full week in July, there are both indoor and outdoor performances with related classes and events. Call 24-hour phone for free brochure, concert locations and tickets. Partially funded by the Oregon Arts Commission. Limited edition poster available. Visa/MC.

25 **Playwrights' American Conservatory Theatre (P.A.C.T.)**
226 S. Broadway, Coos Bay, 97420 (Hwy. 101 southbound in Coos Bay, directly across from Egyptian movie theater).
Tel: 269-2501
Located on the waterfront in an intimate setting, the Playwrights' American Conservatory Theatre offers a wide variety of exciting theater designed to serve a constantly changing summer community. Visiting theater artists complement the resident company. Classes offered regularly for both children and adults. Open year around, performances weekends only. Box office open 1-4 daily.

26 **Seaborne Art Gallery/Studio**
1656 Sherman Ave. (Hwy. 101), North Bend, 97459 (4 blks. south of the North Bend bridge). Tel: 756-3451
Owner-artist Sandy Kretzschmar welcomes visitors to view the gallery selection of "coastal impressions" in stoneware, porcelain, watercolor, fiber, glass, and wood by 50 Northwest artists. Visitors are also invited to watch Sandy and her apprentices at work producing stoneware seafood platters along with a variety of wheel-thrown pottery. Visa/MC/AmEx. 10-5 daily (summer), 10-5 Mon-Sat (winter).

COQUILLE

27 **Danielson Sweet Home**
965 N. Collier. Mailing address: 967 N. Collier, Coquille, 97423. Tel: 396-2945
This is not a bed and breakfast, but a completely furnished, remodeled older home which offers a private, relaxed "home away from home" by the day or week. Guests may prepare their own food in the completely equipped kitchen or eat in nearby restaurants. Close to period-style summer theater. Owners Phil and Sharon Aman live next door. No pets. Open year around.

GOLD BEACH-WEDDERBURN

28 **Catch of the Day**
P.O. Box 228, Wedderburn, 97491.
Tel: 247-7694 or 247-7593
Kay and Don Jenson and Robin Terrett make Japanese-style fish prints of primarily locally caught fish. Rock fish, steelhead, salmon, and perch are some of the species available. The prints are available unmatted, matted, or matted and framed. Shipping via UPS FOB Gold Beach. Call or write for more information or for an appointment.

o **Clay Hill Lodge**
See AGNESS AND BEYOND for listing.

29 **Fair Winds Bed and Breakfast**
3 mi. from Gold Beach, P.O. Box 1274, Gold Beach, 97444. Tel: 247-6753
A delightful home set high in the foothills of the Siskiyous with a distant view of the ocean. Five acres of wooded trails and a jacuzzi hot tub are for guests to enjoy along with one double and one single room, a library, guest bath and TV room. Call or write for reservations and a map. No pets, but children welcome. Smoking outside. Open year around.

30 Jerry's Rogue Jets

South end of Rogue River Bridge, port of Gold Beach, Box 1011, Gold Beach, 97444. Tel: 247-4571 (local) or 800-451-3645 (nationwide)
These are the longest trips available on the Rogue River. Overnight trips to rustic lodges upriver, to Paradise Lodge, or day trips that include meals can be arranged. Passengers see deer, bears, otters, eagles, osprey, sea lions, heron et al. in their natural habitat. Excellent narration by experienced guides. Visa/MC/Discover. Office: 7 AM-9 PM daily (May 1–Oct 30).

○ Lucas Pioneer Ranch and Lodge

See AGNESS AND BEYOND for listing.

○ Paradise Bar Lodge

See AGNESS AND BEYOND for listing.

31 Tu Tu'Tun Lodge

96550 North Bank Rogue, Gold Beach, 97444 (7 mi. up the north side of the Rogue River). Tel: 247-6664
Dirk and Laurie Van Zante's four-star lodge on the Rogue River takes its name from the Tu Tu'Tun Indians who lived on the very same site. Guests find a relaxed atmosphere, sophisticated service and a nationally acclaimed dining room serving regional specialties. Sixteen rooms with private baths, decks and fresh flowers, private dock, heated pool, library and lounge with massive stone fireplace. Visa/MC. May 1-Nov 1.

HARBOR

See BROOKINGS-HARBOR

NORTH BEND

See COOS BAY-NORTH BEND

PORT ORFORD

32 The Art Hatchery

Hwy. 101, P.O. Box 197, Port Orford, 97465. Tel: 332-4011
Vicki and Robert Courtright's friendly gallery displays the work of 35 professional Oregon artists. Five large showrooms feature oils and watercolors, crystalline glaze porcelain, and a large selection of stoneware pottery, plus wood and metal sculpture. Sandblasted driftwood and many other unusual items are also offered for purchase or viewing year around. Visa/MC. 9-5 daily or by appointment.

33 Rick Cook Wood Studio and Art Gallery

705 Oregon St., Port Orford, 97465. Tel: 332-0045
Located in one of Port Orford's historical houses, Oregon designer/craftsman Rick Cook specializes in "one-of-a-kind" handcrafted furniture and wood gift items. Visitors will also discover a collection of contemporary decorative art by other local artists and craftspeople. Both Rick's and the others' work has been shown in major juried and invitational shows around the state. Visa/MC. 9-6 daily.

34 HOME by the SEA Bed and Breakfast HOMESTAY

444 Jackson St. (1 blk. west of Hwy. 101 at south end of town), P.O. Box 606W, Port Orford, 97465. Tel: 332-2855
Alan and Brenda Mitchell's contemporary owner-built home has beach access and dramatic ocean views just out the window. Two bedrooms overlooking Historic Battle Rock Park have private baths, handcrafted myrtlewood queen beds and furniture by Rick Cook, cable TVs, electric blankets, telephones, and laundry privileges. Full breakfast is served. No smoking or pets. Visa/MC. Open all year.

WEDDERBURN

See GOLD BEACH-WEDDERBURN

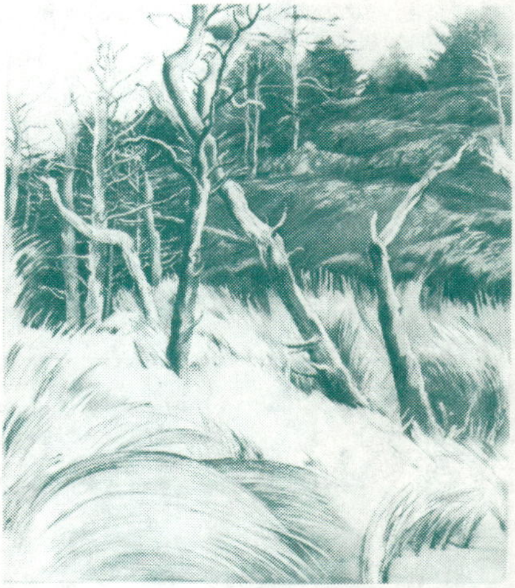

Cape Meares (North Coast), © Liza Jones

South Central Oregon

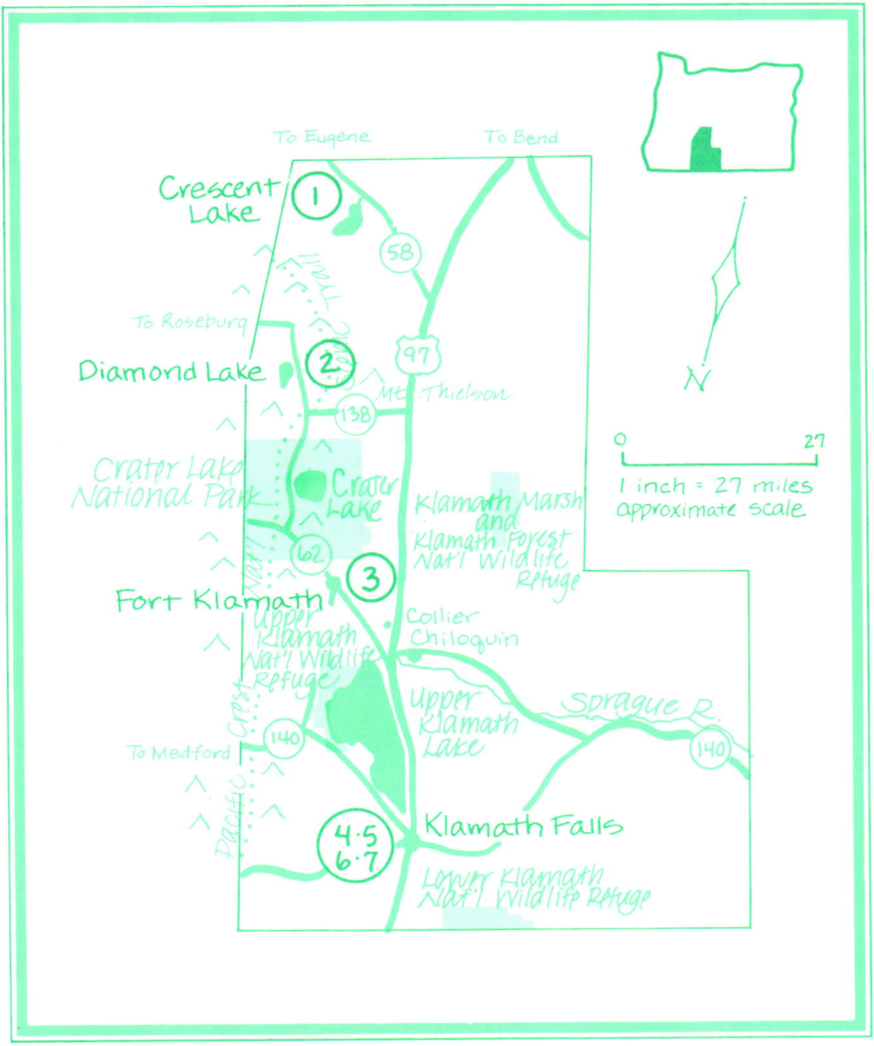

SOUTH CENTRAL OREGON REGIONAL NOTES

For approximately 35 miles from the area about 3 miles south of the junction of Highway 58 to that about 30 miles south, U.S. Highway 97 crosses the thickest part of a vast flat field of **pumice** *erupted from* **Mt. Mazama** *about 6,600 years ago. Indian legends recount a mountain that had been a towering volcano comparable in size to Shasta until it destroyed itself in a great eruption that poured fiery avalanches of hot pumice over the nearby landscape and sent a cloud of volcanic ash as far northeast as central Montana, and buried the area along the highway under a blanket of pumice that averages about 50 feet thick. The pumice field around the volcano is almost perfectly flat and quite variable in thickness, because it filled low spots in the landscape that had existed before the eruption. All that remains of Mt. Mazama is profiled against the skyline west of the pumice field.*

The **Pacific Crest National Scenic Trail** *passes through what is now* **Crater Lake National Park.** *The most outstanding feature of the park is the lake, noted for its brilliant blue color and located in the large volcanic caldera formed when Mt. Mazama blew itself up. The lake is filled entirely from rain and melting snow, and the annual input of water is so small that Crater Lake hardly flushes itself out. For this reason it would be easy to pollute and very difficult to clean up, making it a delicate and vulnerable gem that must be treated with the utmost care.*

A big glacier gouged out what is now **Diamond Lake,** *to the north of Crater Lake, during the last ice age. Trees grow poorly on the rubbly pumice field between Diamond Lake and Crater Lake, because water quickly soaks down beyond the reach of their roots. The pumice is so young and fresh that weathering has hardly begun to reduce it to soil, so the trees are growing on what is essentially a rubble of freshly broken rock. Pumice will float on water because basically it is a frozen foam of rhyolite glass so full of air bubbles that it is very light. It is used for making lightweight concrete aggregate, insulating, and soundproofing. It is not mined extensively in this part of Oregon, however, since there is little local demand for building materials.*

Upper Klamath Lake *is emerald green during the summer months because of the fantastic growth of a blue-green algae. There are only three other lakes in the world where algae grows in such abundance. It is 60% protein with an almost perfect amino acid balance. This particular balance is almost identical to the amino acid balance in the human body and is the highest known source of beta carotene and chlorophyll. As such, this algae growing in Klamath Lake is probably the richest natural source of nutrients for humans in the world.*

Klamath County has six wildlife refuges, 180 lakes and streams and an abundant supply of geothermal energy. Klamath Falls' hospital, Oregon Institute of Technology and many private homes in Klamath Falls are heated by it. The steam literally comes out of the cracks in some of the streets!

Collier State Park *features an open-air historic logging museum and 1880s-era pioneer cabin. Collier State Park has water and a day-use hitching area for horses. The Winema National Forest Supervisor's Office, Post Office Building, 2nd Floor, 7th and Walnut Street (P.O. Box 1390), Klamath Falls, Oregon 97601 (Tel: 883-6714), has maps and information on national forests in the area.*

The **Pacific Flyway** *funnels through the Klamath Basin, creating a haven for wildlife. More than 250 species of birds have been observed in the three national wildlife refuges in Klamath County (***Klamath Forest National Wildlife Refuge [Klamath Marsh],** *and* **Upper** *and* **Lower Klamath Wildlife Refuges),** *including the largest wintering population of bald eagles in the contiguous 48 states and the largest nesting population of bald eagles in Oregon.*

Oregon has an incredible variety of **wildflowers** *throughout the state. Please enjoy them, and please leave them undisturbed for others to enjoy. "A picked wildflower is a thing of beauty, but a joy for only one person for a few minutes." Some wildflowers grow in incredibly delicate environments and can take as long as seven years to bloom again.*

The Nature Conservancy owns and manages a large system of natural preserves throughout the state of Oregon. Call 228-9561 or visit the conservancy's offices in Portland (see Statewide Resources section) for information about preserves the public may visit in this region.

CRESCENT LAKE

1 Crescent Lake Lodge

On Crescent Lake at Crescent Lake junction off Hwy. 58 (Willamette Pass). P.O. Box 73, Crescent Lake, 97425. Tel: 433-2505

Built in the twenties, this is a place where family traditions are made. Seventeen cabins with rustic, knotty pine interiors, living rooms and modern kitchens; a grocery store; cross-country ski and boat rentals; bait, tackle, and a restaurant and lounge. Hosts are Larry and Fran Souza. Visa/MC. Open year around.

DIAMOND LAKE

2 Diamond Lake Resort

Diamond Lake, 97731 (on Hwy. 138, 20 mi. north of Crater Lake). Tel: 793-3333

Built in 1921, this lakeside mountain retreat has 40 motel units, 10 housekeeping units, 42 housekeeping cabins with fireplaces or wood stoves, three restaurants, camping and RV spaces. Year around recreation includes sailing, board sailing, snowmobiling, cross-country and snowcat skiing. Visitors can catch their own rainbow trout and have it prepared by the lodge chef. Open year around.

FORT KLAMATH

3 Fort Klamath Frontier Military Post

Fort Klamath (on Crater Lake Hwy. 62, 44 mi. north of Klamath Falls)

Originally established and garrisoned in 1863 to protect settlers from Indian attack and to maintain peace during the Civil War, the Fort played an important role in the 1864 Peace Treaty of "Council Grove" and in the Modoc War of 1872-1873. Eight acres of the original post are now a Klamath County Park, with historical interpretations and exhibits provided by the Klamath County Museum. 10-6 daily (June-Sept).

KLAMATH FALLS

4 Alice's Saddle Rock Cafe

1012 Main St., Klamath Falls, 97601. Tel: 884-1444

Alice and Nancy Kilham named their restaurant in the Pelican Hotel after the original restaurant located there when the hotel was built in 1928. (The faint outline of the original sign painted on the building is still visible.) All the food is cooked on the premises and includes homemade pastries and desserts, steamed milk and espresso drinks, imported beers, cocktails, Oregon wines, and Sunday brunch with Eggs Benedict and freshly squeezed juice. Live music Fri-Sun. Visa/MC. 7:30 AM-2 PM Mon-Fri (breakfast and lunch), 5:30-9 PM Wed-Sun (dinner), 9AM-2 PM Sun (brunch).

5 Cell Tech

1300 Main St., Klamath Falls, 97601. Tel: 882-5406 or 800-321-1303 (out-of-state)

Daryl and Marta Coleman harvest, freeze-dry, and market the blue-green algae from Upper Klamath Lake. Composed mostly of proteins and minerals, it is sold powdered, in capsules, and as a liquid drink mix. It seems to provide those nutrients that help prevent such degenerative diseases as heart disease, cancer, arthritis, and many allergies. Visa/MC. 8:30-4:30 Mon-Fri.

6 Favell Museum of Western Art and Indian Artifacts

125 W. Main, Klamath Falls, 97601 (97 freeway interchange at Link River Bridge). Tel: 882-9996

The largest public display of miniature firearms in the world, plus over 60,000 mounted arrowheads and other artifacts, pottery, baskets, 800 realistic original paintings, dioramas, sculptures, carvings, and miniatures. Original art sales gallery with many well-known and selected local artists. Limited edition print gallery, gift and book shop. Visa/MC. 9:30-5:30 Mon-Sat.

7 Klamath County Museum Complex

1451 Main (Klamath Co. Museum), Tel: 883-4208; 31 Main (Baldwin Hotel Museum), Tel: 883-4207; Klamath Falls, 97601

The complex operates three museums and a restored 1906 trolley car. The county museum has artifacts, wildlife, life-size rooms depicting the settlement of the Klamath area and Native American heritage. Research library offers materials on local history. Open 9-5 Tues-Sat (June-Oct), 11-5 Tues-Sat (Nov-May). Baldwin Hotel Museum, built in 1906, still contains its original furnishings. Now a state and national landmark. Viewed by tour only, 11-5 Tues-Sat (June-Sept). Trolley connecting downtown and two museums, summer only. (See Fort Klamath Frontier Military Post listing in Fort Klamath.)

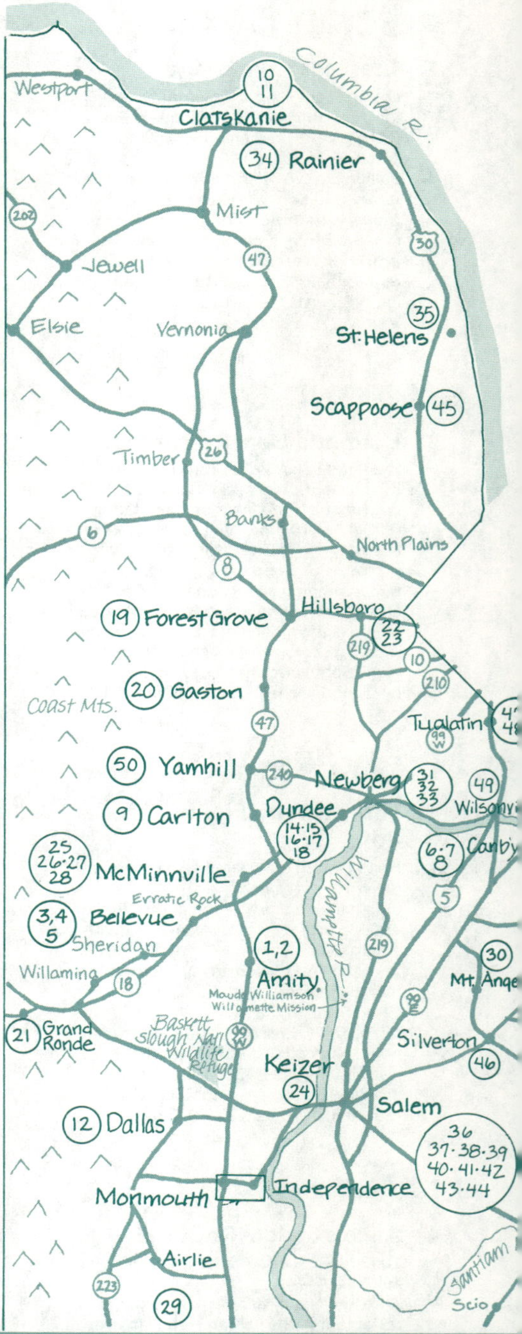
Columbia R.
Westport
10
11
Clatskanie
34
Rainier
Mist
202
Jewell
47
30
35
St. Helens
Elsie
Vernonia
Scappoose
45
Timber
26
Banks
North Plains
6
8
19
Forest Grove
Hillsboro
22
23
219
10
210
20
Gaston
Coast Mts.
47
Tualatin
99W
50
Yamhill
240
Newberg
31
32
33
49
9
Carlton
Dundee
14·15
16·17
18
6·7
8
25
26·27
28
McMinnville
Erratic Rock
5
3,4
5
Bellevue
Sheridan
Willamette R.
1,2
219
30
Amity
Willamina
18
Maude Williamson
Willamette Mission
99E
21
Grand Ronde
Baskett Slough Nat'l Wildlife Refuge
99W
Silverton
46
Keizer
24
Salem
12
Dallas
36
37·38·39
40·41·42
43·44
Independence
Monmouth
Santiam
Airlie
223
29
Scio

Northern Willamette Valley

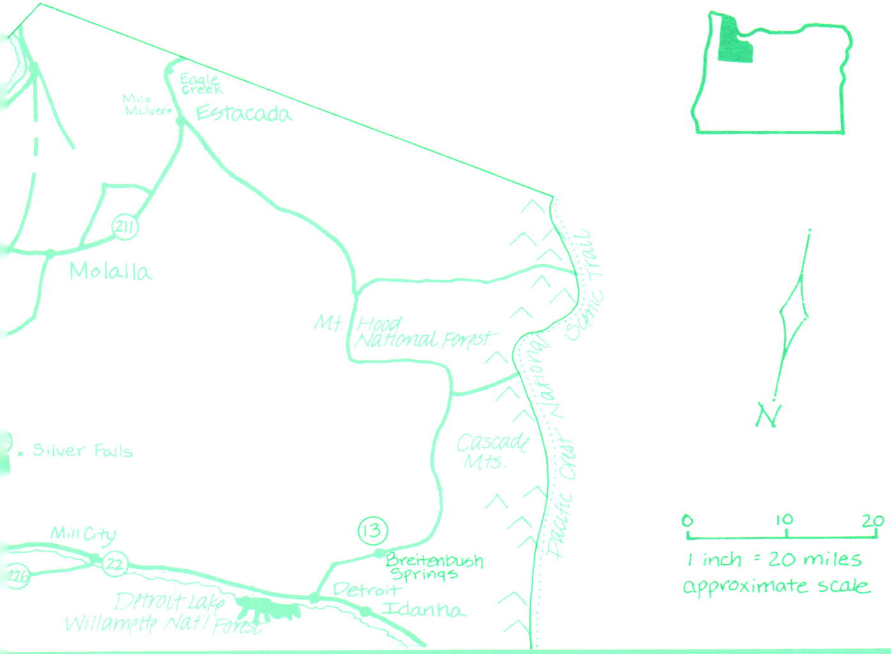

NORTHERN WILLAMETTE VALLEY REGIONAL NOTES

It was its **rich, fertile farmland** *that made the Willamette Valley the destination of the early pioneers following the Oregon Trail and the area around Oregon City (Portland Metro map), Canby, Molalla, Salem, and St. Paul are rich in history about the original settlers. There are even remains of early potteries and brick yards established by potters from the Midwest. Temperatures seldom fall below 25 degrees Fahrenheit in the winter or rise above 80 degrees Fahrenheit in the summer. The Coast Range stops enough of the Pacific weather to allow just the right amount of rainfall to fall between the Coast Range to the west and the Cascade Mountains to the east. Most of what moisture is left in the eastward-moving clouds is dropped as the clouds try to get over the Cascade Mountains. It is an ideal farming situation.*

Around Canby, where seeds and bulbs are grown, there are fields of blooming iris, dahlias, and other flowers in the spring and summer. More than **90 percent of the nation's filberts (hazelnuts)** *are grown in Yamhill County, and numerous vineyards and wineries have located throughout the valley. All manner of fruits and vegetables from berries to beans are grown throughout the area, and although migrant workers are a common sight, many an Oregonian can remember "picking" as a summer job in his youth. The area is still known for its plentiful "u-pick" farms.*

Champoeg State Park *commemorates the site where residents of the "Willamette Settlements" met in 1843 to vote on whether to establish pro-American provisional government or remain under the rule of the Hudson Bay Company. By a 52-to-50 vote, the settlers elected to form a provisional government of Oregon, making the valley the center of the first American commonwealth on the Pacific Coast. From here begins the 40-mile French Prairie Loop through farmland and old pioneer settlements. The land here is mostly flat and easily cultivated yet with Mt. Hood towering in the distance to the east. North of* **Dallas** *on Highway 22 is the* **Baskett Slough National Wildlife Refuge**. *At Bellevue on Highway 18 is* **Erratic Rock** *on a hilltop to the west. It is a large, erratic boulder from Canada that was deposited from a melting ice raft about 10,000 years ago.*

The **North Santiam River Highway** *is one of the Willamette Valley's main connecting routes to Central Oregon and passes by Detroit Lake, between the* **Jefferson** *and* **Mt. Washington Wilderness Areas** *in the* **Willamette National Forest**. **The Pacific Crest National Scenic Trail** *crosses Highway 20 just east of where it connects to Highway 22. For information regarding trailheads, wilderness areas, maps, trail and fire conditions, etc., contact the Willamette National Forest Supervisor's Office, Federal Building, 211 E. 7th Avenue (P.O. Box 10607), Eugene, Oregon 97440 (Tel: 687-6522); or stop in at Willamette Ranger Station across from the entrance to Detroit Lake State Park.*

Many **state parks** *in the Willamette Valley have trails for hiking, including Champoeg, Mary S. Young, Molalla River, Silver Falls, and Willamette Mission. Bicycle paths are located at Champoeg, Silver Falls, and Willamette Mission State Parks. There are equestrian trails at Milo McIver, Silver Falls, and Willamette Mission State Parks. There are boat ramps at Milo McIver, Molalla River, and Willamette Mission State Parks; a boat dock and ramp at Detroit Lake; and a boat dock on the Willamette River at Champoeg.*

Silver Falls State Park, *with its 7-mile trail leading past a dozen waterfalls in two densely forested canyons, has a swimming area and miles of horse and bike trails. It also has extensive group facilities, including a group tent trailer camp with community buildings, group picnic areas, organizational and youth camp facilities, and the Silver Falls Conference Center. Club camping is available at Detroit Lake; group camping is available at Champoeg and Milo McIver State Parks. Group picnic facilities are located at Champoeg, Milo McIver, and Willamette Mission. Champoeg also has a group meeting hall.*

The **Willamette River Greenway** *extends 255 miles from Cottage Grove Reservoir and Dexter Dam (Southern Willamette Valley) to the Columbia River at Portland. It provides opportunities for boating, picnicking, wildlife study, hiking, and overnight camping on public land. Most land along the greenway is private. The State Parks Division has published a Willamette River Recreation Guide to help direct users to public river-access points and landings. (See Statewide Resources section for this and information regarding The Nature Conservancy's preserves in this area that the public may visit.)*

AMITY

1 Amity Vineyards

18150 Amity Vineyards Rd. S.E., Amity, 97101 (Amity is 6 mi. south of McMinnville on 99W; once in Amity, follow signs). Tel: 835-2362

Ione and Myron Redford and Janis Checchia invite visitors to try their Pinot Noir, White Riesling, Chardonnay, Gewurztraminer, Solstice Blanc and Oregon Blush. Their wines have won 12 gold medals in regional and national competitions. Informal picnic area with spectacular view. Visa/MC. 12-5 daily (June-Oct), 12-5 Sat, Sun (Nov-May, closed Dec 24-Jan 31). (See Bellevue for Amity's Oregon Wine Tasting Room listing.)

2 Hidden Springs Winery

9360 S.E. Eola Hills Rd., Amity, 97101 (Amity is on 99W 6 mi. south of McMinnville; from Amity take Nursery St. in town, or Amity Rd. in the country, east toward Hopewell, 1 mi., go right, south, on Old Bethel Rd. for 1 mi., then turn left, east, on Eola Hills Rd. and wind uphill 4½ mi. to vineyard). Tel: 835-2782

Small premium Oregon winery operated by Don and Carolyn Byard and Alvin and Jo Alexanderson, producing carefully made White Riesling, Pinot Noir, Chardonnay and other wines exclusively from Oregon grapes. Wine tasting, tours and picnicking facilities with stunning view of Cascade mountains, surrounding vineyards and orchards. 12-5 daily except Tues (June-Aug), 12-5 Sat, Sun (Mar-May, Sept-Nov), or by appointment. Closed Dec, Jan, Feb.

BELLEVUE

3 Augustine's

19706 S.W. Hwy. 18, Bellevue, 97128 (halfway between Portland and Lincoln City about 10 mi. west of McMinnville; on top of Lawrence Gallery). Tel: 843-3225

Wines from nearby vineyards in the surrounding Oregon countryside accompany the individually prepared meals here. The freshest ingredients are used, including fresh seafood and pasta. Augustine's make all their own desserts and Sunday brunch pastries. They even churn their own ice cream. 11-9 Wed-Sat, 11-8 Sun.

4 Lawrence Gallery

19706 S.W. Hwy. 18, Bellevue, 97128 (halfway between Portland and Lincoln City about 10 mi. west of McMinnville). Mailing address: P.O. Box 187, Sheridan, 97378. Tel: 843-3633

Represents 200 artists and craftspeople producing a wide variety of some of the finest Northwest work being produced. Monthly exhibitions highlight important new work by selected artists and craftspeople, a number of whom have received fellowship awards from the Oregon Arts Commission and the National Endowment for the Arts. While at the gallery, visitors can enjoy fine wines in the Oregon Wine Tasting Room and fine food at Augustine's upstairs. Visa/MC/AmEx/Discover. 10-5:30 daily.

5 Oregon Wine Tasting Room

19706 S.W. Hwy. 18, Bellevue, 97128 (halfway between Portland and Lincoln City about 10 mi. west of McMinnville).

Operated by Amity Vineyards, this multi-vineyard tasting room features wine from over 30 Oregon wineries, including table wine and fruit and berry wines. All available for free tasting and retail sales. Visa/MC. 12-5:30 daily. (See Amity for Amity Vineyards listing.)

CANBY

6 Filbertreats

356 N.W. First Ave., P.O. Box 612, Canby, 97013. Tel: 266-8172

Oregon is known for its filberts and since 1980 Lester Gahler has been doing fascinating things with them in his candy shop in Canby. Kitchen tours show such filbert delights as chocolate-covered, vanilla, butterscotch and sherry-flavored filberts being made. 9-5 Mon-Sat.

7 Swan Island Dahlias

995 N.W. 22nd Ave., P.O. Box 800 TG, Canby, 97013. Tel: 266-7711

The Gitts family is the nation's largest grower, with 50 acres and over 300 varieties of dahlias in bloom from August until frost. Their free indoor Dahlia Festival and show, where thousands of cut flowers are arranged by professional designers, is the largest of its kind staged by one grower anywhere. 1988 show dates are Sept 3-5 and Sept 10-12 from 11 AM to 6 PM. Visa/MC. Fields open 8 AM-dusk daily (Aug-frost). Office and order desk open 9-4:30 Mon-Fri. Catalog cost refundable with first purchase. Gift certificates available.

8 Tall Talk Dairy

11961 S. Emerson Rd., Canby, 97013 (approx. 6 mi. southwest of Canby, 25 mi. south of Portland). Tel: 266-1644
Esther and Harlen Peterson's goat dairy produces milk and related dairy products, including raw and pasteurized goat milk and cheeses (feta, plain jack, jalapeño jack, caraway jack, and eight varieties of soft cheeses). Products are delivered to retail outlets throughout the Portland area, e.g. Strohecker's, Nature's, some Thriftway stores, and Fred Meyer Nutrition Centers, and through a distributor to other locations. Some items are only available seasonally. The Petersons hope to be producing yogurt and ice cream in the near future. Visitors are welcome by appointment. A Neiman-Marcus selection.

CARLTON

9 Chateau Benoit

6580 N.E. Mineral Springs Rd., Carlton, 97111 (just southwest of Lafayette on Hwy. 99W, go north on Mineral Springs Rd. for 1½ mi. to winery on right. Note: if you take Hwy. 18 bypass to avoid McMinnville you will miss it).
Tel: 864-2991 or 864-3666
Founded in 1979 and owned and operated by Fred and Mary Benoit with winemaker Gerard Rottier, it produces award-winning varietal table wines, notably Sauvignon Blanc, and Müller-Thurgau and hand-done sparkling wines in the Champagne method. Some of its Pinot Noir, Chardonnay and Riesling grapes come from its 15-year-old vineyard near Eugene. Picnic tables with beautiful view. Groups of more than 15, please phone ahead. Visa/MC. 11-5 Mon-Fri, 12-5 Sat, Sun.

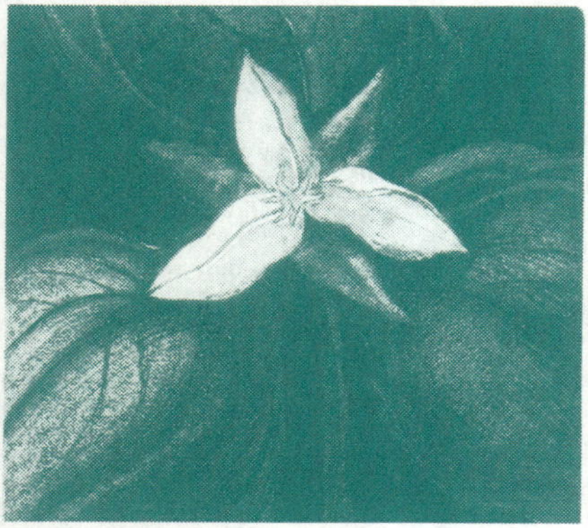

Trillium, © Liza Jones

CLATSKANIE

10 City of Clatskanie

95 S. Nehalem St., P.O. Box 9, Clatskanie, 97016. Tel: 728-2622
Office: 8-5 daily.
The City of Clatskanie nestles along the Clatskanie River and is a good stopping place on Highway 30 between the coast and Portland. Near the downtown area visitors can picnic at the city park, which has a heated pool, camping facilities, and a boat ramp. Also popular are tours of the historic Flippin House, a restored, turreted, Queen Anne-style home built in the 1890s. For old-fashioned fun, the hometown Fourth of July celebration with canoe races, a parade, logging show, and, of course, fireworks, is a classic. Clatskanie is also becoming a favorite with sailboarders because of the wide sand beaches and excellent winds about four miles from town at Jones Beach.

1988-89 Clatskanie Area Events include:

July 4: Old-fashioned Fourth of July Celebration

11 Hump's Restaurant

50 W. Columbia River Hwy., Clatskanie, 97016. Tel: 728-2626
What Forris Humphrey started 30 years ago as a candy shop and soda fountain has grown to a restaurant and lounge with coffee shop. Forris's daughter Pamela, her husband, and teen-age daughters carry on the tradition of family service. Travelers stop for homemade peanut brittle, special homemade desserts, or Sunday brunch. Columbia River boaters can follow signs up Clatskanie River at high tide to Hump's own dock. Visa/MC/AmEx/Diners. 6 AM-10 PM daily.

LOOK AT A MAP

Before setting out even on a marked trail, **orient yourself.** *Take note of drainages and ridges, and when out walking continually take note of where you are. An eight-year-old boy was able to find his way back to his parents' campsite after 24 hours because he had paid attention to which way the stream flowed, the position of the sun and the configuration of the hills. Always* **tell someone where you are going** *and when you plan to return.*

DALLAS

12 Cherry Knoll Creations

3945 Mistletoe Rd., Dallas, 97338.
Tel: 623-6169
Cathy Van Ess's cherry creations grew out of a large Christmas show she has in her house every year. Her cherry sauce is great for topping cheesecake, ice cream, and French toast, and the cherry syrup is thicker by far than maple syrup. She makes cherry and cherry/berry jellies, cherry honey (a thick, reddish honey with chunks of cherries in it), and even cherry vinegar! A Neiman-Marcus selection. Also available at the Prancing Pony in Independence and Guy's Hardware Store in Dallas. Write or call for Christmas gift pack brochure.

DETROIT

13 Breitenbush Retreat Center

P.O. Box 578 (Mile 10, Route 46), Detroit, 97342. Tel: 854-3501 or 854-3314
Located at Breitenbush Hot Springs, 60 miles east of Salem in the Cascade Mountains near Mt. Jefferson Wilderness and Lake Detroit, this is a beautiful setting for conferences, workshops, and personal retreats. Restored and renovated, the historic 1930s mineral springs resort provides year-around rustic, cozy cabin accommodations, hearty vegetarian meals, mineral spring baths, hot tubs, steam sauna, and direct access to hiking and cross-country skiing in nearby old-growth forests. Call or write for information and calendar of events. Office: 9-1 and 2-6 daily. Reservations necessary.

DUNDEE

14 Dundee Orchards

P.O. Box 327, Dundee, 97115.
Tel: 538-1063
Oregon produces nearly 98% of the nation's hazelnuts (filberts). In 1984 two farm families with small orchards joined forces to create delicious hazelnut butters: creamy, crunchy, walnut, and chocolate. They intend to continue expanding their contribution to Northwest cuisine. Send for retail price list. A Neiman-Marcus selection and also available at Made in Oregon Shops in Portland and Salem, Josephson's in Astoria, Blue Heron Cheese in Tillamook, Oregon Store in Ashland, Placesetters in Medford, and at Knudsen Erath Winery.

15 Elk Cove Dundee Wine Cellar

575 S.E. Hwy. 99W, Dundee, 97115. Tel: 538-0911
Winemakers Pat and Joe Campbell, owners of Elk Cove Vineyards, invite visitors to taste their fine wines at the Dundee Wine Cellar in the heart of Oregon's wine country. Over 100 different wines from Oregon's premier wineries are available here, as well as deli items and bread for assembling a "wine country picnic." Visa/MC. 11-6 daily (May-Nov), 11-5 daily (Dec-April). (See Gaston for Elk Cove Vineyards listing.)

16 Knudsen Erath Winery

17000 N.E. Knudsen Lane, Dundee, 97115 (blue state highway sign marks turn-off at 9th St. from center of Dundee on Hwy. 99W, then 2¼ mi. up hill to winery). Tel: 538-3318
Founded by Oregon winemaking pioneers Dick Erath and Cal Knudsen, this is the state's largest vineyard-winery operation, with over 100 acres of grapes, and one of the largest producers of Pinot Noir in America. The award-winning winery, overlooking the rolling Red Hills of Dundee, also produces Chardonnay, White Riesling, and limited quantities of Cabernet Sauvignon and Gewurztraminer, using time-honored, uncompromising wine-making practices, with a minimum of processing. Picnic sites and facilities for private parties. Large group tours are welcome by appointment. Visa/MC. 10-6 daily (summer), 11-5 daily (winter).

17 Sokol Blosser Winery

5000 N.E. Sokol Blosser Lane, Dundee, 97115 (at southwestern end of Dundee, turn north on Sokol Blosser Lane off Hwy. 99W just 1 mi. east of east end of Hwy. 18 bypass around McMinnville).
Tel: 864-2282
Owned and operated by the Sokol and Blosser families, the winery and tasting room overlook the Willamette Valley and surrounding orchards and vineyards. Award-winning winemaker Bob McRitchie produces White Riesling, Chardonnay, Pinot Noir, Gewurztraminer, Sauvignon Blanc, Müller-Thurgau and two special blends, Bouquet Blanc and Bouquet Rose. Tasting room available for banquets and meetings for small groups. Group tours by appointment. Visa/MC. 11-5 daily.

18 Tualatin Vineyards Dundee Tasting Room

110 S.W. Hwy. 99W, Dundee, 97115.
Tel: 538-1410
This is Tualatin Vineyards second tasting room. Visitors are invited to sample and purchase White Riesling, Gewurztraminer, Chardonnay, Pinot Noir, and other estate-bottled wines from the 15-year-old winery. Visa/MC. The tasting room is open 9:30-5:30 Mon-Fri, 10-6 Sat-Sun (March-Dec); 9:30-5:30 Fri, 10-6 Sat-Sun (Jan-Feb). (See Forest Grove for Tualatin Vineyards listing.)

FOREST GROVE

19 Tualatin Vineyards

Rt. 1, Box 339, Forest Grove, 97116 (between Banks and Forest Grove; from Hwy. 26 go southwest on Hwy. 6, following blue vineyard signs). Tel: 357-5005
Visitors are welcomed by a spectacular view of Tualatin's 85-acre vineyard and the Tualatin Valley from the winery's new tasting room and picnic area. White Riesling, Gewurztraminer, Chardonnay, Pinot Noir, and other estate-bottled wines are offered for tasting. William Fuller is Tualatin's winemaker. Tours of the 15-year-old winery and group tastings arranged by appointment. Annual Thanksgiving Art Show and 4th of July Barrel Tasting. Visa/MC. Tasting room open 10-4 Mon-Fri, 1-5 Sat-Sun. Closed Jan. (See Dundee for Tualatin Vineyards Dundee Tasting Room listing.)

GASTON

20 Elk Cove Vineyards

27751 N.W. Olson Rd., Gaston, 97119 (just south of Gaston on Hwy. 47—take Olson Rd. 2.8 mi. west to Elk Cove; turn right at mailbox, right beyond new vineyard). Tel: 985-7760
Named for herds of Roosevelt Elk which migrate here each spring and with spectacular views of the coast range, Elk Cove Vineyards is operated by Pat and Joe Campbell and produces estate-bottled, award-winning Rieslings, Pinot Noirs, Cabernet Sauvignon, Gewurztraminer, and Chardonnay wines. Tasting room and picnic area may be reserved for banquets and meetings. Group tours by appointment. Riesling Festival, Memorial Day weekend; Pinot Noir Picnic, Labor Day weekend. Visa/MC. 12-5 daily. (See Dundee for Elk Cove tasting room listing.)

GRAND RONDE

21 Confederated Tribes of Grand Ronde

P.O. Box 38, Grand Ronde, 97347.
Tel: 879-5215
The Confederated Tribes of Grand Ronde is comprised of over 20 tribes and bands from Western Oregon and Northern California, including the Kalapuyan, Shasta, Rogue River, Molalla, and Umpqua.

By Executive Order in 1855, the tribes were relocated from their original homelands onto the Grand Ronde Reservation. Later federal policies gradually reduced the size of the reservation, and in 1954, Congress passed the Termination Act which severed the trust relationship between the government and Tribe.

However, in 1983, the Grand Ronde Confederated Tribes regained their federal recognition, and are working towards establishing tribal self-sufficiency. A nine-member Tribal Council sets policy for programs which provide assistance in education, social services, health services, housing, judicial and cultural development. There are now over 2100 people enrolled in the Grand Ronde Tribes.

Each year, the Confederated Tribes of Grand Ronde observe Memorial Day with various activities, hold an annual Pow-wow on the third week of August and, on or around November 22nd of each year, celebrate the Tribe's Restoration. The public is welcome to participate in these activities, which all take place in Grand Ronde.

HILLSBORO

22 Loughridge Farm

13300 S.W. River Rd., Hillsboro, 97123 (⅛ of a mi. on River Rd. off Scholls Ferry Rd. [Hwy. 210]). Tel: 628-1286
In 1907 Ferd Groner came north to become the "Walnut King of Oregon" with over 400 acres of walnuts. The 50-foot-high barn red dryer he built in 1916 is still in use. The farm's country store features walnuts, filberts (hazelnuts), elephant and Italian garlic, garlic braids, wreaths, and other gift items. Resident sheep and Canadian geese too. 10 AM-dusk daily except Mon. Tours by appointment.

23 Oak Knoll Winery

Rt. 6, Box 184, Hillsboro, 97123 (from Hillsboro go south on Hwy. 219 to Burkhalter Rd. on left and then winery on the right). Tel: 648-8198

Founded in 1970 by the Ron Vuylsteke family, Oak Knoll produces quality, award-winning wines from Oregon-grown fruits, berries and varietal grapes. Oak Knoll features all popular varietal grape wines as well as dry and semi-sweet fruit and berry wines. Awarded Governor's Trophies at 1983 State Fair for Pinot Noir and raspberry wines. Oak Knoll hosts its annual "Bacchus Goes Bluegrass" Wine Festival in mid-May and "Niagarafest" in mid-Aug. 12-5 daily (summer), 12-5 Wed-Sun (winter), or by appointment. Visa/MC. (See Lincoln City, Central Coast, for Shipwreck Cellars—Oak Knoll Wine Tasting Room listing.)

KEIZER

24 Willow Lake Nursery and Farms

5655 Windsor Island Rd. N., Keizer, 97303. Tel: 390-3032

Grandpa Blake started this farm in 1906. Now Jim LaRock, John, Bill and Phyllis Blake and friends grow walnuts and hazelnuts (filberts), and then during November and December put up Oregon gift packs with food items produced all over Oregon including their own chocolate-covered walnuts and filberts. Mail order year-round. Ship UPS. Catalog on request. They also have a 2½ acre retail nursery with complete selection of landscape materials. Visa/MC. 9-5:30 Mon-Sat, 10-4 Sun (closed Jan).

McMINNVILLE

25 Gallery Players of Oregon

Corner of 2nd and Ford St., P.O. Box 245, McMinnville, 97128. Tel: 472-2227

The Gallery Players offer year-round performances of drama, comedy, musicals and full dance programs. Located just off Hwy. 18 to the coast, the Gallery Theatre is surrounded by Oregon's wine country, award-winning restaurants, and comfortable motels. Programs are partially supported by grants from the Oregon Arts Commission. Tickets available at the Book Shop on 3rd St. or at the theater. Visa/MC. Performances at 7 PM Sun, 8 PM Thurs-Sat.

26 Mattey House Bed and Breakfast Inn

10221 N.E. Mattey Lane, McMinnville, 97128 (between Lafayette and McMinnville turn off Hwy. 99W onto Mattey Lane and go to the oak tree). Tel: 434-5058

This Queen Anne turn-of-the-century house on ten acres in the heart of Oregon's wine country is on the National Historic Register. Decorated with Victorian-style antiques and period wallpapers, it has four guest rooms, one with private bath, overlooking large evergreens, a vineyard and orchard. Gene and Susan Irvin serve full breakfasts with homemade breads and jellies (from their own fruits and berries). No smoking on the premises. No pets. Older children welcomed. Visa/MC. Feb-Dec (closed Jan).

27 Nick's Italian Cafe

521 3rd St., McMinnville, 97128. Tel: 434-4471

Because Nick Peirano has been making meals for the local winemakers for the past ten years, his wine list is extensive. He serves five-course, fixed-price dinners with everything made on the premises, including fresh pasta, pastries and desserts. He uses fresh, local produce whenever available. Reservations suggested. Take-out lunches available. Dinners daily except Mon.

28 Yamhill Valley Vineyards

16250 S.W. Oldsville Rd., McMinnville, 97128 (5 mi. southwest of McMinnville on Hwy. 18 to Oldsville Rd., follow signs ½ mi. to winery). Tel: 843-3100

Founded in 1983, Yamhill Valley Vineyards is owned and operated by the Burger-McCall and Hinrichs families. The winery and tasting room overlook 50 acres of vineyards planted in Pinot Noir, Chardonnay, Riesling, and Pinot Gris. Winemaker Denis Burger produces varietal, vintage-dated wines from these and other Willamette Valley grapes. Tasting room available for banquets and meetings. Groups welcome by appointment. Picnic facilities also available. Visa/MC. 11-5 daily except Mon.

MONMOUTH

29 Airliē Winery

15305 Dunn Forest Rd., Monmouth, 97361 (from Monmouth go 7 mi. south on 99W; 6 mi. west on Airlie Rd. to Airlie; go south on Maxfield Creek Rd. 3 mi.; go east on Dunn Forest Rd. about ½ mi. Follow signs). Tel: 838-6013
Alice and Larry Preedy's winery is located approximately 15 miles southwest of Monmouth and 20 miles northwest of Corvallis, overlooking the Dunn Forest Vineyard. The winery is dedicated to vintage-dated premium quality wines. They produce Pinot Noir, Chardonnay, Müller-Thurgau, Gewurztraminer, White Riesling, and an award-winning Pinot Noir Blanc called "Crimson." Tasting room with picnic area by pond open 12-5 Sat-Sun (Oct-May). Closed Jan. Open 12-5 daily except Mon (June-Sept). Group tours by appointment. Call or write for festival event information.

○ Oregon Elderhostel

See STATEWIDE RESOURCES for listing.

MT. ANGEL

30 Mt. Angel Oktoberfest

P.O. Box 1054, Mt. Angel, 97362.
Tel: 845-9440
"Put a little 'omm-pah' in your life" at the 23nd Annual Oktoberfest, Thurs, Sept 15, through Sun, Sept 18, 1988. Almost 300,000 people are expected to take part in festival activities, which include Bavarian dancing, yodeling, street dancing, art shows, sports events, and tours of Mt. Angel convent and abbey. Free kindergarten, puppet shows, and pony rides for children. Hot-air balloon rides, Bavarian biergarten and weingarten for adults. No admission charge. All proceeds go to local charities. Call for schedule.

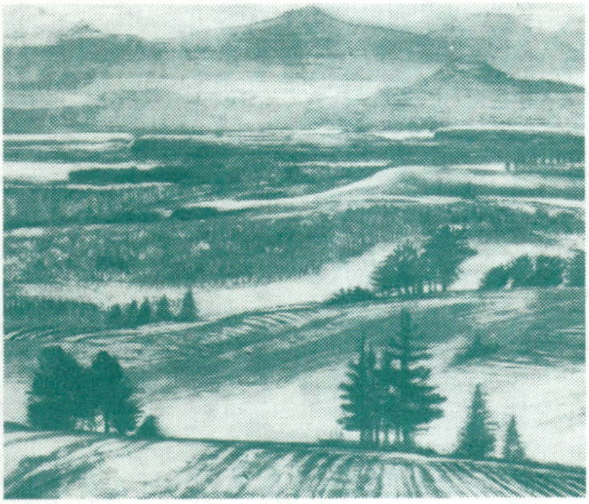

NEWBERG

31 Tourism Council of Yamhill County

115 N. Washington St., Newberg, 97132. Tel: 538-2014
Office: 9-5 Mon-Fri, 10-3 Sat (summer); 9-5 Mon-Fri (winter).
Yamhill County is Oregon's wine country. Fifteen wineries, including the state's two largest and several tasting rooms, are located in this beautiful, fertile valley. Residents and visitors also appreciate the county's small, comfortable towns, fresh produce, antique shops, museums, historical homes and sites, and recreational areas and resorts. Sometimes called "Portland's Country Next Door," Yamhill County has much to offer the busy city-dweller or unhurried traveler.

1988 Yamhill County Area Events include:

- May 28-29: Memorial Day Boat Races, Newberg
- June 16-19: Phil Sheridan Days & Phil Sheridan Rodeo, Sheridan
- July 7-9: Turkey-Rama, McMinnville
- July 16: Yamhill Derby Days, Yamhill
- July 23: Amity County Fair, Amity
- July 23-24: Old Timers Parade, Dayton
- July 28-31: Newberg Old-Fashioned Festival, Newberg
- July 30-31: Carlton Fun Days, Carlton
- Aug 5-8: Yamhill County Fair, McMinnville
- Aug 12: International Pinot Noir Festival, McMinnville
- Nov 24-26: Wine Country Thanksgiving, all Yamhill County wineries

32 Oregon Apiaries

1306 N. Harmony Lane, P.O. Box 1078, Newberg, 97132 (.8 mi. north on 99W past Newberg Springbrook stoplight; on right of road when going north).
Tel: 538-8546
Beekeepers since 1979, John and Marita Trunk founded Oregon Apiaries in 1983. They have perfected the production of honey creme, a smooth, semi-solid form of honey which they mix with other all-natural products such as hazelnuts (filberts), raspberries, and blueberries. All these products, as well as bulk raw honey, are available at their plant and at all Made in Oregon Shops, the Tillamook Cheese Factory, and Sokol Blosser Winery. A Neiman-Marcus selection. Visa/MC. 9-4:30 Mon-Fri, 10-5 Sat.

Mist Country (Willamette Valley), © *Liza Jones*

33 Rex Hill Vineyards

30835 N. Hwy. 99W, Newberg, 97132 (on Hwy. 99W, 2½ mi. east of Newberg). Tel: 538-0666
Established in 1982 on historic Rex Hill, Paul Hart's and Jan Jacobsen's showcase winery in a remodeled nut dryer emphasizes vintage-dated, vineyard-designated bottlings of Pinot Noir, Chardonnay, White Riesling and Gewurztraminer using its own and other Willamette Valley grapes. Picnic facilities available. Groups, meetings and caterings welcome by appointment. Tasting Room: 11-5 daily (May-Dec), 11-5 Fri-Sun (Feb-April), closed Jan. Visa/MC/AmEx/Discover.

RAINIER

34 Bonaventura

71318 Neer Rd., Rainier, 97048. Tel: 556-2126
John Ullman and Marilyn Kennelly make fine gourmet products celebrating the essence of Oregon at their family-operated commercial kitchen. Dessert Conserve is a magnificent blend of raspberries, orange, and bittersweet chocolate—like fine chocolates in a jar—for topping desserts. Bonaventura Biscotti, "The Dipping Cookie," in filbert or orange, is made to be dipped in coffee/tea or wine. A Bloomingdale's "Oregon, the Natural Resource" selection. Free catalog: Bonaventure, P.O. Box 763, Rainier, OR 97048.

ST. HELENS

35 Oregon Hill Farms

61160 Skeet Ave., St. Helens, 97051. Tel: 397-2791
Dan and Joe Luttrell not only make their all-natural syrup the old-fashioned way, they also farm and process most of the berries used in it. This versatile topping made with whole fruit is great on ice cream, waffles, and cheesecake. Flavors include marionberry, apple cinnamon, raspberry, apricot, and strawberry. "A taste of Oregon to serve or give as a gift." Available at Strohecker's in Portland, Wizer's in Lake Oswego, Made in Oregon Shops in Portland, Salem, and Eugene, Osbornes at Cannon Beach, Maiden Bend, et al. Gift packs and shipping available. Call or write for more information.

SALEM

36 . . . And Old Lace

320 Court St., Salem, 97301 (in downtown Salem, 2 mi. off I-5 from Exit 253, north or south). Tel: 585-6010
Elizabeth Southwell's store is a replica of an early Salem linen and lace shop selling doilies, textiles, heirloom embroideries, fancywork and quilts—many made by early Oregon settlers. Also featured is the work of textile artists as well as clothing supplies, old buttons, edgings and keepsakes. Visa/MC. 10:30-5:30 Mon-Sat.

37 Croissant Co. Bakery and Café

190 High St. S.E., Salem, 97301. Tel: 36-BREAD
Fred Schneider's famous "Salem French Ficelle" is Oregon's only version of the thin, crusty bread prepared for the French Embassy in New York every day. Other items include baguettes, croissants, danish, chocolate decadence, pasta salads, fresh bagels, and ham and cheese croissant sandwiches. Coffee and lunch served in bakery. 7:30 AM-5:30 PM Mon-Fri, 8:30 AM-4:30 PM Sat. Wholesale and retail sales.

38 Et Cetera Antiques

3295 Triangle Dr. S.E., #110 (out South Commercial; turn west at Safeway to Triangle Square Plaza Bldg.), P.O. Box 3444, Salem, 97302. Tel: 581-9850 or 581-2127
Specializing in the Oregon in Oregon, Cynthia Day buys from Oregon families, always looking for historical pieces having to do with early Salem and early Oregon and the state government, since she is located in the capital city of Oregon. Also carries Oregon Native American artifacts such as coastal baskets, etc. Write for newsletter. Visa/MC. 11-5 Mon-Sat.

39 Made in Oregon

Lancaster Mall, 831 Lancaster Dr. N.E., #117, Salem, 97301. Tel: 371-8614, Toll-free phone orders: 800-4-BUY-ORE (in-state), 800-8-BUY-ORE (out-of-state)
Conveniently located in the Lancaster Mall, the "Made in Oregon" shop showcases the same rich selection of things made, caught, or grown in Oregon as found in its Portland and Medford stores. The "Made in Oregon" catalog, available at all locations, provides the convenience of mail-order shopping. (See Portland and Medford for other locations). Visa/MC/AmEx/Discover. 10-9 Mon-Fri, 10-6 Sat, 12-5 Sun.

40 Made In Salem

189 Liberty St. N.E., Salem, 97302 (corner of Liberty and Court in historic Reed Opera House, downtown Salem). Tel: 399-8197

A co-op run by Dave and Cheri Posedel (Mud-Pie); B. Taylor, P. Powers and N. Blackburn (Colored Light Stained Glass); and H. McManus (Oregon Exotic Wood) with forty additional craftspeople consigning their work: pottery, wood, stained glass, photography, country crafts, soft sculpture and more. There is usually an owner/artist working on site. Visa/MC. 10-9 Fri, 12-5 Sun, 10-6 all other days.

41 Mirassou Cellars of Oregon—Pellier

6785 Spring Valley Rd. N.W., Salem, 97304 (from West Salem bridge go 6 mi. northwest on Hwy. 221 to Lincoln Corner, then west on Zena Rd., and north 1.2 mi. on Spring Valley Rd.; follow signs). Tel: 371-3001

The Mirassou family is America's oldest winemaking family and Mitch and Bev Mirassou are proud to be producing fine varietal wines from the Willamette Valley. Their vineyard was established in 1981, and they are dedicating their label to Pierre Pellier, the great-great-grandfather and founder of the family tradition of fine winemaking. The winery is located nine miles northwest of Salem in the historic Eola Hills region, and seven miles east of 99W. Tasting Room open 11-5 daily except Mon, year around. Tours by appointment. Picnic facilities available.

42 Mission Mill Village

1313 Mill St. S.E., Salem, 97301 (exit at Hwy. 22 off I-5, go west on Mission to 14th St., north on 14th and west on Mill St.). Tel: 585-7012

Includes Jason Lee House and Parsonage (1841), Boon House (1847), Pleasant Grove Presbyterian Church (1858), Thomas Kay Woolen Mill building (1889) with two floors of exhibits, "Fleece to Fabric" and "The Finishing Room." Mill has original water power system in operation. Tours, textile classes, 4½ acres of parks and specialty shops with antiques, miniatures, dolls, candles, quilting supplies, children's apparel, knitting machines, Oregon books, Oregon products, and handcrafted gifts. Deli and picnic area. The activities of Mission Mill Museum Association are often supported by grants from the Oregon Arts Commission and the National Endowment for the Arts. Visa. 10-4:30 Tues-Sat.

43 Salem Art Association

600 Mission St. S.E., Salem, 97302 (in Bush's Pasture Park off Mission, High, and Bush streets in downtown Salem). Tel: 581-2228

Visitors will find plenty to see and do here. There's the Bush Barn Art Center with an arts and crafts gift shop, two exhibition galleries, (holiday show in December); Bush House Museum (1878) (Victorian decorations in December); Bush Conservatory Greenhouse (1882) and Rose Gardens; Salem Art Fair and Festival (third weekend in July) showcasing 200 artists, performing arts, food, children's activities, 5K run; art education classes; and special events. Some of the activities of the Salem Art Association have been supported by grants from the Oregon Arts Commission and the National Endowment for the Arts. Visa/MC. Bush Barn Art Center: 10-5 Tues-Fri, 1-5 Sat, Sun (extended hours in Dec). Bush House: 12-5 Tues-Sun (June-Aug), 2-5 Tues-Sun (Sept-May).

44 State Capitol Gift Shop

State Capitol Building, Salem, 97310 (Main State Capitol Bldg. with gold pioneer on top). Tel: 373-1006 (shop), 378-4423 (information).

A state gift shop offering a variety of Oregon-made gifts is located right in the state capitol building. Also upstairs in the governor's Ceremonial Office open to the public is an ongoing exhibition of work by outstanding Oregon artists. Visa/MC. 9-4:30 Mon-Fri, 10-4 Sat, 12-4 Sun.

○ Willow Lake Nursery and Farms

See KEIZER for listing.

SCAPPOOSE

45 TransWestern Helicopters

53894 Airport Way (take Hwy. 30 from Portland, then follow airport signs from Scappoose), P.O. Box R, Scappoose, 97056. Tel: 226-4731 (Portland number)

Betsy Johnson's full-service helicopter company provides charter, contract flight and maintenance to a wide range of customers throughout the western United States. Her helicopters have served the USGS since pre-eruption in the Mt. St. Helens event area and provide "one-of-a-kind" experiences for those wanting to see a volcano "up close." Other work includes major motion picture support services. 8-5 daily (24 hr. service also).

SHERIDAN

See BELLEVUE

SILVERTON

46 The Goldworks Custom Jewelry

206 E. Main St., P.O. Box 822, Silverton, 97381. Tel: 873-4757
John Osborn and Jean Witte do all their goldsmithing on the premises. They make original designs in gold and platinum, specializing in colored stones and colored diamonds. Remounting, repairs, appraisals and gemological services also available. Small gallery featuring local artists here too. Visa/MC/Discover. 11-7 Tues-Sat.

TUALATIN

47 Rich's

18810 S.W. Boones Ferry Rd., P.O. Box 1024, Tualatin, 97062. Tel: 692-1460
"Buildings are the most visible indication of the history of a community," says Carol Tittel. Though built in 1912, its history and the history of Tualatin go back at least 120 years. The century-old mellow brick walls of Rich's Kitchen provide a genuine historic atmosphere for a gourmet restaurant serving fresh Oregon products and Northwest wines, such as Pacific Oysters Dundee. Visa/MC/AmEx/Diners. 11-2 (weekday lunches), 5-10 Mon-Thurs (daily dinners), 5-11 Fri- Sat (weekend dinners), 10-2 Sun (brunch), 5-9 Sun (dinner).

48 Wilhelm Farms

6001 S.W. Meridian Way, Tualatin, 97062 (Take Tualatin/Sherwood Exit off I-5 onto Nyberg Rd. Go east ¼ mi. and then south uphill by Meridian Park Hospital. Continue south over the hill until road turns into "65th." Continue south approx. 2 mi., following Rainbow signs to farm). Tel: 638-5387
This 100-acre u-pick berry farm has been in the Wilhelm family for over 40 years. Strawberries, raspberries, boysenberries, marionberries, blueberries, plus a ten-acre u-pick vegetable garden. Six acres of pumpkins available beginning three weeks before Halloween. There is also a full produce stand, open April 25-Dec 23, and a small commercial kitchen producing jams and syrups. Gift packs, Christmas trees, wreaths, and greens available during Christmas season. Catalog and shipping available. 8 AM-dusk (Mon-Fri), 10 AM-6 PM (Sat, Sun).

WILSONVILLE

49 Larsen Farm Nursery

25935 S.W. Stafford Rd., Wilsonville, 97070 (Stafford Rd. Exit off I-5, east 2 mi. to Stafford Rd., or Stafford Rd. Exit off I-205, west 4 mi.). Tel: 638-8600
A large selection of annuals and perennials is located here, as well as a perennial display garden and gift shop with houseplants, antiques, baskets, local crafts, and gourmet foods. Fresh cut flowers are available all summer and u-pick filberts in the fall. The first two weeks in May the farm hosts the annual Spring Gallery, a large arts and crafts fair with thousands of jury-selected, handmade items from hundreds of craftsmen. Visa/MC. 10-6 Wed-Sat (April-Dec).

YAMHILL

50 Flying M Ranch

23029 N.W. Flying M Rd., Yamhill, 97148 (10 mi. west of Yamhill, follow Flying M signs toward Fairdale and Oak Ridge Rd.—or fly in and land on 2,200-foot turf strip). Tel: 662-3222
After a devastating fire, the Flying M Ranch has once again become one of the Northwest's finest rustic "getaways." A 30' section of a 36"-diameter Douglas fir log is now the bar, and the original massive stone fireplace crackles in the dining room of the new 17,000-sq.-ft. log lodge. Overnight trail rides, picnics, hayrides, tennis, a swimming pond, banquet facilities, cabins and "Bunk House" with 24 rooms. Visa/MC/AmEx. 8-8 Mon-Thurs, 8-10 Fri-Sun. Closed Dec 24, 25.

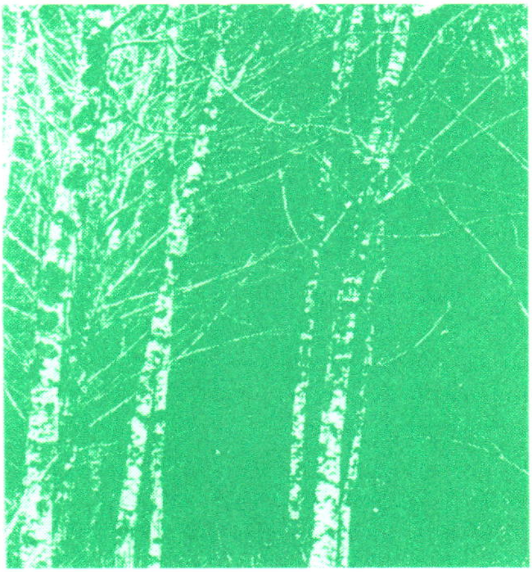

Alders, © Paul Miller

Southern

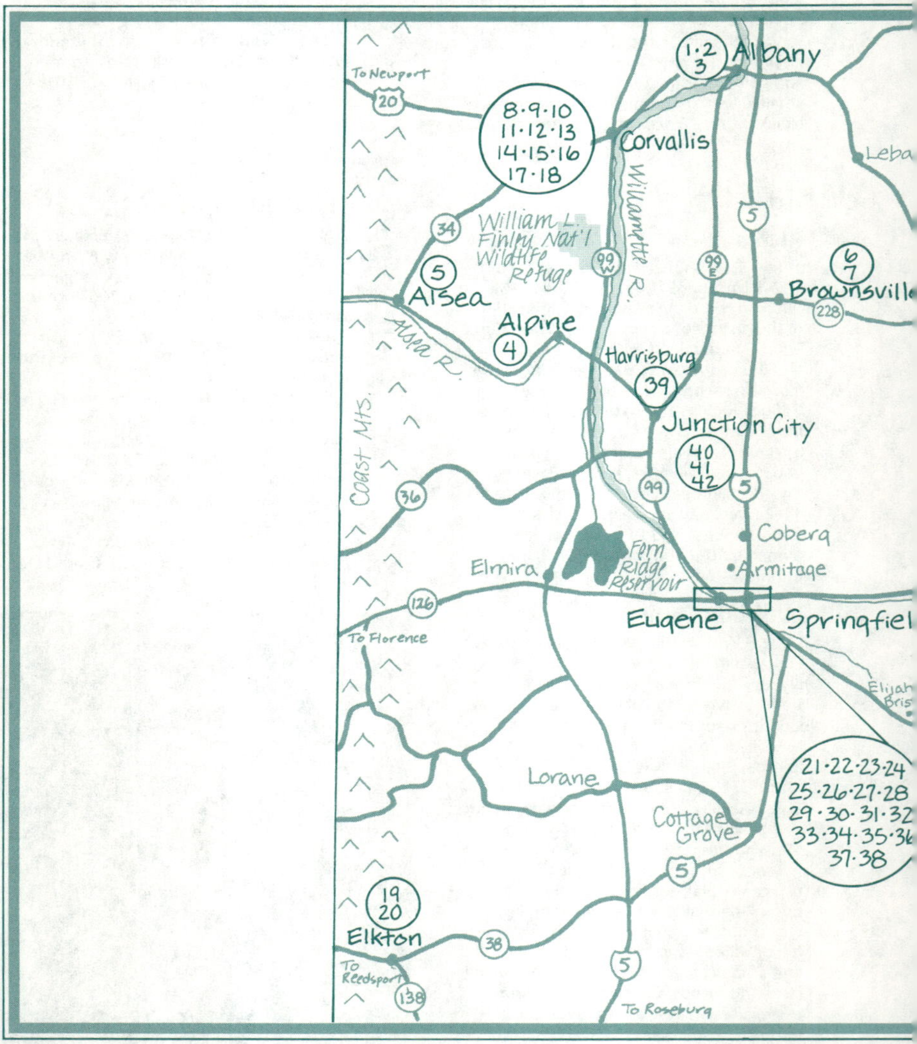

To Newport
20
1·2 3
Albany
8·9·10 11·12·13 14·15·16 17·18
Corvallis
Leba
Willamette R.
5
34
William L. Finley Nat'l Wildlife Refuge
99W
99E
6 7
5
Alsea
Brownsvill
228
Alpine
4
Alsea R.
Harrisburg
39
Junction City
Coast Mts.
40 41 42
36
99
5
Cobera
Elmira
Fern Ridge Reservoir
Armitage
126
Eugene
Springfiel
To Florence
Elijah Bris
21·22·23·24 25·26·27·28 29·30·31·32 33·34·35·36 37·38
Lorane
Cottage Grove
5
19 20
Elkton
38
To Reedsport
5
138
To Roseburg

Willamette Valley

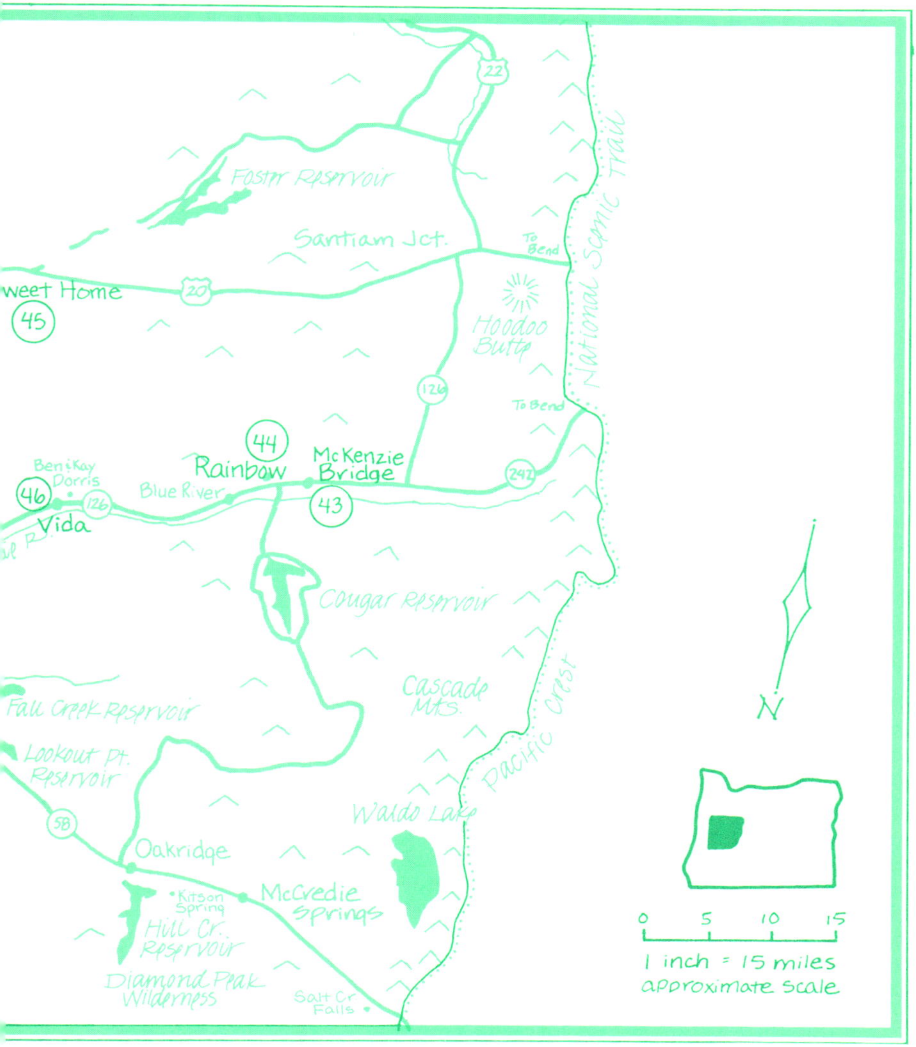

SOUTHERN WILLAMETTE VALLEY REGIONAL NOTES

It was its **rich, fertile farmland** *that made the Willamette Valley the destination of many of the pioneer wagon trains following the Oregon Trail. Many covered bridges, especially around* **Albany** *attest to the pioneers' solution to icy winter bridges.*

Although similar to the Northern Willamette Valley, the Southern Willamette Valley is perhaps a little warmer, and there are a number of nurseries that ship shrubs and herbs and seeds all over the world. Temperatures seldom fall below 25 degrees Fahrenheit in the winter or rise above 80 degrees Fahrenheit in the summer. The Coast Range stops enough of the Pacific weather to allow just the right amount of rainfall to fall between the Coast Range to the west and the Cascade Mountains to the east. Most of what moisture is left in the eastward-moving clouds is dropped as the clouds try to get over the Cascade Mountains. It is an ideal farming situation.

East of **Eugene** *the* **McKenzie River** *passes through several resort communities and rustic river lodges. It is one of the rivers that feeds the* **Willamette River** *and is the namesake for the "McKenzie Riverboat" used by many fishermen. Thundering waterfalls on the Upper McKenzie are accessible by short trails from Highway 126.*

Above **Oakridge**, *near the* **Diamond Peak Wilderness Area** *in the Deschutes National Forest, are Waldo Lake, the second-largest natural lake in Oregon; McCredie and Kitson Hot Springs; Salt Creek Falls; and Diamond Peak itself. For trailhead locations, maps, and fire conditions, contact the Deschutes National Forest Supervisor's Office, 1645 Highway 20E, Bend, Oregon 97701 (Tel: 382-6922); or stop by the ranger station just west of Oakridge. The* **Pacific Crest National Scenic Trail** *crosses Highway 58 at Willamette Pass in the Diamond Peak Wilderness. This area is especially popular with cross-country skiers.*

Sweet Home *in the foothills of the Cascade Mountains has an abundance of silicified fossil wood left from a prehistoric forest.*

South of Corvallis, off Highway 99W, is the **William L. Finley National Wildlife Refuge**; *and often driving up and down I-5 one can see flocks of birds overhead.* **Mary's Peak** *in the* **Siuslaw National Forest** *just west of Corvallis is the* **highest peak in the Coast Range**. *For maps and fire conditions in the Siuslaw National forest, contact Siuslaw National Forest Supervisor's Office, 4077 Research Way (P.O. Box 1148), Corvallis, Oregon 97333 (Tel: 757-4480).*

Since **Corvallis** *is the seat of the state land grant agricultural college (Oregon State University) and 80 percent of its faculty is involved in research, a number of very interesting projects go on here. Field burning (the process of burning the fields before planting more grass) is accepted by residents as representing one of the essences of the area—the area is one of the nation's largest producers of grass seed.*

There are a marina and a half-dozen parks at Fern Ridge Reservoir west of Eugene, group picnic facilities at Cascadia and Elijah Bristow, equestrian trails at Elijah Bristow, and boat ramps at Armitage, Ben and Kay Dorris, and Hendricks State Parks.

The **Willamette River Greenway** *extends 255 miles from Cottage Grove Reservoir and Dexter Dam (Southern Willamette Valley map) to the Columbia River at Portland. It provides opportunities for boating, picnicking, wildlife study, hiking, and overnight camping on public land. Most land along the greenway is private. The State Parks Division has published a Willamette River Recreation Guide to help direct users to public river-access points and landings. The guide is available from state park offices (see Statewide Resources section in this book). The author, her husband, and an entourage of friends once canoed the Willamette River from Eugene to near Portland. It is a very enjoyable trip that takes several days and has only a few areas with rapids that even an 11-year-old can handle—and did.*

The Nature Conservancy owns and manages a large system of natural preserves throughout the state of Oregon. Call 228-9561 or visit the conservancy's offices in Portland (see Statewide Resources section) for information about preserves the public may visit in this region.

ALBANY

1 Albany Convention and Visitors Commission

435 W. First Ave., Albany, 97321 (in downtown Albany in Chamber of Commerce Bldg.). Tel: 926-1517 Office: 8-5 Mon-Fri

There are three historic districts listed on the National Register of Historic Places in Albany, a city where "history lives with today." Famed for its Victorian homes, it offers visitors charming tours through old neighborhoods filled with historic homes and gardens. Free walking or driving tour guides may be picked up at the Gazebo Information Center at 8th and Ellsworth or at the Chamber of Commerce. Three museums: the 1849 Monteith House, the Albany Regional Museum, and the Albany Fire Museum, also bring back the flavor of turn-of-the-century life.

1988 Albany Area Events and Tours include:

July 1-4: World Championship Timber Carnival
July 3–Sept 11: Gibson Girl Horse-drawn Carriage Rides
July 7–Aug 18: River Rhythms 88 (free summer concert series)
July 9: Garden Tour
July 14-17: Midsummer Jazzfest, Crazy Days
July 22-24: Great Balloon Escape (hot air balloon festival)
July 24: Slack Water Drift on Willamette River
July 30: Historic Interior Homes Tour
Sept 6: Oregon Championship State Chili Cook Off
Nov 11: Linn County Veterans Day Parade
Dec 11: Old-Fashioned Christmas Parlour Tour of Historic Homes
Dec: Albany Victorian Christmas

2 Lilla's House: Cafe and Bed and Breakfast Inn

206 S.W. 7th, Albany, 97321 (3 blks. from Amtrak in historic Monteith District). Tel: 928-9437

Everything to eat in this restored, historic 100-year-old house is "made from scratch" on the premises. Owners Nancy and Chuck Gilliam serve full breakfasts every day to overnight guests and brunches to walk-ins, Sun 10-2, plus lunches Tues through Fri 11-2 and dinners Wed through Sat 5:30-9. Three guest rooms plus one suite with private bath. Children OK. No pets. Visa/MC/AmEx.

3 Nichols Garden Nursery

1190 North Pacific Hwy., Albany, 97321 (parallel to I-5 north of Albany; take I-5 South Exit 235 at Millersberg or I-5 North Exit 234 at Knox Butte). Tel: 928-9280 The Nichols family has been in the seed and nursery business since 1950. Their garden store has the Northwest's largest selection of vegetable, herb and flower seeds (developed specifically for this climate) plus ingenious garden aids and a rural bookstore. Herb, vegetable and flower display gardens open to the public. Catalog available. Visa/MC. 9-5:30 Mon-Sat.

ALPINE

4 Alpine Vineyards

25904 Green Peak Rd., Alpine (Monroe), 97456 (just north of Monroe on Hwy. 99W between Corvallis and Eugene—take shortcut turnoff going west to Alsea for 4 mi. to Alpine, then go 1.4 mi. to Green Peak Rd. and 1.5 mi. northwest along it to vineyards). Tel: 424-5851 Established in 1980 by Dan and Christine Jepsen when the vineyards were four years old, this winery is nestled in spectacular foothills of Coast Range southwest of Corvallis. Dan is the winemaker, assisted by Kerry Norton. All wines are estate bottled and include Chardonnay, Pinot Noir, White Riesling, Gewurztraminer, Cabernet Sauvignon and Pinot Noir Blanc. Picnic facilities overlooking vineyard are available. Group tours by appointment. Visa/MC. 12-5 daily (June 15-Sept 15); 12-5 Sat, Sun (Sept 16-June 14). Closed Jan.

ALSEA

5 Farmer's Kitchen Restaurant and Herb Garden

185 W. Main, Alsea, 97324 (on scenic Hwy. 34 to the coast). Tel: 487-4384 Meals with "that homemade touch fresh from the garden" are a specialty at Janet and Rolfe Hagen's Farmer's Kitchen. Guests are invited to enjoy the beauty and fragrance of the surrounding herb gardens after a meal in the rustic dining room. Containing over 140 varieties of herbs, the gardens provide herbs and edible flowers for the restaurant. The Hagens also support local potters, basketmakers, and other craftsmen, as well as honey producers, by offering their products for sale too. 7 AM-7 PM Mon-Thurs, 7 AM-8:30 PM Fri-Sun (summer); 6 AM-3:30 PM Mon-Thurs, 6 AM-7 PM Fri-Sat, 6 AM-5 PM Sun (winter).

BLUE RIVER

O Holiday Farm Resort

See RAINBOW for listing.

BROWNSVILLE

6 City of Brownsville and Chamber of Commerce

255 Main St., Brownsville, 97327, Tel: 466-5880.
Office: 8-5 Mon-Fri.
Brownsville, in the foothills of the Cascades, is one of Linn County's oldest settlements. The city was settled in 1846 and since 1887 it has hosted the Linn County Pioneer Picnic, Oregon's oldest continuous celebration. Pioneer Park, on the Calapooia River, is open from April 15 through October 15 and has camping, picnicking, fishing, a BMX track, horseshoe pits, and a baseball area. There is also a kitchen at the park which can be rented by large or small groups. Other points of interest in the Brownsville area include covered bridges, shops with handcrafted items, convenient motels, restaurants, art and photo galleries, antique stores, and a museum and library which have genealogical information. Visitors may also tour the local paper plant and fabricated-construction-board plant.

1988-89 Brownsville Area Events include:

1988

3rd weekend in April: "Carriage Me Back," an historical presentation with carriage rides, local actors in period costumes
June 17-19: Linn County's Pioneer Picnic, honoring Linn County's pioneers, and Chamber of Commerce Wagon Train Breakfast, 6-9 AM Sat-Sun, City Park
July 4th: Family celebration with fireworks at dusk, City Park
Nov 11: Veterans Day Breakfast honoring Linn County's veterans, 6-9 AM, City Park
3rd weekend in Oct: Oktoberfest, 10-5, Recreation Center

1989

3rd weekend in March: Flea Market, 10-5 Fri-Sun, Recreation Center

7 Linn County Historical Museum

101 Park Ave., Brownsville, 97327. Tel: 466-3390
The original Brownsville railroad depot and connecting boxcars housing pioneer artifacts; Moyer House, an historic mansion built in 1881; and a rock museum exhibiting the lifetime collection of Howard Taylor are all open to the public. Wagon rides into the past, re-enacting domestic life, fashion, and personalities of early Linn County, are staged the third weekend in April. Office: 11-4 Tues-Sat, 1-5 Sun (summer); 11-4 Thurs-Sat, 1-5 Sun (winter).

CORVALLIS

8 Corvallis Convention and Visitors Bureau

420 N.W. Second, Corvallis, 97330. Tel: 757-1544
Office: 8-5 Mon-Fri, 10-5 Sat.
Nestled between the Coast Range mountains and the picturesque Willamette River, Corvallis is full of exciting things to do for travelers and convention delegates alike. Contact the Corvallis Convention and Visitors Bureau for information about local points of interest (museums, galleries, bike paths, parks, wineries, fishing, Oregon State University), tour suggestions, events calendars, accommodations and dining. It also provides professional meeting planning assistance for conventions and conferences of all sizes and invites visitors to discover the charm of Corvallis.

1988 Corvallis Area Events include:

April 7-9: Oregon Dance Theatre (concert)
April 22-24: Hoolyeh Folk Dance Festival
May 20-21, 26-28: "Hair" musical production
June 16: "Summerfest 88" Celebration with circus and parade
June 17–July 16: "Inherit the Wind" Première, Courthouse Centennial Celebration
June 25-26: Folklife Festival
July 8-10 Benton County Courthouse Centennial Celebration
July 12-27 Festival Corvallis
Aug 2-6: Benton County Fair & Rodeo
Sept 24-25: Corvallis Fall Festival
Nov 25: 4th Annual Corvallis Community Christmas Parade
Sept-May: OSU Pac-10 Sports

9 Corvallis Arts Center

700 S.W. Madison Ave., Corvallis, 97333. Tel: 754-1551
Offers a variety of handmade crafts from Oregon artists and craftspeople in its shop, plus monthly exhibitions in its gallery. Also sponsors performances and festivals and gives classes and workshops. Its programs are often supported with grants from the Oregon Arts Commission. Visa/MC. 12-5 daily except Mon.

10 Corvallis Fall Festival

c/o Corvallis Area Chamber of Commerce, 420 N.W. Second, Corvallis, 97330 (in Central Park, between 6th and 8th, Monroe and Madison). Tel: 757-1505
This renowned crafts fair, now in its 16th year, features high-quality artists' and craftsmen's wares ranging from pottery to stained glass to hand-woven clothing: 150 booths in all. Also featured are continuous and diverse entertainment, a block-long food booth area, and Oregon wine garden. 10-6, Sept 24-25, 1988.

11 ECRU (handcrafted garments)

221 S.W. 2nd, Corvallis. Mailing address: P.O. Box 1354, Corvallis, 97339. Tel: 753-3300
Quality handcrafted garments and jewelry produced by Oregon artists and craftspeople are featured at Ecru. This interesting gallery/shop specializes in garments of original contemporary design as well as those of a classic timeless design representing the tradition of ethnic garments. Visa/MC. 10-5:30 Mon-Sat.

12 Garland Nursery

5470 N.E. Hwy. 20, Corvallis, 97330 (at 5 mi. marker halfway between Albany and Corvallis on Hwy. 20). Tel: 753-6601
Donald and Sandra Powell operate one of Oregon's largest retail nurseries with five acres of quality plants, a garden store and gift shop. They have a good selection of ornamental trees and shrubs, berry plants, herbs, perennials and bonsai. Visa/MC. 9-6 Mon-Fri, 9-5 Sat, 10-5 Sun.

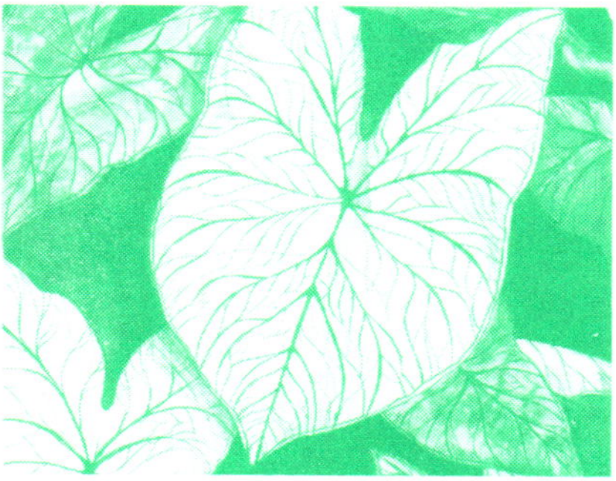

Caladium, © Liza Jones

13 Horner Museum

Gill Coliseum, Oregon State University, Corvallis, 97331 (in lower level of Gill Coliseum, at 26th and Washington, OSU campus). Tel: 754-2951
Assembled here is the largest single collection of historical properties in state ownership as well as many other objects from the cultural and scientific heritage of Oregon and a few other cultures. Permanent and temporary exhibits, an oral history collection, films, bus tours and a gift shop also featured. 10-5 Mon-Fri, 2-5 Sun (June through Aug); 10-5 Tues-Fri, 12-4 Sat, 2-5 Sun (Sept through May).

14 Madison Inn Bed and Breakfast

660 S.W. Madison Ave., Corvallis, 97333 (walking distance from OSU and downtown). Tel: 757-1274
The Brandis family operates this five guest-room inn built in 1897 and now on the National Historic Register. Guests appreciate the colorful quilts, books and flowers, two cozy lounge areas, and front parlor. Breakfasts feature treats such as cheese strata or maybe Dutch babies and scones with butter and homemade preserves. Visa/MC. Open every day, all hours.

15 New Morning Bakery

231 S.W. Second St., Corvallis, 97333. Tel: 754-0181
A popular place with locals, Ann and Joel Weinstein's small, downtown bakery makes everything from scratch including pecan sticky buns, wholewheat and honey cinnamon rolls, carrot cake with honey cream cheese frosting, over fifteen cookie varieties, an assortment of chocolate delights, croissants with Oregon-made jams . . . and homemade soups. Limited seating in bakery. Nearby riverfront park good for take-out picnics. 7-6 Mon-Fri, 7:30-5 Sat, 8-2 Sun.

16 Northwest Botanical Notecards

3200 N.W. Garfield Ave., Corvallis, 97330. Tel: 757-1632
Barbara Weber produces notecards and letter paper with local flowers, leaves, weeds, grasses, ferns, and lichens using a hand-print "softset" technique. Each is unique and suitable for framing. Work available at Corvallis Art Center and Pegasus Gallery in Corvallis, Bush Barn Art Center in Salem, Rogue Gallery in Medford, Lithia Creek Arts in Ashland, or by writing for price sheet.

17 Pegasus Gallery and Frame Studio

341 S.W. 2nd St., Corvallis, 97333 (in the Old Town Center, S.W. 2nd and Adams, 1 blk. from river bike path). Tel: 757-0042
Offering one-of-a-kind and limited edition originals as well as reproductions, posters, and catalog sales. More than 150 Northwest contemporary and Native American artists represented, some of whom have received grants from the Oregon Arts Commission and the National Endowment for the Arts. Annual costume party the Friday following the summer solstice. Studio owners personally assist clients with out-of-the-ordinary designs for presentation of two-dimensional and three-dimensional artwork. They also offer more than 30 years experience in restoration and archival framing. Bankcards accepted. 10-5:30 Mon-Sat minimum hours.

18 Tyee Wine Cellars

26335 Greenberry Rd., Corvallis, 97333 (7 mi. south of Corvallis; 2.3 mi. west of Hwy. 99W on Greenberry Rd.).
Tel: 753-8754
Established in 1985 on a third-generation Willamette Valley farm, the winery is owned and operated by Dave and Margy Buchanan, Nola Mosier, and Barney Watson, winemaker. Limited production of fine varietal wines, including Pinot Noir, Chardonnay, Pinot Gris, Gewurztraminer, and Pinot Noir Blanc. ("Tyee" is a traditional Northwest Indian word for "chief" or "best" and is used today to describe large Chinook or King Salmon). Visitors may picnic in the vineyard near the ancient Indian campgrounds with a view of Mary's Peak. Call or write for information re: celebrations and releases of new wines. Visa/MC. 12-5 Sat, Sun (May-Sept) or by appointment. Closed Oct-April except by appointment.

ELKTON

19 Elkton Pastry Mill Bakery

14834 Hwy. 38 (right next to cafe in Elkton on the south side of Hwy. 38), P.O. Box 485, Elkton, 97436. Tel: 584-2855
Travellers should believe their eyes because it is true. There is a bakery that makes handmade pastries, cookies, breads, cakes (and incredible pizzas with fresh ingredients to order on Fri, Sat and Sun) in this community on Hwy. 38 halfway between Eugene and the coast. 5 AM-6 PM daily.

20 Hiroshi Ogawa—Potter

1264 Wells Rd., Elkton, 97436 (2 mi. south of Elkton; Wells Rd. is reached from Hwy. 138). Tel: 584-2857
Although Hiroshi Ogawa's pottery is marketed all over the U.S., Hiroshi chooses to live and work in Elkton, Oregon. Functional and non-functional stoneware, plus his specialties, tea ceremony utensils, custom orders and dinnerware, are all available at his gift gallery and studio in Elkton. Visa/MC. 10-5 Tues-Thurs, or by appointment.

EUGENE-SPRINGFIELD

21 Eugene-Springfield Convention and Visitors Bureau

305 W. 7th, Eugene. Mailing address: P.O. Box 10286, Eugene, 97440.
Tel: 484-5307 or 800-452-3670 (in-state)
Office: 8-5 Mon-Fri, 9-4 Sat (summer); 8-5 Mon-Fri (winter).
Located at the junction of the Willamette and McKenzie Rivers, surrounded by farm land, forests, and mountains, Eugene is a dynamic city. It is the home of the University of Oregon, the world-class Hult Center for the Performing Arts, numerous restaurants, bistros, cafes, shops, and department stores. Public parks stretch for acres—one of them along a lush river bank. Possibilities for recreation include everything from wild, whitewater rafting to a relaxing round of golf. People who live here enjoy it so much that for a few days each September they rope off the downtown area and throw a party . . . the Eugene Celebration. And you're invited.

1988-89 Lane County Area Events include:

May: Rhododendron Festival, Florence (997-3128)
May: Oakridge Tree Planting Festival
June: Oregon Bach Festival, Eugene
June/July: Prefontaine Classic, Eugene
July: Art in the Vineyard, Eugene
July: Oregon Country Faire, Veneta
July: Bohemia Mining Days, Cottage Grove
Aug: Springfield Broiler Festival
Aug: Scandinavian Festival, Junction City
Aug: Lane County Fair, Eugene
Sept: Eugene Celebration
Oct: Fall Festival, Florence

22 Campus Cottage Bed and Breakfast Inn

1136 E. 19th Ave., Eugene, 97403 (close to the U of O campus). Tel: 342-5346
This first bed and breakfast in Eugene has three guest rooms with private baths, furnished with antiques, down comforters and fresh flowers. Living room with fireplace and deck are for guests' enjoyment. Full breakfasts served by innkeeper Ursula Bates include special egg dishes, fresh fruits, juices and pastries. Older children welcome. No pets. Open year around.

23 Duggan's Ingredients

N-M

1365 Interior St., # A, Eugene, 97402. Tel: 343-8697
Duggan's Ingredients, the ultimate in taste. Featuring a full-scale condiment line that includes salad dressings, mustards, herbed oils and vinegars, fudge sauces, chutneys, and smoked salmon. Robert and Duggan Peak use the freshest ingredients available, all from Oregon. Having gained national distribution in the past year, they are now selling in France, Switzerland, and Japan. Available in Oregon at Strohecker's, Nordstrom, Meier & Frank, and Crane & Co. Tours by appointment only.

24 Eugene Saturday Market

Park Blocks, 8th and Oak, P.O. Box 427, Eugene, 97440. Tel: 686-8885
This weekly open-air marketplace is now a tradition in Eugene. The market grew out of Lotte Streisinger's Christmas crafts sales in the '60s which benefited the anti-Vietnam War effort. Located in a lovely park setting, it draws craftspeople, farmers, and cooks from surrounding areas who bring their work to town to be sold. Great food, fresh produce, and entertainment. Some vendors honor charge cards. 10-5 Sat (April to Christmas).

25 Eugene's Fall Creek Bakery

881 E. 13th St., Eugene, 97401 (on U of O campus next to U of O Bookstore). Tel: 484-1662
Everything in Kimberly Murphy's retail bakery is made on the premises. She uses quality ingredients and no preservatives and works in the classic European and American traditions. Winner of the local cinnamon roll and chocolate chip cookie contests, the bakery came in 2nd in the Eugene Celebration cake contest in 1985. 7:30-6 Mon-Fri, 8-3 Sat.

26 Excelsior Café

754 E. 13th Ave., Eugene, 97401 (1 blk. west of U of O). Tel: 485-1206 or 342-6963
Stephanie Pearl and Phillip Kimmel's menu changes monthly, highlighting what is in season. Three-course dinners feature fine seafood, veal, poultry, game and produce prepared in delicious ways. Lighter, "bistro dinners," hors d'oeuvres and a large selection of Oregon wines also available. Pastries and ice cream made on the premises. Elegant coffees, teas, and cocktails. Visa/MC/AmEx/Diners. 11:30 AM-midnight Mon-Fri, 5:30-12:30 Sat, 10-2 Sun brunch, 5:30-midnight Sun dinner.

27 Excelsior Charcuterie

901 Pearl St., Eugene, 97401 (corner of Broadway and Pearl in old Eugene Hotel Bldg.). Tel: 342-3110
Makes all its own fresh sausages and patés, cow and goat milk cheeses, French-style breads, pastries, ice cream, vinegars, mustards, chutneys, preserves with local fruits and herbs, salads, soup, roast chicken, gourmet pizza, et al. Wine and beer (with emphasis on Oregon), soft drinks, mineral water. All "to go" or to eat in the urban cafe setting. Visa/MC/AmEx. 7:30 AM-9 PM Mon-Thurs, 7:30 AM-11 PM Fri, 11-11 Sat, 12-4 Sun.

28 Fenton and Lee Confections

N-M

135 E. 13th, Eugene, 97401. Tel: 343-7629
Named after the owners' two sons, Fenton and Lee specializes in manufacturing fine, hand-dipped and molded chocolates. All ingredients are pure and natural with an emphasis on fruits, berries and nuts indigenous to the Pacific Northwest. Janele Smith, her family and four employees hand-make and hand-pack each individual chocolate. Mail order shipping between Oct and May. 10-5 Mon-Sat. Closed in July.

29 Fifth Street Public Market

296 East 5th, Eugene, 97401 (corner of 5th and High in downtown Eugene). Tel: 484-0383
Amidst the everyday hustle and bustle of Market activity, artists create, music is made, and bakers bake. Lamps to leatherwork. Wool, wine, wood and whale bone. Mindgames to marigolds. Inlay and au lait. Earthenware and running wear. Art to artichokes. Amazing glazes, jewelry cases and exquisite vases. Literally soup to nuts . . . and mostly made in Eugene. 70 shops and restaurants. Shops: 10-6 daily. Food: 7-10 Mon-Sat, 9-6 Sun.

30 Hinman Vineyards

27012 Briggs Hill Rd., Eugene, 97405 (from Eugene go west on 11th to Bertelsen; go 5 mi. south to Spencer Creek Rd. and then 2½ mi. west to Briggs Hill Rd; winery is on left 3½ mi. south). Tel: 345-1945
The philosophy at Hinman Vineyards, established in 1979, is to provide individual attention to each of its premium wines and consistently to create quality wines it is proud to share. The picturesque setting offers an ideal place for an afternoon picnic. An addition completed in October 1987 provides a full rental facility and a large visitors' reception room. Visa/MC. 12-5 daily. Closed Thanksgiving and Christmas through Jan 1.

31 Leah's Restaurant and Lounge

720 Willamette St., Eugene, 97401 (corner of 7th and Willamette, across from Hult Center, on ground floor of parking structure). Tel: 484-4041
Fresh Northwest cuisine with a continental flair is featured at Leah's. Seasonal Pacific coast seafood, Chinook salmon, crab, and scallops can be grilled or sauteed to order. Oregon poultry is served here too and rack of Oregon lamb is the house specialty. Chef Robert Davidson prepares all foods in-house, including desserts, soups, and sauces, using locally grown herbs. Extensive wine list with Oregon wines by the glass. Visa/MC/AmEx/Discover. 11:30 AM-2 PM Tues-Sat (lunch). Opens for dinner at 5 PM Tues-Sun. Open for dinner after theater.

32 Made in Oregon

295 E. 5th, Eugene, 97401. Tel: 343-5051
Joanne McAdam's gallery/shop is a Eugene showcase for elegant Oregon crafts: baskets, jewelry, paper, pewter, porcelain, stoneware, textiles and wood, including unusual Myrtlewood gifts. In 1985 Made in Oregon began to carry delicious non-perishable Oregon-made gourmet food products, suitable for gift baskets and boxes. Daily UPS service. Visa/MC. 10:30-5:30 Mon-Sat.

33 Monster Cookie Company

27 W. 5th Ave., Eugene, 97401 (1 blk. north of Hult Center in 5th Ave. Historical District). Tel: 687-1064
Children of all ages know where to find Maggie Ortiz' Monster Cookie Company. Its cookies, brownies and bars are all made from scratch and can be found along with an ice cream and espresso bar in the restored Palace Hotel. Used earlier this century to house railroad workers, the hotel is now called the Lane Building. 7:30-6 Mon-Fri, 9-5:30 Sat, 11-5 Sun.

34 Oregon Bach Festival

Office: Rm. 263, School of Music, University of Oregon, Eugene, 97403. Performances at Hult Center for the Performing Arts and Beall Concert Hall, U of O. Tel: 687-5000 (for tickets), 686-5666 (for brochure)
"A jewel of a festival . . . Brilliant!" June 19–July 3, 1988, Helmuth Rilling conducting. Now in its 19th season, the nationally acclaimed Oregon Bach Festival will feature 30 different concerts ranging from Bach to Penderecki, from classical music to jazz. More than 200 artists from around the world will congregate to make the city of Eugene an international musical showplace. In 1988 the festival will feature Poland's composer Krzysztof Penderecki, who has become a legend in his own time. Also unique to the year's program will be the popular Canadian Brass. The Festival's programs are supported by the National Endowment for the Arts, the Oregon Arts Commission, the Eugene Arts Foundation, and many corporate sponsors. Visa/MC/AmEx.

35 Springfield Museum

590 Main St., Springfield. Mailing address: 225 N. 5th St., Springfield, 97477. Tel: 726-2300
The museum is located in a restored 1908 PP&L transformer station. The upstairs gallery has the permanent Historic Springfield display, and the main galleries feature rotating exhibits. The museum shop has traditional crafts, dolls, baskets, books, and cards. Parking adjacent is handicap accessible. Visa/MC. 11-5 Wed-Sat.

36 Suzette's Marvelous Mustard

P.O. Box 5117, Eugene, 97405. Tel: 484-4834 or 484-0142
Selected by both Bloomingdale's and Neiman-Marcus for their promotion of Oregon products, Suzette's Marvelous Mustard is also available throughout Oregon and in fine gourmet stores and delicatessens. It is salt-free and made without preservatives. Not just for sandwiches, this marvelous mustard can also be used in cooking. New to the Suzette's family of fine foods is a sensational cranberry chutney. Call or write for more information.

37 University of Oregon Museum of Art

University of Oregon, Eugene, 97403 (in the middle of the U of O campus, next door to the main library). Tel: 686-3027
Offers changing exhibitions and permanent collections devoted to Oriental art and contemporary American art and photography. Guided tours every Sunday at 2 PM and by arrangement. Its Visual Arts Resources department packages and circulates work by Oregon artists throughout the state. Gift shop and rental sales gallery. Visa/MC. 12-5 Wed-Sun.

38 Willamette Science and Technology Center (WISTEC)/ Lane ESD Planetarium

2300 Centennial Blvd., Eugene, 97401 (next to Autzen Stadium). Tel: 484-9027 or 689-6500, ext. 227
Both adults and children can explore science, astronomy, and technology in depth here. WISTEC creates hands-on exhibits and hosts traveling shows (e.g. Kaleidoscopes: Reflections of Sound and Art, July 2—Sept 25, 1988, and Dinosaur Families, Oct 8, 1988—Jan 2, 1989). Lane ESD Planetarium produces original multimedia programs. WISTEC has received support from numerous foundations and the National Endowment for the Humanities, the Oregon Committee for the Humanities, the National Science Foundation, Institute of Museum Services, et al. Visa/MC. Museum: 12-5 daily except Mon. Planetarium shows: 3 PM daily during Dinosaur Families show, 1 PM and 3 PM Sat, Sun. Groups by reservation, 9-9 daily except Mon.

STATE ANIMAL

The American Beaver (Castor canadensis) was named Oregon State Animal by the 1969 Legislature. Prized for its fur, the beaver was overtrapped by early settlers and eliminated from much of its original range. Through proper management and partial protection, the beaver has been reestablished in watercourses throughout the state and it remains an important economic asset. The beaver has been referred to as ''nature's engineer'' and its dam building activities are important to natural water flow and erosion control. Oregon is known as the ''Beaver State'' and Oregon State University's athletic teams are called the ''Beavers.''

HARRISBURG

39 Detering Orchards

30946 Wyatt Dr., Harrisburg, 97446. (Going south on I-5 take the Halsey Exit 216 and go into Halsey, then about 9 mi. south on 99E to Harrisburg. In Harrisburg, take the last turn to the left off 99E, cross two railroad tracks and go right [south] on the Coburg-Harrisburg Rd. Turn right about 5 mi. down the road onto Wyatt Dr. [across from the Wyatt Schoolhouse] and go about ¼ mi. to the orchard. Going north on I-5 take the Coburg Exit 199 into Coburg and then turn right and go 7 mi. north on the Coburg-Harrisburg Rd. to Wyatt Dr. on the left [opposite the Wyatt Schoolhouse] and go about ¼ mi. to the orchard.) Tel: 995-6418
Established by Gerald and Marie Detering in 1934, this third-generation farm is now run by Roger Detering. It produces all kinds of fruits and vegetables including 75 acres of rhubarb; pears; peaches (available July 20—Sept 15); over 30 varieties of apples; Montmorency, dark sweet, and many other kinds of cherries; filberts (hazelnuts) and walnuts; as well as apple cider (Sept-March). The Deterings can also pit customers' cherries with their big old cherry pitter. ''Sharon's'' butters, syrups, preserves, jams, and jellies, including rhubarb jelly (which we think is the only such jelly in the U.S.), are now famous. A Neiman-Marcus selection. 7-7 daily (July-Sept), 8-5 daily (winter).

JUNCTION CITY

40 The Acorn Tree

264 W. 6th, Junction City, 97448. Tel: 998-8031
Mary Lou Finigan's Acorn Tree is both a full-service florist and a gift shop featuring Oregon crafts, wines, candy, non-perishable gourmet foods, antiques, Norwegian Rosemaling, and her own tole and decorative art. All of the jams and jellies at the Acorn Tree are made in Junction City and Harrisburg. Even the bags in which the popcorn is packaged are made in Harrisburg. Mary Lou teaches classes and workshops September to May. Visa/MC/Discover. 9-5:30 Mon-Fri, 9:30-4 Sat.

41 Harwood Farms

91984 River Rd., Junction City, 97448 (halfway between Junction City and Beltline on west side of River Rd., signs on antique farm machinery). Tel: 688-1846 or 688-4091

Featuring an antique horse-equipment display, an early Oregon kitchen with 1800s utensils, old-time farm tools and a fine collection of logging and hand-forged blacksmith tools (items not for sale), Leslie and Geneva Harwood, Oregon State Family Farm winners three times, are proud to offer the highest quality produce at the lowest possible prices. 8-7 daily. June 10-July 10 for strawberries, raspberries, blueberries and early broccoli. Aug 7-Nov 15 for fall fruit and vegetables.

42 Scandinavian Festival

P.O. Box 5, Junction City, 97448. Tel: 998-3300 or Chamber of Commerce 998-6154

Junction City has a strong Scandinavian heritage, and 1988 will be the 28th year that the festival has transformed downtown into a charming old-world village. Ethnic foods, traditional handcrafted items, colorful costumes, lively music, folk dancing and bright flowers abound. Demonstrations. Tours. Only cost is for food or craft items. 1988 Festival dates are Aug 11-14, Thurs-Sun, from 10 AM-10 PM.

McKENZIE BRIDGE

43 Log Cabin Inn

56483 McKenzie Hwy. McKenzie Bridge, 97413 (50 mi. east of Eugene on Hwy. 126). Tel: 822-3432

Tony and Jean Puddefoot operate this historic coach stop that looks much the same (except for furnishings) as it did in 1906 when it was rebuilt after a fire. The log structure has a full-service restaurant and lounge with meals served on the porch in the summer and rustic cabins on the McKenzie River. Bed and breakfast. Visa/MC. 9-9 in season, call in winter.

MONROE

See ALPINE

RAINBOW

44 Holiday Farm Resort

On the McKenzie River Dr. at Rainbow (¼ mi. off Hwy. 126, 50 mi. east of Eugene, 80 mi. west of Bend). Mailing address: 54455 McKenzie River Dr., Blue River, 97413. Tel: 822-3715

This secluded 90-acre resort along the bank of the beautiful McKenzie River has cottages both along the river bank and in the woods. There are 750 feet of river frontage, two private lakes for swimming and fishing, trails and streams to explore, two restaurants (one a former stage coach stop), a cocktail lounge, and a game room. Guides are available for rainbow trout, steelhead, and salmon fishing. An 18-hole championship golf course is a half-mile away. Open 7 AM to midnight.

SPRINGFIELD

See EUGENE-SPRINGFIELD

SWEET HOME

45 East Linn Museum

746 Long St., Sweet Home, 97386. Tel: 367-4580

This is a museum of pioneer artifacts, primarily of local origin, displayed in and around an old church building and separate blacksmith shop. There are exhibits of farming, medical, logging, and mining equipment as well as period rooms: kitchen, parlor, bedroom. Other exhibits display china, dolls, clothing, jewelry, guns, maps, photos, books, cameras, and musical instruments. 11-4 Tues-Sat, 1-4 Sun (May-Labor Day); 11-4 Thurs-Sat, 1-4 Sun (Sept-April).

STATE FISH

The Chinook Salmon (Oncorhynchus tshawytscha), also known as spring, king and tyee salmon, is the largest of the Pacific salmons and the most highly prized for the fresh fish trade. Declared State Fish by the 1961 Oregon Legislature, the Chinook Salmon is found from southern California to the Canadian Arctic. Record catches of 52 inches and 126 pounds have been reported.

VIDA

46 McKenzie River Bowl Works

90986 Leashore Dr., Vida, 97488 (from I-5 in Eugene go east on Hwy. 126 to covered bridge on right; cross bridge onto Good Pasture Rd. and go about ¼ mi.; go right again onto Leashore Dr. and keep your eyes peeled for a sign and two, cedar modified "A"-frame buildings).
Tel: 896-3402
Larry Peterson used to be a newspaperman. Then he built a shop, ordered his first lathe from England, and since 1984 has been turning wooden bowls (with natural edges) and making bud vases, corkscrews, little covered boxes, sake cups, ball point pens, and all manner of objects from interesting, distressed pieces of wood of all kinds. His work has been sold to customers from as far away as Japan, Canada, southern California, and Michigan. Open daily most of the day unless he's out hunting wood, or by appointment.

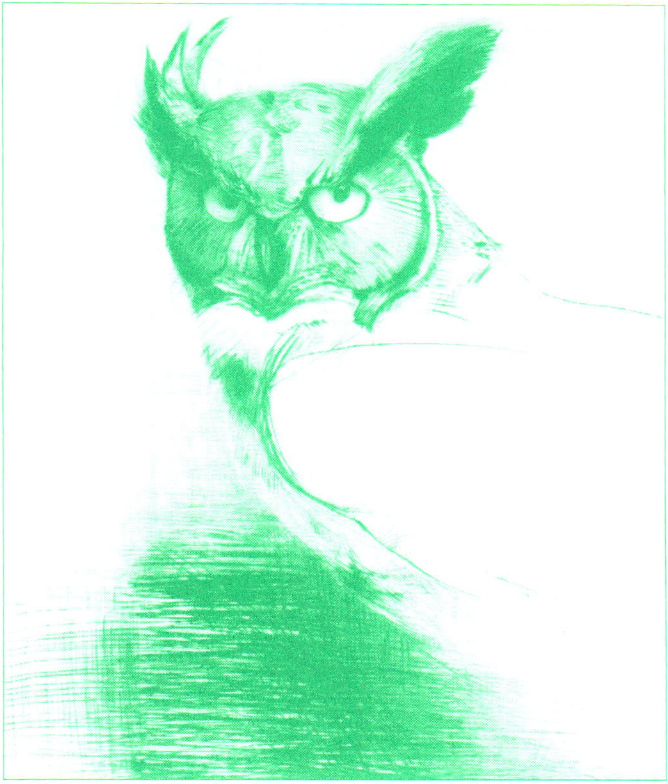

Great Horned Owl, © Liza Jones

Southern

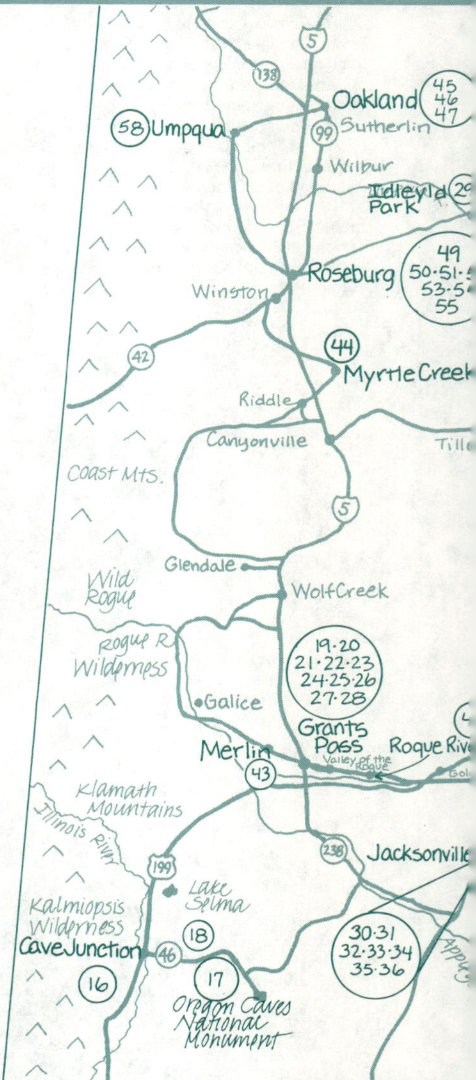

5
138
Oakland
45
46
47
58
Umpqua
99
Sutherlin
Wilbur
Idleyld Park
Roseburg
49
Winston
55
44
42
Myrtle Creek
Riddle
Canyonville
Coast Mts.
Glendale
Wild Rogue
Wolf Creek
Rogue R Wilderness
19·20
21·22·23
24·25·26
27·28
Galice
Grants Pass
Merlin
Roque River
Valley of the Rogue
43
Klamath Mountains
Illinois River
238
Jacksonville
199
Lake Selma
Kalmiopsis Wilderness
18
Cave Junction
46
30·31
32·33·34
35·36
16
17
Oregon Caves National Monument

Oregon

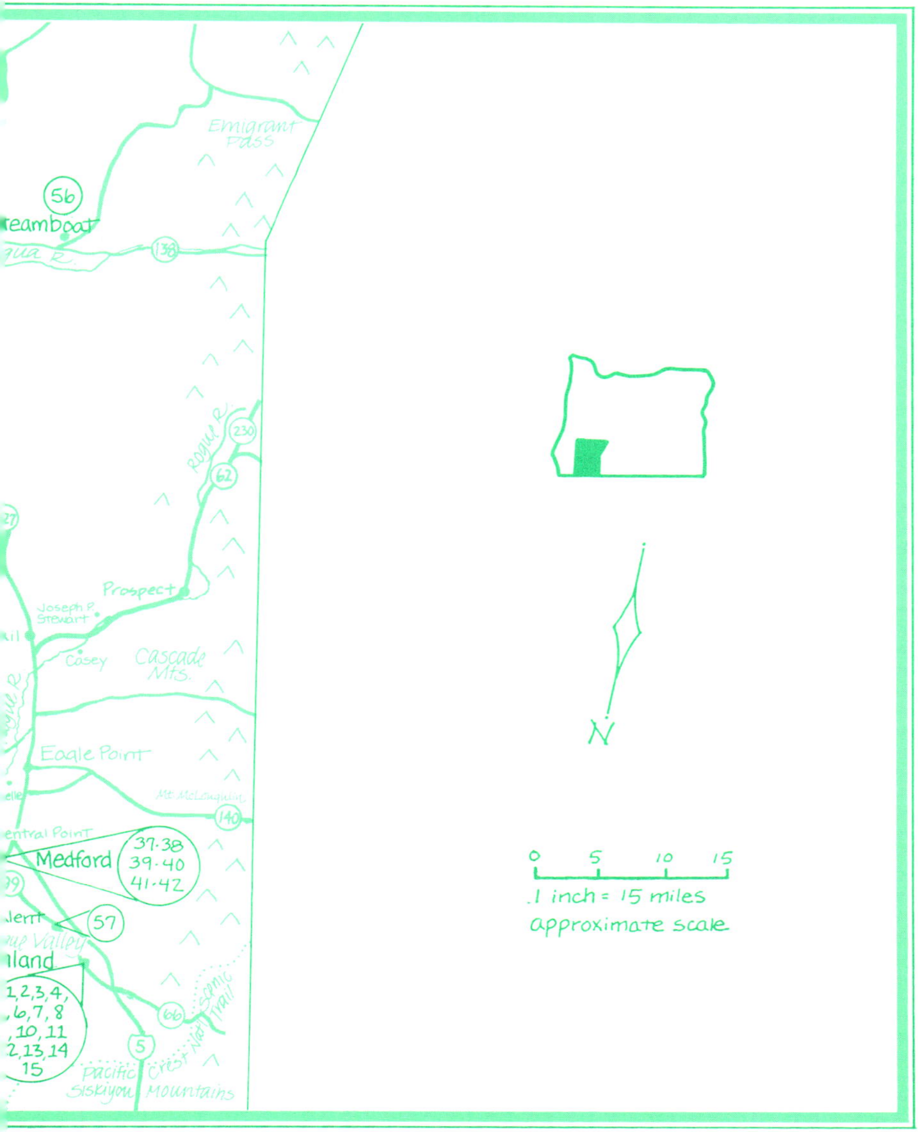
Emigrant Pass
56
138
Rogue R.
230
62
Prospect
Joseph P. Stewart
Casey
Cascade Mts.
Eagle Point
Mt. McLoughlin
140
Medford
37·38
39·40
41·42
57
66
5
Scenic Trail
Pacific Crest Nat'l
Siskiyou Mountains
N
0
5
10
15
.1 inch = 15 miles
approximate scale

SOUTHERN OREGON REGIONAL NOTES

Sheltered from the Pacific Ocean by the Klamath and Siskiyou Mountains, Southern Oregon has dry weather conditions and more extreme temperature ranges than those of the Willamette Valley to the north.

Oregon's oldest known rocks *(maybe 425 million years old) are in the* **Siskiyou Mountains** *along the California state line about 20 miles west of Interstate 5. However, they are almost inaccessible due to the very rugged mountains in the area. The* **Klamath Mountains** *between* **Grants Pass** *and Crescent City also have some of the oldest and most interesting rocks in the Northwest. However, again, the dense forests covering these very old mountains make them difficult to survey. The Kalmiopsis Wilderness Area west of Cave Junction is known for its interesting botanical and floral phenomena; however, it is mostly impenetrable, even to determined bush-whacking geologists.*

Myrtlewood *and the objects made from it are rapidly becoming a thing of the past as the older craftsmen are dying and the trees are being cut as slash. Northern California, the South Oregon coast, and Southern Oregon are the only places in the Americas where myrtlewood is grown. It takes one hundred years to "get the right grain," yet no one is planting myrtlewood for future generations.*

The Redwood Highway that connects Grants Pass to Crescent City on the north California coast passes near this area. At Lake Selma, there are horses and boats. The **Illinois River**, *as it flows north to Agness (South Coast map), and the* **Rogue River** *between Agness and Galice are designated* **Scenic Waterways**. *People here are fiercely independent and have more than once threatened to secede from the Union.*

At the **Oregon Caves National Monument**, *(see Southern Oregon listings) one can see caves of marble formed from folded limestone when a nearby mass of igneous rock from the Klamath Mountains heated and recrystallized it about 150 million years ago. Rain seeping into the rocks along fractures slowly dissolved holes that have created the actual caves. The original limestone was deposited in seawater about 200 million years ago. It is difficult to tell when the actual caves were formed.*

Southern Oregon contains a lot of serpentine and a lot of red soil, which is often associated with nickel, and specific kinds of plants. The **only nickel mine in the United States** *has operated in one of these serpentine areas at Nickel Mountain, just west of Riddle. The deposit was discovered in 1865, and the Riddle Mine has been known to produce up to 25 million pounds of refined nickel in a year.*

The **Rogue River** *[a designated* **Scenic Waterway** *between Agness (South Coast map) and Galice] is famous for its white-water trips and a hiking trail along its bank. For more information on the Wild Rogue Scenic Waterway, the Kalmiopsis Wilderness, and the Siskiyou National Forest, contact the Siskiyou National Forest Supervisor's Office, 200 N.E. Greenfield Road (P.O. Box 440), Grants Pass, Oregon 97526 (Tel: 479-5301).*

There are a number of historic towns in Southern Oregon that follow the original **North-South Stagecoach route**. *Built in the 1870s and originally a stage stop, Wolf Creek Tavern is believed to be Oregon's oldest hostelry.*

The **Umpqua River** *is one of the nation's most famous fly-fishing streams. The* **Roseburg** *area (see Southern Oregon listings) has attracted a number of vineyards and wineries, and the* **Rogue Valley** *(see Medford listings) has long been known as a fruit-producing area, with some of the largest direct-mail gift fruit companies in the country.*

Near Medford is the Table Rock Preserve and Area of Critical Environmental Concern (ACEC). These 2,820 acres are cooperatively manged by The Nature Conservancy and the U.S. Bureau of Land Management (BLM) to protect special biologic, geologic, historic and scenic values. Visitors are invited to walk the trails, taking care to respect the land and its living treasures.

The Preserve was established in 1979, when The Nature Conservancy purchased portions of the John Day Ranch with assistance from the Elmer Feldenheimer Land Preservation Fund, the Carpenter Foundation, the Cheney Foundation and many individual donors. The preserve adjoins an additional 300 acres along the Rogue River at Kelly Slough managed by Jackson County (as part of the Bear Creek Greenway) and the Oregon Department of Fish and Wildlife. The BLM designated its land on Upper and Lower Table Rocks as an ACEC in 1984. Day-to-day management of the Table Rocks is the responsibility of the Table Rocks Stewardship Committee, a group of local citizens, scientists and Bureau of Land Management and Nature Conservancy representatives.

"The basalt that forms the scenic rimrock

on both Table Rocks is remant of intracanyon lava flows that filled the portions of the ancient Rogue River an estimated 4.5 million years ago. During the subsequent millennia, the surrounding softer geologic formations eroded away, leaving the two conspicuous flat-topped mesas standing some 800 feet above the Rogue Valley. Erosion continues today, slowly splitting great blocks of basalt from the cliffs. The broad 'skirts' of the Rocks are made up of a much older sandstone formation.

"The variety of parent material, slope and aspect on the Table Rocks leads to a mosaic of soil types and conditions that support several plant communities. Oregon white oak, madrone and ponderosa pine dominated woodlands, and oak savannas flank the Rocks. Rogue Valley chaparral mixes with the woodlands and savannas on the slopes and includes shrub species such as wedgeleaf ceanothus, deerbrush, poison oak, and sticky manzanita. Grasslands on the lower slopes and in the bowls of the Rocks were dominated by native bunchgrasses including California oatgrass, Lemmon's needlegrass, Idaho fescue and rough bluegrass prior to changes resulting from extensive grazing. Vegetation on top of the Rocks was dominated by the same grasses and numerous wildflowers. Here the land exhibits "patterned ground," a distinctive combination of low, grassy mounds, stony intermound areas, and vernal (springtime) pools. From March to June this grassland is strewn with colorful wildflowers: goldfields, grass widows, poverty clover, miniature lupine, and many others. An endemic species of meadowfoam grows nowhere else in the world—only here on the tops of the two Table Rocks.

"The Rocks host many wildlife species. Some common species include blacktail deer, dusky-footed woodrats, valley pocket gophers, western meadowlarks, rufous-sided towhees, and mountain quail and western rattlesnakes. This also is home to striped whipsnakes and the California kangaroo rat—here occurring east of their principal range—and blue-gray gnatcatchers—nesting here at the northern edge of their range.

"For thousands of years before European contact, the Rogue River Valley and the Table Rocks had been occupied by bands of Takelma Indians. During the tragic Rogue River Wars of the 1850s, the Takelmas skirmished with the U.S. Army in this area, and Lower Table Rock became part of the short-lived Table Rock Reservation.

"In keeping with the objectives of The Nature Conservancy and the Bureau of Land Management, the Table Rocks are carefully managed as a natural area. Its flora, fauna and other natural values are protected so that scientific research, education and compatible forms of recreation may continue.

"Visitors to the Preserve are asked to please observe the following guidelines: Obey all signs. Stay on trails. The interior valleys or 'bowls' of the Table Rocks are not open to public use. Do not walk on the soft ground near vernal pools. Avoid wearing vibram soled shoes. Do not pick flowers or disturb vegetation and wildlife. Do not disturb scientific study plots. No fires, no litter, no dogs. Pick up any trash you may encounter. Thank you for your help." (From The Nature Conservancy's materials. See Statewide Resources section.)

For hikers, the Joseph P. Stewart State Park has 8 miles of hiking and bicycling trails. From the park, the U.S. Forest Service's Upper Rogue River Trail connects with the **Pacific Crest National Scenic Trail** *at Crater Lake National Park (South Central Oregon map). Boat ramps are available at Casey, Joseph P. Stewart, Tou Velle, and Valley of the Rogue State Parks. There are a marina and boat docks on the reservoir at Joseph P. Stewart State Park.*

ROAD SENSE

On extended car trips, especially over mountains or in Eastern Oregon, carry a sleeping bag, boots, water, wool hat, mittens and socks and a suitable jacket—even in summertime. (Food would be nice, too.) **Weather conditions,** *mechanical problems or deer in the path of speeding vehicles* **can stop a car for hours or even days** *. . . and it can get miserably cold. There may not be a town for miles and it may be the middle of the night.*

The author's husband once spent two days on a mountain pass on Interstate 5 near Grants Pass when two semi-trucks jackknifed (one in front of him and the other on the north-bound side), immobilizing 500 cars before the state police could stop the oncoming traffic. Meanwhile a storm dumped three feet of snow on the unprepared travelers, and it was two days before snow removal equipment could extract everyone.

ASHLAND

1 Archibald's Tasting Room/ Rogue River Vineyards Ltd.

297 S.E. Main St., Ashland, 97520.
Tel: 488-1467
This is a cooperative effort between the Rogue River Vineyards and the Quality Meat Company, both from Grants Pass. Wines from Rogue River Vineyards include varietal wines, Chardonnay, White Riesling, Early Muscat, Gewurztraminer, Pinot Noir Blanc, Pinot Noir, Cabernet Sauvignon, Silver Springs White Blush, Red Table Wine, apricot and strawberry-flavored Chablis, and the ever-popular Very Berry Wine Cooler. In addition, there is an astounding selection of hardwood-smoked meats, cheeses, and breads. The experienced and friendly staff at Archibald's can help put together meats, cheeses, and wines that complement each other. Visa/MC. 10 AM-12 PM daily. (Additional tasting rooms at Rogue River Vineyards in Grants Pass and Archibald's in Beaverton, Portland Metropolitan section.)

2 Ashland Bakery and Cafe

38 East Main St., Ashland, 97520 (off the Plaza). Tel: 482-2117
Five years ago Steve Sachs thought Ashland needed a casual, but cosmopolitan, cafe. In 1985 his dream received Oregon Magazine's "Best Place to Wake Up in Ashland" award. Its eclectic cuisine is composed of fresh foods made on the premises with whole grain breads, croissants, fresh-baked pastries, espresso and cappuccino being specialties. Visa/MC. 7 AM–9 PM daily (summer); 7 AM–8 PM Mon-Fri, 7 AM–9 PM Sat, Sun (winter).

3 Chanticleer Bed and Breakfast Inn

120 Gresham St., Ashland, 97520 (4 blks. from Shakespearean Theater in a residential neighborhood). Tel: 482-1919
Jim and Nancy Beaver's fabulous breakfasts incorporating Dutch Babies with apple fillings, cheese-baked eggs, fresh pastries, smoothies and more complement their luxuriously restored 1920 American Craftsman Bungalow home with large living room, country French interiors, mountain views and beautiful gardens. Antiques, fluffy comforters, fresh flowers and imported soaps fill seven guest rooms and private baths. Children by prior arrangement. Smoking outside. Open all year.

4 Chappell-Swedenburg House Museum

990 Siskiyou Blvd., Ashland, 97520 (corner of Mountain Ave.). Tel: 488-1341
Located on the campus of Southern Oregon State College and operated by the Southern Oregon Historical Society, the museum occupies the first floor of the restored Swedenburg Home. Exhibits feature the history of Ashland and southern Jackson County. Summer walking tours of downtown Ashland and railroad district. 1-5 daily except Mon.

5 Greenleaf Delicatessen

49 N. Main St., Ashland, 97520 (on the Plaza). Tel: 482-2808 or 482-2835
Daniel Greenblatt and the folks at Greenleaf Delicatessen take pride in offering a variety of freshly prepared gourmet foods, daily specials of traditional deli fare, desserts and ethnic specialties. Seating on their deck by the creek or specially packed meals to go. Visa/MC. 9-9 daily.

6 Hanson Howard Galleries

82 N. Main St., Ashland, 97520.
Tel: 488-2562
H.H.G. has moved uptown. Owned and operated by Judy Howard and Marie Baxter, artists themselves, the gallery features monthly exhibitions of contemporary art work by Oregon and West Coast artists plus a selection of finely crafted items and posters published by Ashland Editions. A number of the artists represented have received Fellowship Awards from the Oregon Arts Commission. Visa/MC. 10:30-6 daily.

7 The Morical House Bed and Breakfast

668 North Main St., Ashland, 97520.
Tel: 482-2254
Surrounded by more than an acre of lawns and flower gardens with a putting green and views of the mountains and valley, this 1880s Victorian farmhouse was carefully renovated in 1982 by Joe and Phyllis Morical. Furnished throughout with antiques and decor that evokes an earlier, more graceful time, the five guest rooms have private baths and are centrally air-conditioned. Full breakfast, including fresh baked goods. Children welcome. No pets. Visa/MC. Open year around.

8 Oregon Shakespearean Festival

P.O. Box 158, Ashland, 97520. Box office: 482-4331/Other: 482-2111
Eight-month repertory of classic and modern plays presented in two indoor theaters and on one outdoor Elizabethan stage. The festival, around which Ashland revolves in the summer, draws visitors from all over the world. Its programs are partially supported by grants from the Oregon Arts Commission and the National Endowment for the Arts. Season runs Feb to Oct. Closed Mondays. Other attractions include backstage tours and exhibit center. Visa/MC/AmEx. Tickets may be ordered in advance by mail.

9 Festival Exhibit Center of the Oregon Shakespearean Festival Association

15 S. Pioneer St. P.O. Box 158, Ashland, 97520. Tel: 482-2111
The festival's past and present can be seen in photographs, costumes, designs, props and on videotape. Visitors are invited to try on costumes, pose for pictures and strut the stage in the Fantasy Gallery. Open every performance day (season Feb-Oct). Closed Mondays. Visa/MC/AmEx.

10 Tudor Guild of the Oregon Shakespearean Festival

15 S. Pioneer St. P.O. Box 1210, Ashland, 97520. Tel: 482-0940
The place for unique festival souvenirs, including old costumes and props, plus the books, guides, synopses and programs needed to make a knowledgeable playgoer. Visa/MC/AmEx. 10-8 during festival season.

11 Parkside Bed and Breakfast

171 Granite St., Ashland, 97520.
Tel: 482-2320
Conveniently located, overlooking Lithia Park near the Plaza and theaters, are Susan and Rod Reid's cottage with private entry, bath, and patio and their two-bedroom suite with private entry, bath, living room, front porch, and swing. Both have kitchenettes with the makings for continental breakfasts. Open year around.

12 Rising Sun Farm

2300 Colestin Rd., Ashland, 97520 (I-5 south to first exit in Calif., take a right; farm is 3.2 mi. north on Colestin Rd., on the left; follow signs; large white gate).
Tel: 482-5392
The picturesque Rising Sun Herb Farm is nestled in the Siskiyou Mountains south of Ashland, 5 minutes from I-5. Hosts Richard and Elizabeth Fujas invite visitors to come and learn about the growing of herbs and sample their 29 specialty herb products. Herb plants, fresh and dried herbs, gifts, and one-of-a-kind items are available throughout the year. Children welcome, but please leave pets at home or in the car. Call or write for group tour arrangements. A Neiman-Marcus selection. 9-5 Mon-Sat.

13 Romeo Inn Bed and Breakfast

295 Idaho St., Ashland, 97520 (on Idaho between Iowa and Holly, 8 blks. from theaters). Tel: 488-0884
Innkeepers Margaret and Bruce Halverson invite guests to relax in quiet elegance in their lovely Cape Cod house set amid towering pines overlooking the Rogue Valley. There's a new, luxurious, completely detached suite with whirlpool bath and kitchen, and four spacious guest rooms with central air-conditioning, king-sized beds, and private baths, plus a reading room with fireplace, baby grand piano, pool and spa, and colorful gardens. Delicious full breakfasts. No children, pets, or smoking. Open year around.

14 Valley View Tasting Room

52 East Main, Ashland, 97520.
Tel: 482-8964
Valley View Vineyard operates a third tasting room, located in the heart of downtown Ashland, where guests can taste and purchase its award-winning wines. 12-5 daily except Mon. Closed Jan and Feb. (See Jacksonville for Valley View Vineyard listing.)

STATE FLOWER

The legislature designated the Oregon Grape (Berberis aquifolium) as the Oregon State Flower in 1899. A low growing plant, the Oregon Grape is native to much of the Pacific Coast and found sparsely east of the Cascades. Its year-round foliage of pinnated, waxy green leaves resembles holly. The plant bears dainty yellow flowers in early summer and a dark blue berry that ripens late in the fall. The fruit can be used in cooking.

15 Winchester Inn

35 S. Second St., Ashland, 97520 (2 blks. south of Shakespearean Theater, Lithia Park, and 1 blk. above Main St. shopping). Tel: 488-1113 (inn), 488-1115 (restaurant)

The Gibbs family welcomes guests to its century-old, renovated Queen Anne-style home in Ashland's downtown historic district. Now on the National Register of Historic Places, the home's gracious charm, quiet parlor, and seven guest rooms with private baths create an atmosphere of sophisticated country living. Full gourmet breakfast served to overnight guests on patio or in picturesque dining room overlooking tiered gardens. Dining room open to public for dinner 5:30-8:30 Tues-Sun until May 31, then 5-9 daily. 10-2 Sun brunch. Reservations welcome. Visa/MC. No pets.

CAVE JUNCTION

16 Chocolate Affair

333 Redwood Hwy. (Hwy. 199S), P.O. Box 418, Cave Junction, 97523 (on the corner of Redwood Hwy. and Caves Hwy. [Hwy. 46]). Tel: 592-4186

Gary and Donyne Bell say that their fresh chocolate desserts could be the best reason to visit Cave Junction! They use only pure chocolate and other natural ingredients in making their handmade, hand-dipped chocolate truffles. They invite travelers to stop in for a memorable treat on the way to the Oregon Caves or the coast. 10-5 Mon-Sat. Mail-order truffles available Oct-April. Call or write for more information.

17 Oregon Caves Chateau (Inn)

20000 Caves Hwy., Cave Junction, 97523 (Cave Junction is 29 mi. SW of Grants Pass on Hwy. 199 and the Oregon Caves and Chateau are 19 mi. east of Cave Junction on Hwy. 46). P.O. Box 128. Tel: 592-3400

Built over 50 years ago, this rustic chateau-style lodge rises six stories from Cave Creek Canyon. Guests are lulled to sleep by rushing water outside their restful rooms after an enjoyable meal and relaxing evening in the lodge's charming old dining room and lobby. Susie Weisberg is the lodge's chef. Full bar, large selection of Oregon wines, old-fashioned soda fountain, and gift shop. Visa/MC (gift shop only). About mid-June to early Sept.

18 Siskiyou Vineyards

6220 Caves Hwy., Cave Junction, 97523 (6 mi. east of Cave Junction along Hwy. 46, gateway to the Oregon Caves National Monument). Tel: 592-3727

At the foot of the Siskiyou National Forest in the scenic Illinois Valley flourishes one of the state's most charming additions to the Oregon wine industry. Suzanne (C.J.) David's new winery, tasting room, picnic area, nature trail and annual spring and fall festivals welcome all who enjoy fine table wines, art, and music. Sales and tasting room open 11-5 daily. Visa/MC.

GRANTS PASS

19 Growers' Market

Market: between 6th and 7th St. at "L" St., Oregon Bank parking lot, Grants Pass. Mailing address: P.O. Box 573, Grants Pass, 97526. Tel: 476-5375

From Easter to Thanksgiving, one can partake of the bounty of Josephine County and the Rogue Valley. Fresh produce in season, bedding plants, houseplants, herbs, homebaked cookies, cakes, pies, breads; homemade candies, and handcrafted items are all available directly from the creators. "We grow what we sell," is the market's motto. It is the longest-running and largest open air agricultural market in Oregon. 9-1 Sat (Easter to Thanksgiving). Call for additional summer markets, times, and locations. There is now another Growers' Market, in Medford.

20 The Handmaidens' Inn

230 Red Spur Dr., Grants Pass, 97527 (5 mi. outside of Grants Pass). Tel: 476-2932

Bette and Jody Hammer's inn in the foothills of the Siskiyou Mountains overlooking the Rogue River Valley has three rooms including a spacious suite, all with beautiful views. Breakfasts include homebaked breads and pastries. Dinner and picnic baskets available upon request. Central air conditioning. Hot tub on back deck. No pets or children. Smoking outside. Visa/MC. 7 days a week.

21 Hellgate Excursions/Rogue Jet Boat Excursions

953 S.E. 7th St., Grants Pass, 97526 (by the Riverside Inn in downtown Grants Pass). Tel: 479-7204 or 476-2628
Excursions daily from mid-May through September down the beautiful Rogue River. Four trips available: two-hour Scenic Hellgate Tour, five-hour Whitewater Excursion, four-hour Country Dinner Excursion with dinner at OK Corral or Doubletree Place, and Champagne Brunch Delight with breakfast served on deck at OK Corral. Reservations suggested. 8-6 daily.

22 Jerry's Rogue Rafts

2750 Cloverlawn Dr., Grants Pass, 97527. Tel: 476-2941 or 479-1504
Second-generation licensed river guide Jerry Briggs offers 3- and 4-day raft trips on Rogue River with overnight stops in rustic lodges (Maria Lodge, Black Bar Lodge, et al.) along the way. Trips start in Grants Pass every Tues, June-Aug. Fishing tackle, food and lodging and return trip to Grants Pass provided. Write or call for brochure.

23 Lawnridge House Bed and Breakfast Inn

1304 N.W. Lawnridge, Grants Pass, 97526. Tel: 476-8518
This stately 1909 home sports guest-only living room with beamed ceilings, large fireplace, VCR, two private dining rooms, and shady deck for al fresco breakfasts. Two suites, each with private bath, TV, and books. (Honeymoon suite has handmade, curtained, canopied bed.) Air-conditioned. Breakfasts feature treats like fresh seasonal dungeness crab, salmon or steelhead (yours or theirs), and freshly baked pastries. Smoking on balcony or covered porch. Children by arrangement. Barbara Head, innkeeper. Open year around.

24 Mt. Baldy Bed and Breakfast

678 Troll View Rd., Grants Pass, 97527. Tel: 479-7998
John and June Gustafson's new, air-conditioned, ranch-style home in a quiet, out-of-town area was built to be shared. It has a deck, beautiful views, and two guest rooms, each with queen-sized bed, private entrance, and bath. Covenient to fishing, rafting, jet boats on the wild and scenic Rogue River, Oregon Caves, Jacksonville, and Ashland. Full breakfast. No pets. Smoking outside. Open all year.

25 Paradise Ranch Inn

7000 Monument Dr., Grants Pass, 97526 (Exit 61 [Merlin] off I-5, then 2 mi. on Monument Dr.). Tel: 479-4333
Oliver and Matilda Raymond offer fishing, all-weather, lighted tennis, Rogue River rafting, golf, tranquil walks, bicycling, a heated pool and spa, cocktails in their barn and meals prepared by Chef Billy Dunn, featuring Oregon food and wine, to guests in search of a "gentleman's white-fence, picture-book ranch" experience. An 18-hole golf course is under construction.Visa/MC. Rooms available year around (dining room closed Mon, Tues during winter).

26 River Adventure Float Trips

2407 Merlin/Galice Rd., P.O. Box 841, Grants Pass, 97526. Tel: 476-6493
Mel and Diane Norrick have been running trips on the Rogue River for 27 years. Three-day raft trips through June, July, and August start on Tuesday and Friday of each week. Each night is spent in a different rustic lodge. Three-and-a-half day fishing trips from September 1 through mid-November. All fishing tackle, food, and lodging furnished. Write or call for brochure. Office: about 7 AM–7 PM daily.

27 Rogue River Vineyards Ltd.

3145 Helms Rd., Grants Pass, 97527 (7 mi. southwest of Grants Pass, just off Hwy. 199 on the way to the Oregon Caves). Tel: 476-1051
Established in 1984 and owned and operated by Albert Luongo, Dan Solowy, Gail Tanabe, and winemaker Bill Jiron, Rogue River Vineyards produces varietal wines, Chardonnay, White Riesling, Early Muscat, Gewurztraminer, Pinot Noir Blanc, Pinot Noir, Cabernet Sauvignon, Silver Springs White Blush, Red Table Wine, apricot and strawberry-flavored Chablis, and the ever-popular Very Berry Wine Cooler. The tasting room is open year around for wine tasting and tours, 10-6 daily except Monday. Visa/MC. (Additional tasting rooms at Archibald's in Ashland and Beaverton, Portland Metropolitan section).

28 The Washington Inn Bed and Breakfast

1002 Washington Blvd., Grants Pass, 97526 (Exit 58 from I-5; then take Savage to Washington Blvd.). Tel: 476-1131
Maryan and Bill Thompson's 1883 historical Victorian home is now a nostalgic bed and breakfast. One suite with balcony, fireplace, private bath. Two guest rooms, one with fireplace, private bath, and one with shared bath. All have queen-sized beds. An "enhanced" continental breakfast includes fresh-baked pecan muffins and a fresh fruit sculpture that looks like a banana split! Bicycle built for two available. Smoking outside. No pets or children. Visa/MC. Open all year.

IDLEYLD PARK

29 Mazama Outdoors

North Umpqua Hwy. 138; HC 60, Box 64-A, Idleyld Park, 97447 (47 mi. east of Roseburg on North Umpqua River, Hwy. 138, about halfway between Crater Lake National Park and Roseburg).
Tel: 498-2235
The North Umpqua River offers thrilling whitewater rafting trips for experienced and beginning boaters. Winding through a scenic canyon in the Umpqua National Forest, the river has nearly continuous rapids that are challenging but forgiving. Mazama Outdoors provides experienced guides, equipment, transportation, and a riverside picnic lunch. Trips depart daily at 9 AM from March through October. Half-day and overnight trips and private instruction in canoeing, kayaking, and rafting also available. Visa/MC.

JACKSONVILLE

30 Peter Britt Music Festivals

Jacksonville (theater); P.O. Box 1124, Medford, 97501 (office).
Tel: 800-33-BRITT (in-state), 800-88-BRITT (out-of-state)
Britt, the oldest outdoor music and performing arts festival in the Northwest, is also in one of the most beautiful outdoor concert settings. A wooded hillside offers festival-goers an opportunity to picnic on benches or picnic blankets. Five different festivals feature world-class artists in classical music, jazz, bluegrass, dance, and musical theater. James DePreist, conductor. Classes offered in most art forms presented. Visa/MC. Call or write for more information.

31 Jacksonville Inn

175 E. California, Jacksonville, 97530.
Tel: 899-1900
Built in 1863 and on the National Register of Historic Places, this inn is maintained by Jerry Evans in the tradition of the Old West. Eight rooms furnished with restored, local antiques. Oregon wines are among the 500 available in excellent dinner house featuring gourmet dishes individually prepared to order by executive chef Diane Menzie, including Oregon Chinook salmon and razor clams in season. Visa/MC/AmEx/Diners/CB/Discover. Gift shop: 9:30-5:30. Restaurant: 11:30-2 daily (lunch), 5-10 daily (dinner), 10-2 Sun brunch.

32 Livingston Mansion Inn

4132 Livingston Rd. Box 1476, Jacksonville, 97530. Tel: 899-7107
The three spacious but cozy rooms at this inn sitting amid quietly aging oak and madrone trees on the outskirts of century-old Jacksonville each have a private bath and spectacular view. Wally and Sherry Lossing's fabulous breakfasts include their "breakfast cookies," a long-time Lossing tradition. Visa/MC. Open all year.

33 McCully House Inn and Cafe

240 E. California St. (in the historic core area, within walking distance of dining, shopping, and Peter Britt Music Festivals), P.O. Box 387, Jacksonville, 97530.
Tel. 899-1942
This 1861 Classical Revival home on the National Register of Historic Places has three guest rooms with private baths, and a special parlor for guests. Full breakfasts featuring fresh fruits and dairy products are served by innkeeper Sanda Collegio. Gourmet lunches include homemade soups, biscuits, muffins, salads, sandwiches, and desserts, which are a real specialty. Breakfasts for overnight guests year around. Breakfasts and lunches 8 AM-4 PM for walk-ins in summer, lunches only for walk-ins in winter. Banquets year around. No smoking or pets. Older children only. Visa/MC. Open year around, by reservation.

POET LAUREATE

In 1974 Governor Tom McCall, at the recommendation of the Oregon Arts Commission, appointed William E. Stafford, Lake Oswego, as Oregon's Poet Laureate.

34 Pinnacle Orchards' Store

115 W. California St., Jacksonville, 97530. Tel: 899-1481
A picnic take-out and retail store and mail-order outlet for Pinnacle Orchards, one of Medford's oldest pear-packing companies, sending out thousands of gift boxes and baskets through colorful catalogs. (This year it is celebrating its 50th anniversary.) The Comice, Bosc, and Bartlett pears and red and yellow Delicious apples are all grown in Rogue Valley orchards. Other items for sale include smoked salmon, smoked trout, Tillamook cheese and ice cream, Oregon wine cookies, hazelnut butters, and Pinnacle's own jams, jellies, and syrups. Visa/MC/AmEx. 10:30-5:30 daily (summer).

35 Southern Oregon Historical Society

5 mi. west of Medford on Ore. Hwy. 238, P.O. Box 480, Jacksonville, 97530. Tel: 899-1847
Founded in 1851 following the discovery of gold in Rich Gulch, the entire town of Jacksonville is an historic landmark! (There are only eight such towns in the nation.) Located here are a museum in the old Jackson County Courthouse, where there's currently the exhibit "Making Tracks," celebrating the Oregon and California Railroad Centennial; a Children's Museum in the old jail; and the restored Beekman Bank, Beekman House, Catholic Rectory, and U.S. Hotel. A research library and gift shop are in the main museum. Living History programs at Beekman House and costumed greeters at Beekman Bank: 1-5 daily (Memorial Day to Labor Day). Museums: 10-5 daily (Memorial Day to Labor Day). Closed Mon, Labor Day to Memorial Day.

36 Valley View Vineyard

1000 Applegate Rd., Jacksonville (Ruch), 97530 (the Applegate Valley is about 8 mi. SW of Jacksonville). Tel: 899-8468
The Wisnovsky family planted the modern-day Valley View Vineyard in 1972, in the unique fog-free microclimate of Southern Oregon's beautiful Applegate Valley. Nestled at 1,500 feet elevation in an area justly nicknamed "Sunshine Village," the winery produces award-winning Cabernet Sauvignon, Chardonnay, Gewurztraminer, Pinot Noir, and Merlot. Tasting room and informal tours. Visa/MC. 11-5 daily. (See Ashland for Valley View Tasting Room listing.)

MEDFORD

37 Farrago Chocolates

301 West 6th, Medford, 97501 (at the corner of 6th and Holly). Tel: 772-8532 or 800-FAR-RAGO (nationwide)
Timothy McClure and Daniel Kempfer brought the art of fine chocolate making to Southern Oregon in 1984. Their truffles (incorporating fine liqueurs, glacéed fruits and freshly roasted nuts), tortes and gateaux are some of the finest in Oregon. Nothing artificial used. Also available are espresso and cappuccino. Farrago chocolates are available at various locations around the Rogue Valley. Mail-order corporate catalog available to everyone. Visa/MC. 10-5 Mon-Fri.

38 Growers' Market

Market: between Bartlett and Central on 5th St. in the heart of Medford. Mailing address: P.O. Box 573, Grants Pass, 97526. Tel: 476-5375
Fresh produce in season, bedding plants, houseplants, herbs, homebaked cookies, cakes, pies, breads; homemade candies, and handcrafted items are all available directly from the creators. "We grow what we sell," is the market's motto. 9-1 Thurs (April-Nov). Call 899-8081 for additional market hours and locations. The original Growers' Market is in Grants Pass, the longest-running and largest open air agricultural market in Oregon.

39 Harry and David's® Original Country Store

2836 S. Pacific Hwy., Medford, 97501 (1 mi. south of Medford on Hwy. 99). Tel: 776-2277
There really was a Harry and a David, and they started shipping pears nationwide in the forties. Now one of the nation's leading shippers of fine food and fruit gifts, Harry and David's® has a restaurant, deli, gift shop, floral shop, mail order counter, fruit stand, and specialty foods department—all under one roof. Free plant tours available. Call ahead please. Visa/MC/AmEx. 8-6 daily. Restaurant: 8-6 daily.

40 Made in Oregon

Rogue Valley Mall, 1600 N. Riverside, #2061, Medford, 97501. Tel: 779-8114. Toll-free phone orders: 800-4-BUY-ORE (in-state), 800-8-BUY-ORE (out-of-state) Conveniently located in the Rogue Valley Mall, the "Made in Oregon" shop showcases the same rich selection of things made, caught, or grown in Oregon as found in its Portland and Salem stores. The "Made in Oregon" catalog, available at all locations, provides the convenience of mail-order shopping. (See Portland and Salem for other locations.) Visa/MC/AmEx/Discover. 10-9 Mon-Fri, 10-6 Sat, 11-6 Sun.

41 The Rogue Gallery/Art Association and Center for Visual Arts

40 S. Bartlett, Medford, 97501.
Tel: 772-8118
Features monthly exhibitions of regional, national and international works and runs seminars and classes year around. Its programs are partially sponsored by grants from the Oregon Arts Commission and the National Endowment for the Arts. Also sells local art and craftwork including exceptionally fine pottery by members of "The Clay Folk" (a potters' cooperative), some of whose members have studied, exhibited and taught in nationally acclaimed ceramic institutions but prefer to live and work in surrounding area. Visa/MC. 9-4 Tues-Sat (June 15–Aug 31); 10-5 Tues-Fri, 10-4 Sat (Sept 1–June 14).

42 Under the Greenwood Tree Bed and Breakfast Inn

3045 Bellinger Lane, Medford, 97501 (at Exit 27 in Medford go west 3 mi. on Stewart Rd. until it becomes Hull; go one blk. to Bellinger Lane). Tel: 776-0000
This ten-acre estate was homesteaded in 1861. Its park-like ambience with four luxurious, romantic rooms, pastoral views, queen-sized beds, private baths, croquet lawn, willow swing, gazebo by the rose garden, orchard, antique farm buildings, and collection of professionally curated museum-quality textiles provide the perfect backdrop for Renate Ellam's sense of style. Three-course breakfasts, high tea, truffles by the beds. Centrally located between festivals. Smoking on porches. No pets. Horses and older children welcome. Visa/MC. Year around.

MERLIN

43 Morrison's Rogue River Lodge

8500 Galice Rd., Merlin, 97532 (located 16 mi. outside of Grants Pass; take Merlin exit off I-5 north of Grants Pass).
Tel: 476-3825 or 800-826-1963
Accommodations at this river lodge include both separate cabins and rooms inside the lodge itself. There are tennis courts, a pool, putting green, and private beach on the grounds, and 1, 2, 3, or 4-day whitewater rafting trips down the "Wild Rogue," as well as steelhead fishing in the fall. Morrison's is well known for its fine dining and serves excellent food with a family-style touch. Visa/MC. Open from May to mid Nov.

MYRTLE CREEK

44 Country Host Registry

901 N.W. Chadwick Lane, Myrtle Creek, 97457. Tel: 863-5168
This group of farm and rural host families in Southwestern Oregon offers guests a chance to see Oregon agriculture in action. A farmstead experience is a chance to share first-hand in the lives and activities of the host family. Sheep shearing, lambing, calving, or haying might be in progress, depending on the season. Visitors with farm backgrounds are welcomed too, to compare operations and practices. Country breakfasts are the heart of the farmstay experience, and lunches and dinners can often be provided. Visa/MC. Office: 8-4 Mon-Fri.

STATE BIRD

The Western Meadowlark (Sturnella neglecta) was chosen State Bird in 1927 by Oregon's school children in a poll sponsored by the Oregon Audubon Society. The bird, native throughout western North America, has brown plumage with buff and black markings. Its underside is bright yellow with a black crescent on the breast; its outer tail feathers are mainly white and are easily visible when it flies. The Western Meadowlark is known for its distinctive and beautiful song.

OAKLAND

45 The Pringle House Bed and Breakfast

114 N.E. 7th St. (1½ mi. off I-5 at Exit 138), P.O. Box 578, Oakland, 97462. Tel: 459-5038
Jim and Demay Pringle provide satisfying bed and breakfast accommodations to discriminating travelers in their restored 1893 Victorian home overlooking downtown historic Oakland. This is one of many homes and businesses in Oakland on the National Register of Historic Places. Special breakfast. Near fine dining, golf, fishing, boating, picnicking, antiques, six wineries, and Wildlife Safari. No pets or younger children. Smoking in designated areas only. Year around.

46 Tollefsons Antiques

115 Locust St. (in the little tiny historic town of Oakland, just off I-5, a few miles north of Roseburg), P.O. Box 31, Oakland, 97462. Tel: 459-3796
This is an antique store and art gallery specializing in 19th and early 20th century American art. When Carol and Terry Tollefson bought this and the building next door in 1968, everything was boarded up and condemned. Now the whole town of Oakland is proud to be on the State and National Historic Registers as an historic district. Family, friends,and neighbors got involved, and even now one of the best things about this place is the "home-grown attention" and commitment to hiring local people who stay on. The Tollefsons try to buy and exhibit as much Northwest art as they can find and can provide expert appraisals and research and business counseling in antique investments. Visa/MC. 10-6 Mon, 10-10 Tues-Sun.

47 Tolly's

115 Locust St. (in the little tiny historic town of Oakland, just off I-5, a few miles north of Roseburg), P.O. Box 31, Oakland, 97462. Tel: 459-3796
This is a dinner house, ice cream parlor, and luncheon place. The beautifully restored buildings have the entire original soda fountain from Carroll's Drug Store on Willamette Street in Eugene. Everything to eat here is homemade and homebaked with no preservatives. Nothing is fried. One of the nice things about Tolly's is its two dining rooms, one for families and the other for couples upstairs with great wing-back chairs and candlelight. Menus specialize in Oregon foods and wines. Visa/MC. 10-6 Mon, 10-10 Tues-Sun.

ROGUE RIVER

48 City of Rogue River

133 Broadway, P.O. Box 1137, Rogue River, 97537. Tel: 582-4401
City Hall: 9-5 Mon-Fri.
Rogue River is the home of the National Rooster Crowing Contest, held each year on the last Saturday in June. It is also a Tree City, U.S.A. This beautiful city of 1720 citizens has five parks. Anna Classick Bicentennial Park has tennis and handball courts and horseshoe pits. Coyote Evans Park and Fleming Wayside, located on the Rogue River, offer picnic areas, boat launching facilities, and year-round fishing for rainbow and cutthroat trout, steelhead and salmon. Palmerton Park is a beautiful arboretum and Ponderosa Memorial Park has scenic hiking trails. Other attractions include an historical museum, library, large senior center, and artists' association. Visitors always welcome at City Hall.

1988-89 Rogue River Area Events include:

Last Sat in June: National Rooster Crowing Contest

ROSEBURG

49 Callahan Ridge Winery

340 Busenbark Lane, Roseburg, 97470 (take Garden Valley exit on I-5 to Melrose, cross S. Umpqua River, right on Busenbark). Tel: 673-7901
The name has changed, and so have some of the players, but Richard Mansfield and Frank Guido are still there, and Richard's wine is still as good as his sense of humor. Marrying the best of the old world with the innovation of the new, Callahan Ridge Winery produces barrel-fermented Chardonnay, White Zinfandel, a dry and late-harvest Gewurztraminer, and a lusciously sweet Riesling. (The Rieslings from the Umpqua Valley region, by the way, are especially good.) Visa/MC. Tasting room hours 11:30-5:30 daily (April-Oct). Closed in winter except by appointment.

o Country Host Registry

See MYRTLE CREEK for listing.

50 Fallen Leaf—Myrtlewood

1631 S.W. McLain Ave., Roseburg, 97470 (I-5 and McLain Ave., high on a west bank overlooking I-5 at Exit 121). Tel: 673-2747

Among other things, this myrtlewood shop handles the handcrafted work of between 100 and 150 individuals ranging in age between 22 and 86 years old working in their own shops all over Douglas County. In addition to the many unusual smaller items, myrtlewood and willow furniture is now available and specialty items can be made to order. Visa/MC. 9:30-5:30 daily.

51 Girardet Wine Cellars

895 Reston Rd., Roseburg, 97470 (10 mi. west of Winston on Hwy. 42). Tel: 679-7252

Philippe Girardet established this vineyard in 1971. Nineteen acres of varietals and French cultivars dot the southwest slope of a shale hillside, producing intensely flavored wines. The winery makes award-winning Chardonnay, Pinot Noir and Riesling in a classic style plus complex and unique wines produced by artfully blending varieties. Since opening in 1984 the Girardets have won 21 medals, 5 silver and 3 best of show. Tasting, sales, picnicking, and tours 12-5 daily (May-Sept), 12-5 Sat (Oct-April), or by appointment. Closed Dec 20—Jan 30. Tour groups welcome. Visa/MC.

52 HillCrest Vineyard

240 Vineyard Lane, Roseburg, 97470 (from I-5 take Roseburg-Garden Valley Blvd. Exit; go west approx. 3 mi. to Melrose Rd.; bear left on Melrose Rd. approx. 3-4 mi. past Melrose Store and then another ½-¾ mi; bear left on Doerner Rd. and turn right on Elgarose Rd. and go approx. 2 mi.; turn left on Vineyard Lane and go to first driveway on left). Tel: 673-3709

HillCrest Vineyard is the oldest varietal winery in Oregon. Owner Richard Sommer planted vines in 1961 and now has 35 acres of estate grapes. The vineyard specializes in Riesling, bottle-aged Cabernet Sauvignon, Pinot Noir, and small quantities of other varieties. Philip Gale is HillCrest's winemaker. The tasting room offers visitors a view from observation decks both inside and outside the winery. Picnickers are welcome. Visa/MC. Open from 10-5 daily, except major holidays.

53 Jonicole Vineyards

491 Winery Lane, Roseburg, 97470. Tel: 679-5771

Situated ½ mile southwest from I-5 and Hwy. 99-42 and only 3 miles from the entrance to the beautiful Wildlife Safari, Jonicole Vineyards Winery was founded in 1975 and dedicates itself to the production of Cabernet Sauvignon and Chardonnay. The tasting room offers a selection of their own wines plus wines from other Oregon wineries. Jon and Laurie Marker welcome visitors throughout the year. Hours are 11-6 daily (summer), 12-5 daily (winter). Large group tastings and tours welcome by appointment. (See Bandon, South Coast, for Jonicole's Bandon Tasting Room listing.)

54 Main Street Gallery

809 S.E. Main St., Roseburg, 97470 (Exit 124 from I-5, across the South Umpqua River, on the fringe of the Roseburg Town Center). Tel: 673-6694

A warm welcome awaits visitors to this gallery located in a charming 1922 Gothic-style church building. The second oldest church structure in Roseburg, and on the National Register of Historic Places, the restored building is now home to a gourmet luncheon restaurant and five specialty shops. Featuring many items made in Oregon, the shops offer candies, art, children's gifts, linens, antiques, and country collectables in a unique gallery setting. Visa/MC. 10-5:30 Tues-Fri, 10-5 Sat. Closed Sun, Mon, and holiday weekends Christmas through New Year's Day. Restaurant: 11-3 Tues-Sat.

55 Umpqua Valley Arts Center

1624 W. Harvard (Exit 124 off I-5, then west on Harvard), P.O. Box 1542, Roseburg, 97470. Tel: 672-2532

Two galleries and gift shop feature regional artists year around. The summer of 1988, the center will sponsor the 20th Annual Umpqua Valley Arts Festival on June 25 and 26, with over 100 artists, food booths, and performers. Its programs are partially supported by grants from the Oregon Arts Commission. Visa/MC. 12-6 Mon-Fri, 1-4 Sat (summer), 12-5 Mon-Fri, 1-4 Sat (winter).

STEAMBOAT

56 Steamboat Inn

Steamboat, 97447 (on the North Umpqua River 40 mi. east of Roseburg and 40 mi. west of Diamond Lake on Hwy. 138).
Tel: 498-2411 or 496-3495
Fly fishermen have patronized this cozy lodge since 1931. Now owners Jim and Sharon Van Loan and manager Pat Lee triple as guides, innkeepers and sophisticated chefs, serving elegant dinners on a table sawn from a single, six-inch slab of sugar pine. Pine-paneled cabins hidden along the river bank all have private baths and decks. Breakfasts and lunches served 8-5 summer and 9-5 winter without reservations. Dinners served a half-hour past sunset or at 7 PM in the winter to lodge guests and those with reservations. Visa/MC. Year around except holidays.

TALENT

57 Pear Blossom Pottery—Sinks and Tiles

2316 S. Pacific Hwy., Talent, 97540 (halfway between Talent and Ashland on old Hwy. 99). Tel: 535-2955
Now residing in Southern Oregon and making quality handmade round and oval sinks with matching tiles and accessories for bathrooms, kitchens and bars, Dave Cornell has been making pots since 1963. He has studied and taught at and even directed some of America's most respected ceramic institutions. He exhibits internationally. 8-5 daily.

STATE TREE

The Douglas Fir (Pseudotsuga menziesii), designated State Tree in 1939, is a principal timber species in North America. Its great strength and stiffness combined with moderate weight make it invaluable for many uses, particularly as structural timber. In proportion to its dead weight, Douglas Fir is said to be stronger than concrete. On the average, the Douglas Fir grows 180 to 200 feet in height and four to six feet in diameter, although heights of 325 feet and diameters of ten to fifteen feet are not uncommon. The tree is named for David Douglas, a 19th century Scottish botanist, sent by the Royal Horticultural Society of London to study the species.

UMPQUA

58 Henry Winery

687 Hubbard Creek Rd. (winery is exactly 7 mi. from I-5; from Sutherlin Exit go west on Hwy. 9 through Umpqua and over Umpqua River; winery will be on your right), P.O. Box 26, Umpqua, 97486.
Tel: 459-5120
Family-operated estate vineyard located by the scenic Umpqua River near Roseburg is dedicated to producing high-quality, dry varietal wines from Gewurztraminer, Chardonnay and Pinot Noir grapes—all hand picked. Sylvia and Scott Henry invite visitors to personally guided seasonal tours of carefully controlled fermentation of their wine in pungent oak-barrel aging room, bottling and labeling activities, plus free tastes of wine. Picnic facilities available. Tour groups by appointment. 11-5 daily. Closed major holidays.

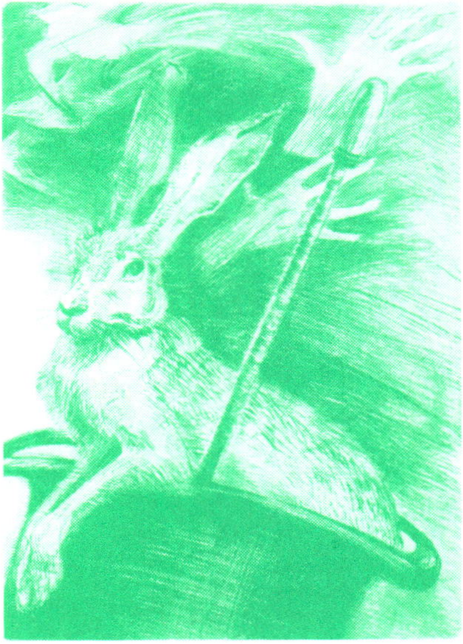

Houdini's Hare, © Liza Jones

Portland

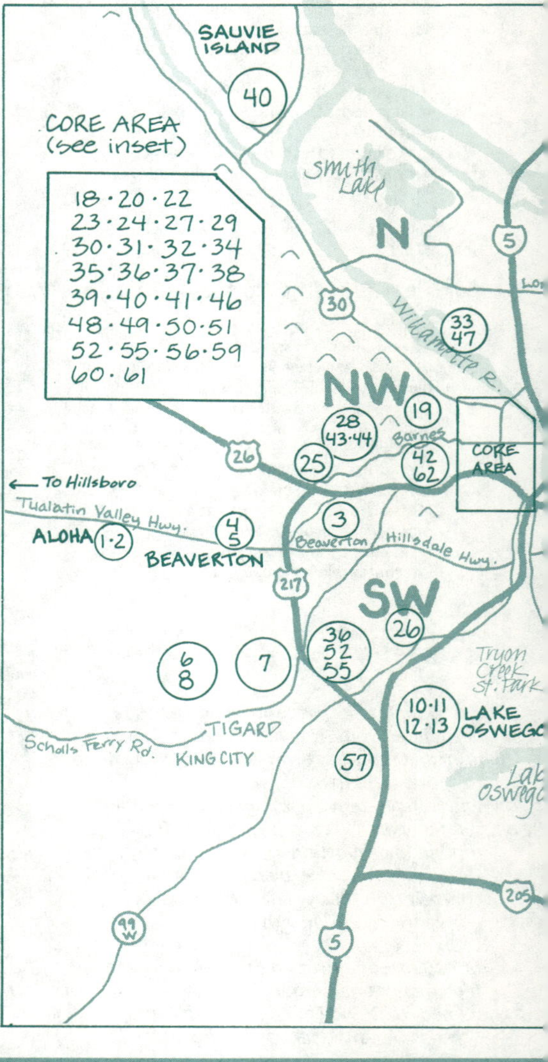

SAUVIE ISLAND
40
CORE AREA (see inset)
18·20·22
23·24·27·29
30·31·32·34
35·36·37·38
39·40·41·46
48·49·50·51
52·55·56·59
60·61
Smith Lake
N
5
30
Willamette R.
33 47
NW
19
28 43·44
Barnes
42 62
CORE AREA
26
25
← To Hillsboro
Tualatin Valley Hwy.
ALOHA
1·2
4 5
3
BEAVERTON
Beaverton Hillsdale Hwy.
217
SW
26
36 52 55
6 8
7
Tryon Creek St. Park
10·11 12·13
LAKE OSWEGO
Lake Oswego
TIGARD
Schalls Ferry Rd.
KING CITY
57
205
99 W
5

Metropolitan

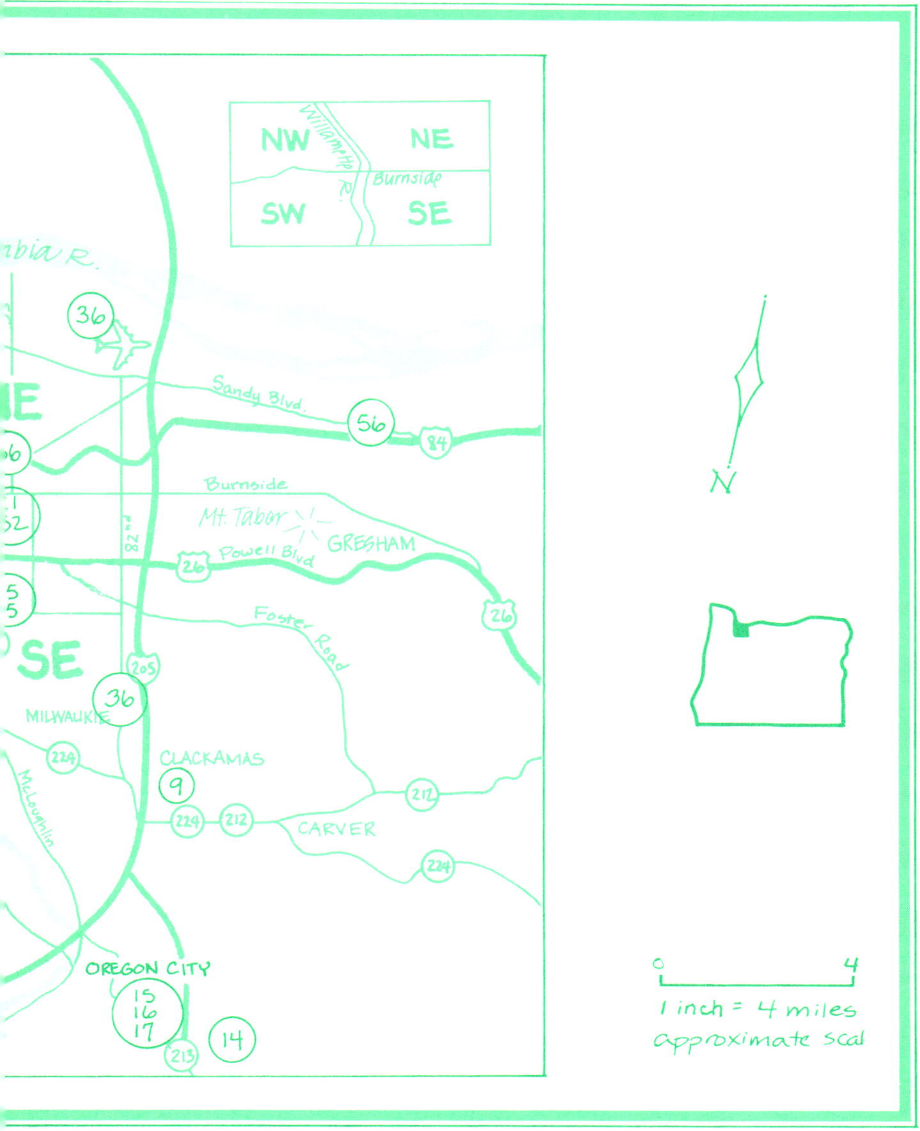

PORTLAND METROPOLITAN REGIONAL NOTES

For people who would prefer to live in the country but need all the amenities of a city, the Portland metropolitan area is a good choice. Juxtaposed against a backdrop of Mt. Hood that can be seen from most parts of the city and its suburbs is a downtown core of **new skyscrapers, restored buildings,** *and a new* **revitalized waterfront** *park where boats can be moored a few blocks from the center of town. There is a* **brand-new light-rail** *system connecting the "East County" to the core and a developing Sunset Corridor to the west, with enough landscaped high-tech business parks to be referred to as Oregon's* **"silicon forest."** *Livable residential areas are scattered equally all over the city, so that it is impossible to say that the "better people" live in any one particular neighborhood.*

An international airport connects businessmen with any city in the world as easily as any other major city in the U.S. does, and camellias bloom in February. On a typical day, while the **mayor bicycles to work** *in the morning, a real estate broker and his* **clients** *are* **delivered by helicopter** *to the top of a 43-floor glass bank building to meet with one of the best lawyers in town, who, in a* **sierra jacket over his Brooks Brothers suit,** *has just driven his old pickup into town from his place 8½ miles and 15 minutes from downtown, after delivering his kids to a rural school.*

In 1903 the Olmsted brothers, the landscape architects who designed Central park in New York City, drew up a master plan for Portland where every public school was situated next to a neighborhood park. The city now has over 175 parks and **8,000 acres of park land.** *(One park, Mt. Tabor in Southeast Portland, is located on the site of a* **dormant volcano where concerts are held**). *People who have made millions of dollars in the lumber, steel, and high-tech industries have over the years donated large sums of money to the Nature Conservancy and have received awards for helping to build art schools and symphony halls. It is no coincidence that Oregon has two voluntary checkoff options on its income tax forms—one for the arts and one for nongame wildlife. The largest percentage of Oregon's voting population lives in Portland, and Portlanders care about such things.*

Art and nature *are* **incorporated into** *the* **urban environment** *almost everywhere a person looks. The people of Lake Oswego recently took it upon themselves to raise $50,000 to hang art on the walls of their brand new city hall. The Beaverton City Council and its Art Commission invited a facilitator in to work with them on ways to involve the arts to improve the quality of life in that part of town. Portland went out on a limb and hired architect Michael Graves to design a great, green-tiled sculpture in which to house its city offices. In the fall of 1985, a* **flotilla of** *literally* **hundreds of** *small* **boats,** *the 499-passenger stern wheeler, and the fireboat ushered the 6½ ton sculpture "Portlandia" up the Willamette River to be hoisted ashore and into place in downtown Portland. Thousands of copies of a poster of the* **mayor "exposing himself" to art** *have been sold nationwide. The statue that elicited his response is only one of many pieces of art that are installed on 5th and 6th Avenues in downtown Portland as part of the city's permanent collection that has been growing over 100 years. Bronze elks, naked ladies, beavers and deer, abstract fountains and sculptures, and colorful banners all have a place in this most livable city. Even the jail has architecturally integrated stained glass, tiles, and light fixtures designed and executed by artists and craftsmen.*

The **official city bird** *is the* **great blue heron,** *because there are so many rookeries within the city limits. Beavers live on an island in the middle of downtown Portland. There is a* **growing number of wildlife refuges throughout the metropolitan area,** *including one next to a business park in the Sunset Corridor, where* **office workers** *have* **binoculars** *in their desk drawers to* **identify birds** *out their windows. The word of a highly respected young man dedicated to the concept of preserving wildlife habitats within the urban area, whose testimony is often required for environmental impact statements, is feared by developers wanting to cover wetlands with asphalt.*

It is this kind of **commitment over the years** *on all levels throughout the Portland metropolitan area that* **has made Portland such a pleasant place to visit, live, and work.**

To find an address in Portland, keep in mind that the city is laid out on a grid, for the most part, and that the **center of the grid** *is where* **Burnside Bridge** *crosses the* **Willamette River,** *N.W., S.W., N.E., and S.E. are all determined from this point. (See map insert.) Numbered streets start at the Willamette River and the numbers get larger as one goes away from the river. Named streets in Northwest Portland are arranged alphabetically.*

ALOHA

1 Little Dipper Chocolates

3735 S.W. 185th Ave., Aloha, 97007.
Tel: 642-3717
This is the home of "Hazelnut Snappers" and other custom candy utilizing Oregon-grown products. Candy makers will find candy molds and supplies here too, as well as custom candy molds for "logo" mints. Retail and wholesale. Shipping daily. Visa/MC. 10-5:30 Mon-Fri, call first on Sat.

2 Prlain's Cheesecakes

3524 E, S.W. 209th, Aloha (west on Tualatin Valley Hwy. to 209th, south on 209th to Industrial Way and Westway Industrial Park). Mailing address: P.O. Box 5802, Aloha, 97006. Tel: 649-1878
"Luscious, creamy cheesecakes table-ready in 12 different flavors, including Oregon hazelnut," are Prlain's Foods' specialties. Made with only Kraft Philadelphia Cream Cheese, graham cracker crust, and all-natural flavorings. David and Jean Prlain say their cheesecakes are a cheesecake lover's dream come true and invite folks to send one to a friend who loves great cheesecakes. Available at most retail markets. Mail order throughout the U.S. 8-6 Mon-Fri or evenings by appointment.

BEAVERTON

3 Archibald's Tasting Room/ Rogue River Vineyards Ltd.

10000 S.W. Canyon Rd., Beaverton, 97225. Tel: 297-2590
This is a cooperative effort between the Rogue River Vineyards and the Quality Meat Company, both from Grants Pass. Wines from Rogue River Vineyards include varietal wines, Chardonnay, White Riesling, Early Muscat, Gewurztraminer, Pinot Noir Blanc, Pinot Noir, Cabernet Sauvignon, Silver Springs White Blush, Red Table Wine, apricot and strawberry-flavored Chablis, and the ever-popular Very Berry Wine Cooler. In addition, there is an astounding selection of hardwood-smoked meats, cheeses, and breads. The experienced and friendly staff at Archibald's can help put together meats, cheeses, and wines that complement each other. Visa/MC. 10-6 daily except Mon. (Additional tasting rooms at Archibald's in Ashland and Rogue River Vineyards in Grants Pass, Southern Oregon.)

4 Beaverton Foods—Gift Factory

4210 S.W. Cedar Hills Blvd., Beaverton, 97005. Tel: 646-8138 (Beaverton Foods), 643-7634 (Gift Factory).
In 1925 Rose Biggi, widowed with three children to support, began growing and selling horseradish. Now her son, Gene, manufactures over 49 kinds of gourmet mustards, plus the original horseradish. Beaverton Foods also produces customized gift packs using other famous Oregon products as well as their own. Visa/MC/AmEx. 10-6 Mon-Sat. Tours of horseradish and mustard plant Mon-Fri until 2:30.

5 Chapin's Fudge

P.O. Box 285, Beaverton, 97075.
Tel: 643-1757
Ceac Chapin's fudge is made with a 70-year-old family recipe which uses the purest ingredients, including whipping cream and butter, to produce a truly unique caramel-based fudge, dipped in pure milk chocolate. Found year around at Chocolate Etc. in John's Landing; Strohecker's, How Sweet It Is, The Arrangement, and Sassafras in Portland; and To Market To Market in West Linn. Also available by mail order. Write for information. A Neiman-Marcus selection.

6 Ponzi Vineyards

Rt. 1, Box 842, Beaverton, 97007 (go 4½ mi. west on Scholls Ferry Rd. after it crosses Hwy. 217 at Washington Square in Beaverton, then go ½ mi. south on Vandermost Rd. to vineyards on left).
Tel: 628-1227
Portland's closest winery/vineyard, Ponzi Vineyards produces award-winning dry table wines of Pinot Noir, Chardonnay, Pinot Gris, and White Riesling. Seasonal events feature a wine-music-food festival on Memorial Weekend, Valley Wine Tour on Thanksgiving Weekend, and Vineyard Jazz Summer Concert Series, performances of the finest Northwest jazz musicians the last Sunday of each summer month. Tasting room open 12-5 Sat-Sun or by appointment. Open Mon-Fri for sales only. Group tours welcome by special arrangement. Visa.

7 Powell's Books

Cascade Plaza, 8775 S.W. Cascade, Beaverton, 97005 (Cascade Ave. between Hall Blvd. and Scholls Ferry Rd.; take Progress/Scholls Ferry Rd. exit off Hwy. 217). Tel: 643-3131
Powell's Books in Cascade Plaza is a slightly down-scaled version of their downtown store, and more convenient for some shoppers. Hundreds of new and used volumes line the shelves on a variety of topics. (See Portland listing for information on Powell's other stores.) Visa/MC. 9-9 daily, including holidays.

8 Scholls Ferry Farm

Rt. 1, Box 822, Beaverton, 97007 (4½ mi. west of Washington Square on Scholls Ferry Rd., Hwy. 210). Tel: 644-3233 or 649-7174
The McFarland farm grows several varieties of apples as well as filberts (hazelnuts) and walnuts. Fresh apple cider (in season), old-fashioned apple butter, apple chutney, apple cider jelly, spiced apple jelly, and mint jelly are specialty products of the farm. They are sold separately or made into gift packs. Other local gourmet items are also available in their country store. Call or write for brochure. Visa/MC. 10-5 Thurs-Sun (Aug 1–Dec 30).

CLACKAMAS

9 McSteven's

15410 S.E. 94th St., P.O. Box 293, Clackamas, 97015. Tel: 657-3055
N-M
Continuing in the pioneer spirit of Oregon, Patricia McCormick creates and produces six "sumptuous" flavors of McSteven's Spicey Cocoa at the Pioneer Grange No. 1, the first grange hall in the state, built c. 1873. McSteven's also offers "Pop Toppers," flavorings for home-popped popcorn, as well as flavored tea and gourmet spice blends with no preservatives. Call or write for wholesale or retail prices or location of nearest retail outlet. A Neiman-Marcus selection. Visa/MC.

LAKE OSWEGO

10 The Gazebo Gallery and Restaurant

11 Mt. Jefferson Terrace, Lake Oswego, 97034 (look for the weathervane atop a tall, peaked roof on top of the knoll, Mt. Jefferson, in Mountain Park).
Tel: 635-2506
Elizabeth Morrow's vision became a reality when her architect husband designed her a charming gazebo atop Mountain Park with windows facing Mt. Hood, where people enjoy pleasant dining in a setting filled with plants and handmade objects made by Oregon and Northwest artists and craftspeople. Visa/MC/AmEx. Restaurant: 11:45-2 Tues-Sat (lunch); 6-8:15 Thurs-Sat (dinner). Gallery: 11:30-6 Tues-Wed; 11:30-9 Thurs-Sat.

11 Lakewood Center for the Arts

368 S. State St., P.O. Box 274, Lake Oswego, 97034. Tel: 635-6338 (center), 635-3901 (theater)
A not-for-profit, volunteer community cultural center with a performing arts emphasis housing Lake Oswego Community Theatre, Lakewood Gallery, Collector Gallery, Systems Fitness, artists-in-residence, art education programs, and numerous festivals during the year. Some of its programs are supported by grants from the Oregon Arts Commission. Visa/MC. 9-5 Mon-Fri, open weekends for special events.

12 Paradigm Chocolate Company

Executive Park, 5775 S.W. Jean Rd., Suite 106A, Lake Oswego, 97035.
Tel: 636-4880
N-M
All Paradigm's products are made on the premises with recipes developed by Lynne Barra. They include 17 different dessert sauces (six liquor-laced fudges, one deep dark fudge, four caramel, four Oregon fruit, and two chocolate cream) plus "Jamaican Pecans" (caramel-glazed pecan candies). Paradigm also distributes fine imported and domestic baking chocolate, including Lindt Couvertures. Gift packs and shipping available. Catalog cost refundable with purchase. Available at Strohecker's and Broadway Coffee Merchant in Portland, Wizer's in Lake Oswego, and all Made in Oregon Shops. A Neiman-Marcus selection. 8-5 Mon-Fri.

13 Gloria Sample and Company

199 "E" Ave., Lake Oswego, 97034.
Tel: 636-5111 or 636-3520
Yes, there really is a Gloria Sample, and she produces a classic fruitcake from a recipe handed down to her by her Great-grandmother Dewey. She also makes English catsup, sweet pickled watermelon rind, and all-natural specialty preserves and jams. Products available at Norm Thompson, Meier & Frank, Strohecker's, and Broadway Coffee Merchant in Portland, Wizer's in Lake Oswego, Made in Oregon Shops in Portland and Salem, and at the Lake Grove Market. Corporate gift packs and shipping available. Call or write for appointment, price list, or to place orders. A Neiman-Marcus selection.

OREGON CITY

14 John Inskeep Environmental Learning Center

19600 S. Molalla Ave., Oregon City, 97045 (on the Clackamas Community College Campus). Tel: 657-8400, ext. 351
This eight-acre outdoor museum and technology center continues its leadership role in blending education activities and the environment with the addition of its new Lakeside Educational Hall and Haggart Memorial Celestial Observatory. A cooperative community project, the center includes over one and one-half miles of paths, bridges, streams, waterfalls, and impressive exhibits and demonstration areas concerning birds of prey, fish rearing and aquaculture, farm forestry wildlife, urban streams and wetlands, and a materials reuse and recycling facility. A one-of-a-kind Northwest resource for education and tourism, it also offers traveling exhibits, classes, workshops, seminars, and retreats. Visa/MC. 10-6 daily except Mon.

15 Dr. John McLoughlin House

713 Center St., Oregon City, 97045.
Tel: 656-5146
Residence of Dr. McLoughlin, father of the Oregon Territory and founder of Oregon City. Built in 1846, it is a national historic site and restored with many original furnishings. Graves of McLoughlin and his wife are located on the grounds. Oregon City is the end of the Oregon Trail. 10-4 Tues-Sat, 1-4 Sun.

16 Oregon City Historic Tours

Start at McLoughlin House at 713 Center St., Oregon City, 97045. Tel: 656-5146
Five "self-guided" walking and driving tours of Oregon's oldest city including: the original McLoughlin Town Plat, Main Street and Canemah National Register Historic District. Oregon City is the end of the Oregon Trail. Obtain tour brochures for a small fee at McLoughlin House, where tours begin.

17 Oregon Trail Visitors Center

500 Washington St. (at 5th), Oregon City, 97045. Tel: 657-9336
Oregon City is the nationally designated end of the 2,000-mile overland trail from Independence, Missouri. The Center interprets and explains the arduous trail journey undertaken by over 300,000 pioneers beginning in the 1840s. 10-4 Tues-Sat, 11-4 Sun.

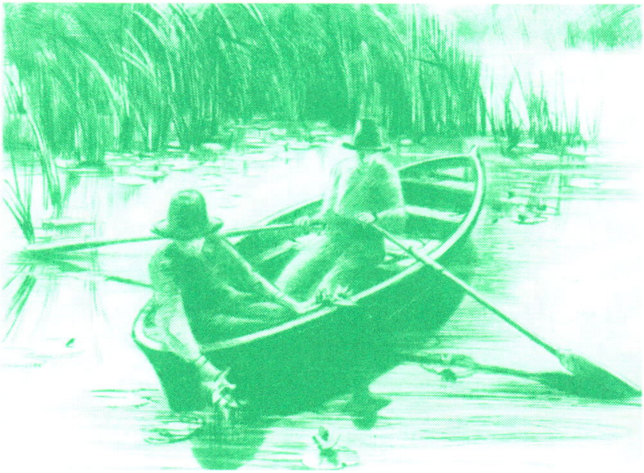

Family Portrait, © Liza Jones

PORTLAND

18 Greater Portland Convention and Visitors Association

26 S.W. Salmon, Portland, 97204.
Tel: 222-2223
Office: 9-5 Mon-Fri
Portland, the "City of Roses" and Oregon's largest city, is one of the country's most livable cities. It lies on the banks of the Willamette River, surrounded by spectacular scenery. The Columbia River Gorge, Mt. Hood, water falls, forests, ski slopes, fishing streams, hunting and camping areas are within easy reach. The International Rose Test Garden is a showpiece with 8,000 bushes and 400 varieties, and the 17-day Rose Festival is Portland's biggest event of the year. Call or write for the Portland Book, a guide to attractions, events, festivals, and restaurants.

1988-89 Portland Area Events include:

1988

April 1-3: Home & Garden Show
June 3-19: 79th Annual Portland Rose Festival
June 26: Cascade Runoff
July 9-31: "Street of Dreams" Homes Tour
July 9-10: State Games of Oregon
July 15-17: 36th Annual Scottish Highland Games & Clan Gathering
July 17: 10th Annual KGW Neighborfair & Folkfest
Aug 5-7: Mt. Hood Festival of Jazz
Sept 2-4: Artquake
Dec 15-23: 33rd Annual Parade of Christmas Ships

1989

Jan 21: PNB Oregon Indoor Track & Field Meet
Feb 18-26: Boat Show

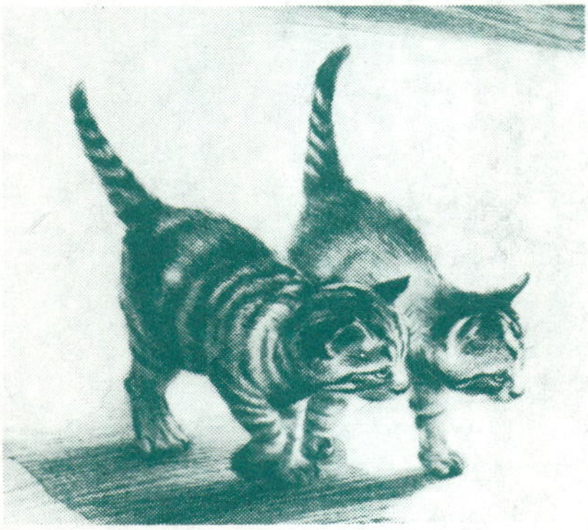

© *Liza Jones*

19 Audubon Society of Portland

5151 N.W. Cornell Rd., Portland, 97210 (from Portland head west on N.W. Lovejoy to Cornell Rd. and keep bearing right. The Audubon Society is just beyond the two tunnels.). Tel: 292-6855
Nestled in Portland's West Hills, the Audubon Society of Portland offers several miles of hiking trails through 110 acres of wildlife sanctuary. The society runs a natural history bookstore and gift shop, a wildlife rehabilitation center for injured and orphaned animals, and offers a wide array of field trips, fund-raising events, and education programs for children and adults. Visa/MC. Trails: dawn to dusk. Bookstore/Gift Shop: 10-6 Wed, 10-4 other days except Mon. Closed Mon and some holidays. Wildlife Care Center: 10-3 daily.

○ Bed and Breakfast Accommodations—Oregon Plus

See STATEWIDE RESOURCES for listing.

20 Bookmerchants (Cafe, Bookstore, Newsstand)

818 S.W. First, Portland, 97204.
Tel: 242-0087
While the bookstore has been open for five years, the lunch restaurant upstairs is new. Bookmerchants carries a wide assortment of magazines and cards, and has a good travel section with lots of maps. The restaurant, with a simpler menu than its parent restaurant, Canyon Way, in Newport, serves hot pastas, pasta salads, sandwiches, its own homemade soups and desserts, espresso, and Oregon and imported beers and wines. "Carry-out" is popular too. Visa/MC. 10-6 Mon-Sat, 10-5 Sun (10-2:30 Sun brunch).

21 Bread and Ink Cafe

3610 S.E. Hawthorne Blvd., Portland, 97214. Tel: 239-4756
Right in the heart of the Hawthorne District, Patricia Hill, Grey Wolfe and Bruce Fishback's Bread and Ink Cafe is a comfortable, welcoming neighborhood restaurant with an eclectic menu reflecting the staff's diverse interests and experience in food. One of Oregon's "ten best restaurants" it is said. Visa/MC. 7-3, 5:30-10 Tues-Fri; 8-3, 5:30-11 Sat; 10-2 Sun; closed Mon.

22 BridgePort Brew Pub/ BridgePort Brewing Company, Inc.

1313 N.W. Marshall, Portland, 97209.
Tel: 241-7179
Portland's original micro-brewery, BridgePort Brew Pub offers freshly made ales, pub-style meals, amiable atmosphere, and a view into the adjacent brewery. Ales include classic English styles, specialty beers, and true cask-conditioned ales—naturally carbonated, full-flavored, and dispensed with beer engines. Handmade pizzas with dough made from beer wort, feta cheese, artichokes, and locally produced sausage. The non-smoking environment makes pub visiting at BridgePort a pleasant experience for non-smokers. Visa. 4-10 PM Tues-Thurs, 2-11 PM Fri, noon-11 PM Sat, 1-8 PM Sun.

23 Briggs & Crampton Caterers, Inc.

1902 N.W. 24th Ave., Portland, 97210.
Tel: 223-8690
Briggs & Crampton's elegant catering, box lunches, and gift and picnic baskets for business meetings and private entertaining are very special. They take great pride in their presentations, using herbs and flowers from their own garden. Lunch for two is served daily in their 1900-era house and is so popular that it is usually reserved six months in advance. Nancy and Juanita's food column in *Northwest Palate* mirrors their own interest in regional, seasonal cooking which includes such delights as fiddlehead ferns and Chinook salmon in spring, berries in summer, pumpkins, nuts and melons in fall, and crab and oysters in winter. Visa/MC. 9-6 Mon-Sat.

24 Cascades

333 N.W. 23rd Ave., Portland, 97210.
Tel: 274-2305
Cascades is more than simply a venue for Portland's finest Northwest regional cuisine. Situated in the heart of exciting Northwest Portland, owners Michael Becker and executive chef Victor Pritzker offer a spectacular, diverse selection of brunch dishes, appetizers, soups, salads, sandwiches, pizzas, entrees, regional wines, and liquor in a magnificent, completely smoke-free environment with outdoor dining. Handicapped access. Visa/MC/AmEx/Diners. 11:30 AM-10 PM Mon-Thurs, 11:30 AM-11 PM Fri, 8:30 AM-11 PM Sat, 8:30 AM-10 PM Sun (summer); 11:30 AM-2 PM Mon-Fri, 5:30-9:30 PM Sun-Thurs, 5:30-10:30 PM Fri-Sat (winter).

25 Chamber Music Northwest

520 S.W. 6th, Suite 1112, Portland, 97204. (Performances at Reed College Campus and Catlin Gabel School on Barnes Rd. next to St. Vincent Hospital.)
Tel: 223-3202
Portland's nationally acclaimed summer chamber music festival is a gathering place for some of the nation's most gifted musicians. The five-week annual season presents 15 concerts at Reed College and 10 at Catlin Cabel School, featuring music of wide-ranging repertoire. Catered pre-concert picnics on the campus lawns are popular with concert-goers. Programs are partially supported by the Oregon Arts Commission and the National Endowment for the Arts. Visa/MC. Office: 9-5 Mon-Fri. Concerts are at 8PM on Mon, Thurs, Sat at Reed and Tues, Fri at Catlin Gabel.

26 Champagne Additions

6728 S.W. Miles Ct., Portland, 97223.
Tel: 222-1045
Guaranteed to change a person's mind about drinking plain champagne, Terri Warren's thick, pureed fruit concentrates can be added to champagne, spumante, soda water, or selzer for an elegant punch. Peach Bellini is a specialty using Oregon fruits made with the Venice, Italy, tradition in mind. Available at Stroheck-er's, Sassafras, and Meier & Frank in Portland, Nature's and Scholls Ferry Farm in Beaverton, and Wizer's in Lake Oswego. A Neiman-Marcus selection.

27 Clear Creek Distillery

1430 N.W. 23rd Ave., Portland, 97210 (off west end of Fremont Bridge, at N.W. 23rd and Quimby). Tel: 248-9470
Specializing in William (Bartlett) Pear Brandy, Stephen R. McCarthy, winemaker and distiller, uses European techniques and stills to make a totally authentic *eaux de vie*. The pears are grown at his orchard in the Hood River Valley. (See Columbia Gorge-Mt. Hood Regional Notes.) This is the only micro-distillery in Oregon and, at 80-proof, Stephen's brandy is sold only in state liquor stores. Tours by appointment.

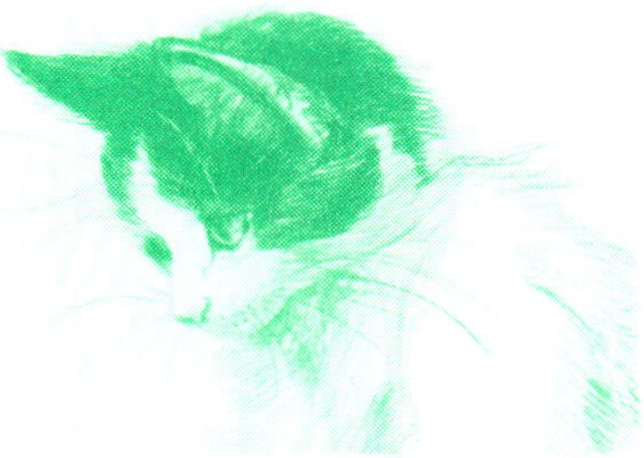

© *Liza Jones*

28 Cornell Farm Nursery

8212 S.W. Barnes Rd., Portland, 97225 (just off Hwy. 26 and Hwy. 217, near St. Vincent Hospital, across Barnes Road from Oregon School of Arts and Crafts). Tel: 292-2939

Ted Blatter and his father before him farmed this place. Ted still tills many of the farms in the area. His son and daughter-in-law recently built a greenhouse in which they grow flowering plants, shrubs and trees to sell to the apartment dwellers that have surrounded their historic Dutch Colonial farmhouse. Their new, retail gazebo is always full of hanging baskets plus fresh cut flowers from their own beds in summer, pumpkins in the fall and Christmas trees in winter. Also available are ornamental planters and a custom potting service.

29 Elephants Delicatessen

13 N.W. 23rd Place, Portland, 97210. Tel: 224-3955

The personalized service and ambience of Elaine Tanzer's fun, fascinating delicatessen featuring picnic foods, salads, main entrees, breads, and desserts, all made with fresh ingredients on the premises, by hand from scratch, always puts customers in a good mood. Also available are local and imported wines, cheeses, smoked fish, gifts, personal catering, and gift packs. Many of the things available here were chosen to be part of the Bloomingdale's promotion of Oregon food and wine products. Visa/MC. 10-6:30 Mon-Fri, 10-6 Sat, 9:30-4 Sun.

30 Heron Haus Bed and Breakfast Inn

2545 N.W. Westover Rd., Portland, 97210. Tel: 274-1846

On Portland's Northwest Hills, Julie Keppeler offers elegant bed and breakfast accommodations in a turn-of-the-century Tudor mansion. Most rooms have panoramic views of the city and mountains, plus spacious sitting areas with private baths. One has a raised whirlpool spa, another has a shower with seven heads. Continental breakfast served in fireplace dining room or overlooking swimming pool. Just two blocks from Northwest Portland's Nob Hill with its shops, boutiques, and eateries. No smoking or pets. Open year around.

31 The Image Gallery

1026 S.W. Morrison St., Portland, 97205. Tel: 224-9629

New owner, Beverly Shoemaker, continues the high standards and special qualities of one of Portland's oldest galleries. It represents some of the area's outstanding painters, printmakers, sculptors, and the estates of highly respected Oregon artists. Some of those represented have received fellowship awards from the Oregon Arts Commission. Known for its Ethnic Art, the gallery has pieces from Africa, Latin America, Thailand, and Poland, as well as Eskimo sculpture and a good collection of modern and traditional prints. Individual and corporate consulting, framing and installation. Visa/MC/AmEx. 10:30-6 Mon-Fri, 11:30-4 Sat-Sun. Open until 8:30 first Thurs of each month.

32 Jake's Famous Crawfish

401 S.W. 12th, Portland, 97205. Tel: 226-1419

Established in 1892, Jake's is a Portland landmark with the largest fresh seafood menu in the Northwest and one of the most extensive Oregon wine lists. Many of Jake's specialties, including its famous chocolate truffle cake, were chosen as part of the Neiman-Marcus and Bloomingdale's promotions of Oregon products. Noted for its traditional turn-of-the-century service and ambience, it has the largest exhibited collection of privately owned fine art works in the Northwest. Visa/MC/AmEx/Diners/CB/Discover. 11-3 Mon-Fri (lunch); 5-11 Mon-Sat, 5-10 Sun (dinner).

33 Jake's Famous Products

4910 N. Basin, Portland, 97217. Tel: 226-1420

Manufacturers of entire line of gourmet seafood products, condiments and desserts including clam chowder, smoked salmon and sturgeon and patés, and chocolate truffle cake made from restaurant's famous recipes and 100% pure ingredients. Selected as part of the Neiman-Marcus and Bloomingdale's promotions of Oregon products. Examples may be tried at restaurant (founded in 1892) at 401 S.W. 12th. Call or write office for wholesale price list or retail availability. Visa/MC/AmEx/Discover. 9-5 Mon-Fri.

34 L'Auberge

2601 N.W. Vaughn St., Portland, 97210.
Tel: 223-3302
Fifteen years ago this was one of only a handful of Portland restaurants which emphasized fresh, regional products. It has remained one of the city's very special places. Bill McLaughlin's fixed menu changes daily. Six-course dinners with a choice of four main dishes and six or seven desserts are served in the dining room. The lounge has a Bistro menu with soups, salads, hors d'oeuvres, light entrees, and desserts. Extensive wine list, with many Oregon wines. Reservations required for dinner. All major credit cards. Dining room: 6-10 Mon-Sat. Bar: 5-12 Mon-Thurs, 5-1 Fri-Sat, 5:30-12 Sun.

o Larsen Farm Nursery

See WILSONVILLE (Northern Willamette Valley) for listing.

35 MacMaster House Bed and Breakfast Inn

1041 S.W. Vista Ave., Portland, 97205.
Tel: 223-7362
Built in 1885 by Englishman William MacMaster, this classic Colonial Revival home has come of age as a bed and breakfast inn operated by Cecilia Murphy. Its colossal portico, seven working fireplaces, and spacious rooms delight guests. Three-room suite, two large bedroom/sitting rooms, and a smaller guest room, all with cable TV. Hearty full breakfast served family style. City parks, gardens, downtown and Northwest Portland within walking distance. No children or pets. Smoking on patio or veranda.

36 Made in Oregon Shops

Nine locations: Portland Airport, 282-7827; downtown Portland: Galleria, 241-3630; Oldtown, 10 N.W. 1st, 273-8354; Tigard: Washington Square, 620-4670; eastside Portland: Lloyd Center, 281-3328 and 282-7636; Clackamas Town Center, 659-3155. (See Salem and Medford for other listings.) Toll-free phone orders: 800-4-BUY-ORE (in-state), 800-8-BUY-ORE (out-of-state). Everything for sale in "Made in Oregon" shops is made, caught or grown in Oregon, including salmon, wine, cheese, jam, ceramics, myrtlewood, and Pendleton blankets. The Portland Airport Shop is particularly convenient for last-minute purchases of authentic Oregon products. The "Made in Oregon" catalog, available at all locations, also provides a full selection of products. Visa/MC/AmEx/JCB/Discover. Mall stores open regular mall hours. Call others for hours.

37 New Rose Theatre

904 S.W. Main St., Portland, 97205.
Tel: 222-2487 (tickets), 222-2495 (admin.)
Portland's only theater committed to the production of modern and classical plays, the New Rose is breathing today's life into the great theater traditions. Located on the Park Blocks in the cultural heart of the city, there is convenient public parking. Newly remodeled, the small, intimate stage will see the end of the 1988 season with "And a Nightingale Sang" by C. P. Taylor and "Misalliance" by G. B. Shaw. Visa/MC. Box office: 3-7 PM Tues-Sat. 8 PM curtain Tues-Sat, 2 PM and 7 PM Sun.

o NW Bed and Breakfast Travel Unlimited

See STATEWIDE RESOURCES for listing.

38 O'Connell Gallery

25 S.W. Salmon St., Portland, 97204.
Tel: 220-0330
Things are happening at the O'Connell Gallery. Located in an all-glass building across from the new waterfront fountain and next to a working antique carousel, this gallery exhibits mobiles, gravitrams, wind chimes, and other kinetic art forms, as well as a wide selection of oils, watercolors, prints, glass, pottery, and sculpture by Northwest artists and craftsmen. Also maps and travel information for tourists. Visa/MC/AmEx/Discover. 10-6 Mon-Fri, 11-5 Sat-Sun. Open until 9 first Thurs of each month.

39 Oregon Art Institute

1219 S.W. Park, Portland, 97205.
Tel: 226-2811
The oldest and largest visual arts institution in Oregon, founded in 1892, it houses the Portland Art Museum, the Pacific Northwest College of Art, the Northwest Film and Video Center with full-time film schedule, a Rental Sales Gallery, and a Museum Shop. Extensive programs of national and international traveling exhibitions plus permanent collections. Programs are often supported by the Oregon Arts Commission, the National Endowment for the Arts, and other organizations. Visa/MC. 11-7 Tues-Thurs, 11-9:30 Fri, 12-5 Sat, Sun. Guided tours Sun at 2. Closed Mon and major holidays.

40 Oregon Historical Society

1230 S.W. Park Ave., Portland, 97205 (Bybee-Howell Pioneer Homestead and Agricultural Museum on Sauvie Island: drive northwest on Hwy. 30 past Linnton to Sauvie Island Bridge, go 1 mi. to Howell Park Rd.). Tel: 222-1741
A major all-new exhibition on Oregon history occupies the entire second floor of the four-story OHS building, which also features other fascinating, nationally recognized permanent and changing exhibitions. No admission charge. Group tours by reservation. Regional research library offers rare books, photographs, films. Publications by Oregon Historical Society Press and gift items available in bookshop. The Bybee-Howell Pioneer Homestead and Agricultural Museum offer a specific rural perspective. Visa/MC. Historical Society: 10-4:45 Mon-Sat year around. Bybee Homestead: 12-5 June-Labor Day.

41 Oregon Mountain Rumcake

0333 S.W. Nebraska St., Portland, 97201. Tel: 246-8875 or 800-237-6047 (nationwide)
Dan Culver says the Culver Family's Oregon Mountain Rumcake is "the state's tastiest year 'round dessert." He calls the "Original Halfway Up The Mountain Cake," created high on the slopes of Mt. Hood, bathed and preserved in rich dark Oregon rum from the Hood River valley, a "visitor's must." Packaged in a miniature souvenir size as well as larger 2 lb. and 4 lb. gift sizes, the cakes are shipped worldwide. Ask for it, or call their toll-free number. A Neiman-Marcus selection.

42 Oregon Museum of Science and Industry (OMSI)

4015 S.W. Canyon Rd., Portland, 97221. Tel: 222-2828
A playground of the imagination, OMSI stimulates and challenges with hands-on exhibits and experiences that prove science is fun and exciting. It is on the leading edge of scientific and technological discovery. Visitors can see, touch and really get to know how things work. Exhibits, classes, planetarium, camps, field trips, gift shop. Visa/MC/AmEx. 9-7 Sat-Thurs, 9-8 Fri (summer); 9-5 Sat-Thurs, 9-8 Fri (winter). Times subject to change, call if possible.

43 Oregon School of Arts and Crafts

8245 S.W. Barnes Rd., Portland, 97225. Tel: 297-5544
Nine-building campus with separate studios for book arts, fibers, wood, clay, metals, photography, drawing and design welcomes visitors to its public spaces enhanced by handmade library furniture, ceramic tiles, gargoyle rain spouts, sculptured fire bowl, architectural glass, iron work, handcarved railings, sculptured fireplace and revolving windship. Year around class/workshop schedule available. The architecturally integrated craftwork and programs of the school have been partially supported by the Oregon Arts Commission and the National Endowment for the Arts. Visa/MC. Hours open to public: see Hoffman Gallery, et al listing. School and studio hours more extensive.

44 Hoffman Gallery, Sales Shop, Bookstore and Lunch Facility at the Oregon School of Arts and Crafts

8245 S.W. Barnes Rd., Portland, 97225. Tel: 297-5544
Sales and exhibition gallery spotlights exceptional contemporary work in monthly exhibitions and represents the work of Northwest craftspeople on an ongoing basis. Bookstore specializes in crafts books. Homemade lunches, dinners, and Sunday brunch, served on handmade dishes, are available to the public in hand-furnished dining room. Hoffman Gallery is partially supported by the Oregon Arts Commission and the National Endowment for the Arts. Visa/MC. Gallery/Shop/Bookstore: 10-5 Mon-Sat, 10-4 Sun. Lunch: 11:30-2 Mon-Fri. Dinner: 5:30-7:30 Mon-Thurs. Sun brunch: 10:30-1:30.

45 Oregon Spice Company

3525 S.E. 17th Ave., Portland, 97202. Tel: 238-0664
The Oregon Spice Company offers more than a hundred packaged gourmet spices and blends plus ice cream and bakery "toppers," gourmet coffees, extracts, and gift items. Tours by appointment. Write for free catalog. 8-5 Mon-Fri, plus 10-2 Sat during holiday season.

46 Pacific Ballet Theatre

1119 S.W. Park Ave., Portland, 97205.
Tel: 227-6867
Sponsored by the 30-year-old Ballet Society of Portland, the city's oldest ballet association, it thrills 65,000 adults and children each season with a number of productions, including "The Nutcracker," which is rapidly becoming a Portland holiday tradition. Meanwhile, the School of Pacific Ballet Theatre offers programs ranging from professional training to novice classes for children and adults in ballet, jazz and modern dance. The return of Artistic Director James Canfield and principal dancer Patricia Miller point toward exciting times for this rising company.

47 The John Palmer House and Carriage Service

4314 N. Mississippi, Portland, 97217.
Tel: 284-5893
This 1890 award-winning Victorian landmark is a memorable retreat into an era gone by. Mary and Richard Sauter say their guests rave about the antique furnishings and wallpapers, breakfasts too beautiful to eat, scrumptious high teas, great beds, and romantic carriage rides. If you are famous, or wish you were, they can offer privacy and elegance. Suites with private or shared bath, double with shared bath. Complimentary high tea and gourmet breakfast. House tours, carriage rides, and high tea available to public by reservation. Visa/MC. Open year around.

48 Plum Hills

525 N.W. 17th, Portland, 97209.
Tel: 224-3749
Jim Bourdin's Plum Hills Barbecue Sauce, which is as legendary as Oregon's own Plum Hills, is a memorable sauce, marinade, or dip for seafood, poultry, pork, beef, and vegetables. With a strong sense of regionalism, Jim uses the finest ingredients available, searching for consistency, purity, and quality. The all-natural, plum-based sauce contains no additives or preservatives. Available at Strohecker's, Nature's, Hartung Meats, Meier & Frank, Made in Oregon Shops, and Zupan's. A Neiman-Marcus selection.

49 Portland Center for the Performing Arts

1111 S.W. Broadway, Portland, 97205.
Tel: 248-4496 (box office), 248-4335 (business office)
The four stages of this award-winning center bring the magic of live performance to diverse audiences. The 3000-seat Civic Auditorium, 2776-seat Arlene Schnitzer Concert Hall, 900-seat Intermediate Theater and 350-seat Dolores Winningstad Theater host performances by the Oregon Symphony Orchestra, Portland Opera, Portland Youth Philharmonic, the Oregon Shakespeare Festival, Portland Center Stage, Ballet Oregon, West Coast Chamber Orchestra, Oregon Repertory Singers, Portland Gay Men's Chorus, Pacific Ballet Theater, Storefront and New Rose theaters; myriad pop, classical, jazz, country and rock concert artists from around the world; and activities as varied as Grand Opera and bodybuilding championships. Visa/MC/AmEx. 10-5 Mon-Sat plus performance times.

50 Portland Civic Theatre

1530 S.W. Yamhill, Portland, 97205.
Tel: 226-3048 (tickets), 226-3040 (admin.)
Portland's oldest and largest live theater offers splashy Broadway musicals, drama and comedy in two separate theaters: the Mainstage and the intimate Blue Room. Active children's theater program too. Programs are partially supported by grants from the Oregon Arts Commission and the National Endowment for the Arts. Visa/MC/AmEx. 8 PM curtain Thurs-Sat, 7 PM curtain Sun.

51 Portland Repertory Theater

25 S.W. Salmon St., Portland, 97204.
Tel: 224-4491
Portland has a theater on a bridge . . . the Portland Repertory Theater. Located downtown in the award-winning Willamette Center on the sparkling waterfront, the Rep offers convenient underground parking and state-of-the-art technical sophistication. As Portland's only professional, resident theater company, the Rep provides an eclectic season of American classic and contemporary plays year around. Visa/MC. 8 PM curtain Tues-Sat, 2 PM and 7 PM Sun.

52 Powell's Books

Main store: 1005 W. Burnside St., Portland, 97209. Tel: 228-4651 (See below for information on other stores.)
Powell's is a Portland tradition, and for some, an addiction. Now owned by Walt's son, Michael, it has grown to fill a full city block. How many books are here? No one seems to know, but there are literally thousands and thousands of new, used, and out-of-print books in hundreds of subject areas, including many on Oregon history and travel. The Anne Hughes' Coffee Room, located in a corner of the store, provides a haven for the weary browser. Powell's now has a second store, in Cascade Plaza in Beaverton (see Beaverton for listing), and three specialty stores: the Technical Store, near the main store, 32 N.W. 11th, Tel: 228-3906; the Travel Store, Pioneer Courthouse Square, downtown Portland, Tel: 228-1108; and Powell's Books for Cooks, 3739 S.E. Hawthorne, Portland, Tel: 235-3802. Visa/MC. Main store: 9 AM-11 PM Mon-Sat, 9-9 Sun. Open holidays. Call specialty stores for their hours.

53 Prescott Street Press

P.O. Box 40312, Portland, 97240-0312
Founded in 1974 and with support from the National Endowment for the Arts, Editor/Publisher Vi Gale's press features poetry and art from nationally known poets and artists, many from Oregon. Notecards, poetry postcards and book collections. Order by mail or through a favorite bookstore.

54 Putney's Specialty Foods

P.O. Box 12651, Portland, 97212.
Tel: 224-4911
Cathy Farley's great-grandmother's recipe for cranberry tangerine chutney launched the business that now boasts a full line of high-quality Northwest fruit products: chutneys, conserves, jellies, plum sauce, and also mustards. Putney's products are available at Norm Thompson and Strohecker's (Portland), the Tillamook County Creamery, the House of Myrtlewood (Coos Bay) and Made in Oregon (Eugene). Call or write for wholesale prices or closest retail outlet. Gift packs (wholesale and retail) available during the holiday season. A Neiman-Marcus selection.

55 The Real Mother Goose

Two locations: 901 S.W. Yamhill, Portland, 97205, and 9610 Washington Square, Tigard, 97223. Tel: 223-9510 (downtown), 620-2243 (Wash. Sq.)
Celebrating its 17th year as a fine-crafts gallery, it consistently shows one of the finest selections of American crafts. Representing over 400 artisans from across the nation, the gallery shows work in all media. Individual artists are spotlighted in regular shows with special emphasis on Northwest craftsmen. Visa/MC/AmEx. Downtown: 10-5:30 Mon-Thurs, 10-6:30 Fri, 10-6 Sat. Wash. Sq.: 10-9 Mon-Fri, 10-6 Sat, 11-6 Sun.

56 Red Wagon Coffee Stores/ Boyd Coffee Company

Two locations: Sandy store, 19730 N.E. Sandy Blvd., Portland, 97225, and Downtown store, 1501 S.W. Taylor, Portland, 97205. Tel: 666-4561 (Sandy), 241-6404 (downtown)
Founded in 1900 by R. P. Boyd, this family-owned business roasts over 20 varieties of coffees. Its active research and development staff creates and manufactures over 500 soups, salad dressings, gravies, beverages and desserts for distribution to restaurants all over the world. Visa/MC/AmEx. Sandy store: 8-4:30 Mon-Fri. Downtown store: 8-6 Mon-Fri, 9-4 Sat.

57 Scimitar Foods

7352 S.W. Durham Rd., Portland (Tualatin), 97224 (Carman Dr. exit off I-5; go south on Upper Boones Ferry 3 blks. to S.W. Durham Rd., turn left into business park, then right, in brick bldg.).
Tel: 684-8073 or 800-553-WINE
Inspired by the variety and quality of Oregon foodstuffs, Terry Horn created Scimitar Foods, which produces a line of smoked, wine-cured meats, game birds, salmon and other seafood, from Oregon resources. Each item is processed in a specific premium Oregon varietal wine (Pinot Noir, Chardonnay, Sauvignon Blanc) and is intended to be consumed with that wine. Available through specialty food and wine retailers or by mail order. Products are vacuum-sealed and shipped refrigerated in insulated containers. A Neiman-Marcus selection. Visa/MC. 8-5 Mon-Fri.

58 Stash Tea Company

P.O. Box 910, Portland, 97207.
Tel: 684-4482
An Oregon company for 15 years, the Stash Tea Company takes great pride in its premium specialty tea line. Stash offers traditional, spiced, decaffeinated, ice tea, and herbal blends, including a delicate, refreshing Oregon Peppermint. The high-quality natural ingredients are collected around the world, cut minutes before blending, and sealed in foil to capture flavor at its peak. Available in finer restaurants and markets or by mail order. Write for catalog. Visa/MC.

○ Sternwheeler "Columbia Gorge"

See CASCADE LOCKS (Columbia Gorge-Mt. Hood) for listing.

59 Strohecker's, Inc.

2855 S.W. Patton Rd., Portland, 97201 (in Portland's West Hills). Tel: 223-7391
A tradition in Portland since 1902, this grocery, bakery, and produce, flower, drug, and liquor store, with gourmet deli and enormous wine selection, was showcasing Oregon products long before it was the fashion. Now run by third-generation Stroheckers, its brand-new building is testimony to the fact that good design pays. Deli features fresh selections daily. Bakery makes its own pies. Demonstrations by Oregon specialty food and wine producers are a weekly occurrence. Visa/MC. 8 AM-8 PM Mon-Sat, 9 AM-8 PM Sun.

60 Thirty One Northwest Restaurant

Uptown Shopping Center, 31 N.W. 23rd Pl., Portland, 97210 (upper level of Uptown Shopping Center off West Burnside). Tel: 223-0106
Conveniently located near Washington Park, Thirty One Northwest provides a warm, comfortable atmosphere for lunch, dinner, or tapas. The innovative menus change every two months and feature ingredients from the Pacific Northwest. Beautifully arranged flowers and art work from the Hoffman Gallery (Oregon's oldest gallery) make this restaurant even more special. Visa/MC/AmEx/Diners/Discover. Tapas are served in the lounge 2:30-10 Mon-Fri and 5:30-10 Sat. Lunch is 11:30-2:30 Mon-Fri and dinner 5:30-10 Mon-Sat.

61 Three Lions' Bakery

1138 S.W. Morrison, Portland, 97205.
Tel: 224-9039
Susan Sumimoto and Fred Hayward have gained a well-earned reputation for their lavish variety of all-butter pastries, cookies, breads and tortes. Charming lunches and espresso are also available in an elegant, classic cafe atmosphere. 7-6 Mon-Fri, 7-5 Sat.

62 Washington Park Zoo . . . and Asian Elephant ZooDoo

4001 S.W. Canyon Rd., Portland, 97221.
Tel: 226-1561
The zoo is world famous for its Asian elephant breeding program, with 24 babies born here since 1962. A by-product of these prolific pachyderms is the potent plant food ZooDoo. Manufactured in large quantities and neatly packaged in attractive cans by the zoo's chapter of the American Association of Zoo Keepers, this garden elixir is sold at the Elephant's Trunk gift shop at the zoo and Made in Oregon stores. The source of this remarkable product, and many other animals of the world and the Northwest, may be viewed daily. Visa/MC/AmEx. 9:30-7 daily (summer), 9:30-4 daily (winter).

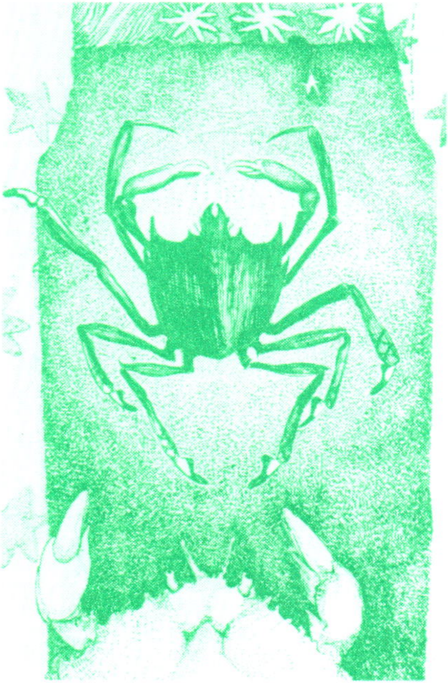

Pas de Deux, © *Liza Jones*

Northeastern

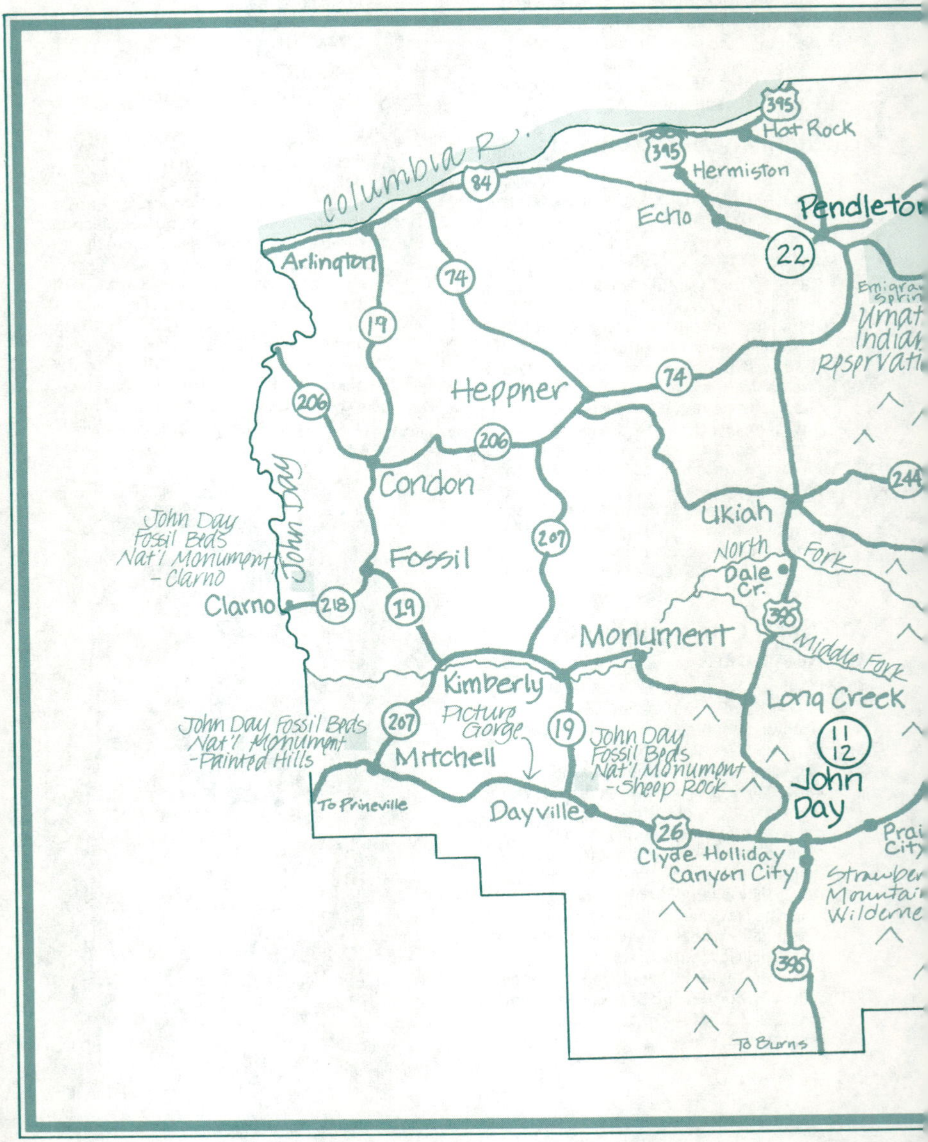

Oregon

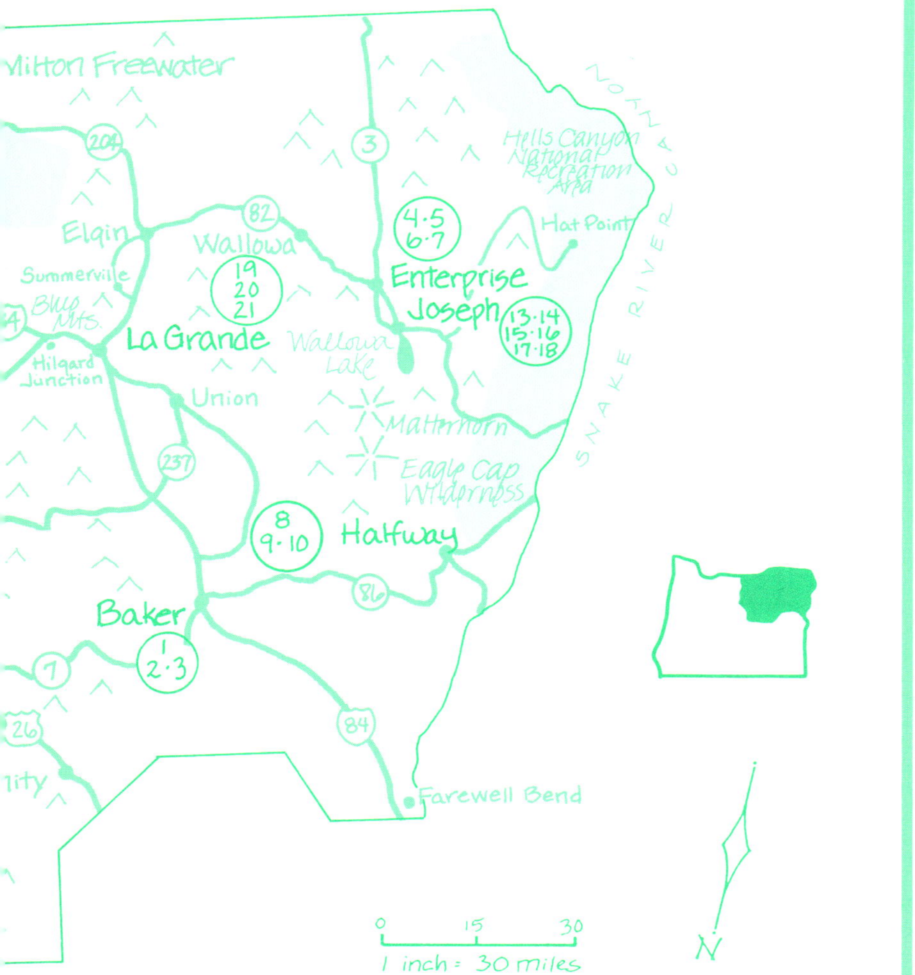

Milton Freewater
204
3
Hells Canyon National Recreation Area
HELLS CANYON
82
4·5 6·7
Hat Point
Elgin
Wallowa
19 20 21
Enterprise
Summerville
Joseph
13·14 15·16 17·18
Blue Mts.
La Grande
Wallowa Lake
Hilgard Junction
SNAKE RIVER CANYON
Union
Matterhorn
237
Eagle Cap Wilderness
8 9·10
Halfway
86
Baker
1 2·3
7
26
84
Farewell Bend
0 15 30
1 inch = 30 miles
approximate scale
N

NORTHEASTERN OREGON REGIONAL NOTES

The old **Oregon Trail** *left the* **Snake River** *at what is now* **Farewell Bend** *State Park and started over the* **Blue Mountains** *to* **The Dalles** *(Mt. Hood-Columbia Gorge Loop map), and I-84 follows close to the path of the Oregon Trail between* **Ontario** *and* **Baker**. *There are Oregon Trail displays at Emigrant Springs, Farewell Bend, and Hilgard Junction State Parks and in safety rest areas at Wetherby, Baker Valley, Charles Reynolds, Deadman Pass, and Stanfield. The Oregon Trail passed through what is now Echo, and crossed the Umatilla River at* **"Emigrants Crossing"** *nearby. Noted in many pioneer diaries, it was considered a good stopover, where animals could rest and graze on the "thigh-high to a horseman" grass of the meadows and where the emigrants could rest up, do their laundry, and trade for the goods needed before hitting the desert lands between Echo and The Dalles.* **Hat Rock,** *a large monolith bearing a likeness to a man's top hat is another landmark often referred to in diaries of early-day explorers and travelers.*

Wallowa Lake *was formed by a glacier at the base of the scenic, rugged* **Wallowa Mountains.** *Had it not been for the many glaciers in these mountains during the last ice age, the Wallowas would not have the ragged, craggy appearance for which they are known.* **Blue Mountain Forest** *and* **Emigrant Springs** *are dominated by* **ponderosa pine forests.**

The Eagle Cap Wilderness Area *is a 220,000-acre forest wilderness of lofty lakes, gushing streams and jagged peaks accessible only by trails. Trails leading into the area begin at Wallowa Lake State Park. The Wallowa Mountains rise out of glacier-sculpted valleys and within them is Oregon's supreme hiking, riding, and fishing country. Since trails receive heavy horse use, they tend to be rocky and dusty, but most hikers and horsemen head for a few well-known areas, particularly Lake Bacon. Other spots such as the 8,200-foot-high Bonnie Lakes, are more private.*

The secondary road from **Enterprise** *to* **Hat Point** *is the only way for road travelers to get a good view of the Hells Canyon of the Snake River, the deepest gorge in the country, and behind that the broken ragged outline of the Seven Devils Mountains. Hells Canyon is in wild and nearly roadless country, so very few people have seen it, and the view from Hat Point is a rare treat. One has to walk to get to any other rim viewpoint on either side of the canyon.*

At Hat Point, **Hells Canyon** *is slightly more than a mile deep and approximately 10 miles wide* **(1000 feet deeper than the Grand Canyon and considerably narrower).** *This part of Oregon gets some rain, and the canyon walls are thinly coated by soil that supports grass and a scattering of bushes and small trees. "The dominant color scheme is in shades of green with the color of the bedrock showing through as an undertone."*

The most famous lakes are reached by trails starting at South Wallowa Lake State Park, which can be reached by a gravel road. One 12-mile track leads to an 8,500-high glacier lake, its pale blue waters reflecting 9,595-foot **Eagle Cap.** *A trail leads to the rocky summit via Mirror and Upper Lakes.*

Ice Lake, beneath the cliffs of the 9,845-foot **Matterhorn,** *is open to horse travel. A rough trail reaches the summit of the Matterhorn, the highest peak in the Wallowas.*

Mountain goats, introduced to the Wallowas a quarter of a century ago, are frequently seen here. At the west end of the **Eagle Cap Wilderness,** *in the middle valley of the Minam River at low elevations, is one of the Northwest's premier* **ponderosa pine forests.** *Higher up, it is decorated with* **Engelman's spruce** *and* **douglas fir.** *Salmon spawn here, and the Minam is a famous trout-fishing stream. Though once threatened by massive logging, the* **Minam Valley** *today remains entirely wild. Only part of it, however, is included in the Eagle Cap Wilderness, and many have urged their congressmen to include these lower reaches of the Minam within the wilderness area.*

The U.S. Forest Service has published a topographical map and guide of the Eagle Cap Wilderness. It can be obtained, along with other guides and stock rules, by contacting the Wallowa-Whitman National Forest Supervisor's Office, 1550 Dewey Ave. (P.O. Box 907), Baker, Oregon 97814 (Tel: 523-6391).

Kam Wah Chung *in* **John Day** *is a Chinese cultural center dating from the 1880s, when many Chinese miners lived in the area. Fifteen miles east of John Day is the* **Strawberry Wilderness Area** *with snow-capped peaks, alpine lakes and over 100 miles of horse and hiking trails. Maps and wilderness permits available at the U.S. Forest Service Ranger Station at Prairie City or at the Malheur*

National Forest Supervisor's Office, 139 N.E. Dayton Street, John Day, Oregon 97845 (Tel: 575-1731).

The **Thomas Condon-John Day Fossil Beds National Monument** *contains fossil beds estimated to be 30 million years old, and has yielded remains of extinct three-toed horses, rhinos, camels, and oreodonts. This national park is divided into three locations:* **Sheep Rock, Painted Hills,** *and* **Clarno.** *The* **Cant Ranch Visitor Center** *has exhibits and picnic facilities just below U.S. Highway 26 junction and Oregon Highway 19, about 5 miles west of Dayville on the John Day River. Park headquarters and displays are also at 420 W. Main in John Day. Fossil collecting and digging are prohibited. From a point just north of the Clarno location, the* **John Day River** *is classified as a* **State Scenic Waterway** *to the Columbia River.*

Picture Gorge *is a spectacular canyon that cuts through a sequence of basalt lava flows, disputing a theory that streams always choose paths of lesser resistance (i.e., softer rocks). There are* **oligo-miocene fossilized leaves** *along the original Oregon Highway 19 near Fossil, in the John Day Formation. Near Mitchell in the Hudspeth Formation, there are* **cretaceous ammonites.** *Two different types of* **thundereggs** *can be found south of Heppner off Highway 207. Material is scarce, and picks, shovels, and bars are needed.*

Petrified wood *is scattered in the Umatilla National Forest. Check at Dale, Ukiah, and Long Creek Ranger Stations and Highland Rock and Gift Shop in Burns (Southeastern Oregon listings) for maps and details.*

There is a boat ramp to the Snake River at Farewell Bend State Park, and a boat ramp to the Columbia River at Hat Rock State Park, as well as a boat ramp and a dock at Unity Lake State Park. Group picnic areas are available at Emigrant Springs State Park, and group tent camping exists at Emigrant Springs, Farewell Bend, and Wallowa Lake State Parks. Club camping is available at Wallowa Lake State Park.

Oregon has an incredible variety of **wildflowers** *throughout the state. Please enjoy them, and please leave them undisturbed for others to enjoy. "A picked wildflower is a thing of beauty, but a joy for only one person for a few minutes." Some wildflowers grow in incredibly delicate environments and can take as long as seven years to bloom again.*

The Nature Conservancy owns and manages a large system of natural preserves throughout the state of Oregon. Call 228-9561 or visit the conservancy's offices in Portland (see Statewide Resources section) for information about preserves the public may visit in this region.

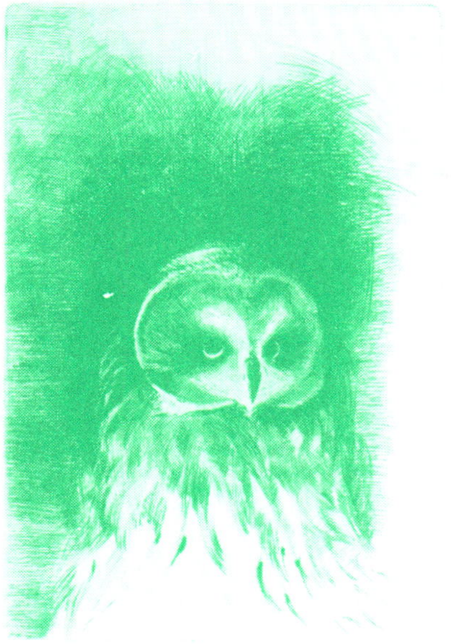

Shorteared Owl, © Liza Jones

STATE ROCK

The Thunderegg (geode) was named State Rock by the 1965 Legislature after rockhounds throughout Oregon voted it first choice. Thundereggs range in diameter from less than one inch to over four feet. Nondescript on the outside, they reveal exquisite designs in a wide range of colors when cut and polished. They are found chiefly in Malheur, Wasco, Jefferson, Wheeler and Crook Counties.

STATE INSECT

In 1979 the legislature designated the Oregon Swallowtail (Papilio oregonius) as Oregon's official insect. A true native of the Northwest, the Oregon Swallowtail is at home in the lower sagebrush canyons of the Columbia River and its tributaries, including the Snake River drainage. This strikingly beautiful butterfly, predominantly yellow, is a wary, strong flier not easily captured.

BAKER

1 Baker County Visitor and Convention Bureau/ Chamber of Commerce

490 Campbell St., Baker, 97814.
Tel: 523-5855
Office open daily from Memorial Day Weekend through Labor Day.
Baker County, on the Old Oregon Trail, welcomes its visitors with "hometown hospitality" and invites them to share the wealth of diversity the scenic county offers. The distinct four-season climate provides ample opportunity for year-around recreation. Baker County is the gateway to unspoiled Hells Canyon and plays host to vertical powder snow at Anthony Lakes. There are top-notch motel, campground, and RV facilities available. Galleries, shops, and museums all contribute to the historic "Baker Image." Call or write for more information.

1988-89 Baker County Area Events include:

1988

2nd & 3rd weekends in April: Championship Bass Tournaments
April 16-17: Anthony Lakes Ski Resort SNODEO
May 11-12: Eastern Oregon Tourism Summit Conference
Memorial Day Weekend: Opening of restored Sumpter Valley Railroad Park (steam train rides, antique show, flea market)
June 18-19: Hells Canyon Junior Rodeo, Halfway
July 4th weekend: Haines, Halfway, Huntington, Sumpter 4th of July Celebrations
3rd weekend in July: Miners' Jubiliee, Baker (festival/parade with mining competition, pub crawl, hot air balloon races, arts & crafts fair, world championship porcupine sprint races, cowbelles' Western breakfast)
2nd weekend in Aug: East-West Shrine All Star Football Game
1st weekend in Sept: Baker County Fair & Rodeo, Halfway

1989

4th weekend in Jan: Elkhorn Crest Sled Dog Championships, Sumpter
3rd weekend in Feb: District B-league Boys & Girls Basketball Tournament, Baker
1st weekend in March: State B-league Boys & Girls Basketball Championship Tournament, Baker

2 Crossroads Creative and Performing Arts Center

2020 Auburn Ave., P.O. Box 235, Baker, 97814. Tel: 523-3704
Baker County's art center presents visual and performing arts in the historic old Carnegie Library where visitors can see new gallery exhibits each month and browse in the gift shop. A number of its projects are supported by grants from the Oregon Arts Commission and the National Endowment for the Arts and it acts as a local arts council. Visa. 12-5 Tues-Fri.

3 Hells Canyon Shoe Manufacturing

1668 Resort St., Baker, 97814.
Tel: 523-5704
The Hells Canyon Packer is only one of the handmade boot styles made by old-line bootmaker George Ziermann, who is currently setting up a bootmaking school in Baker. His boots are guaranteed to fit, and his customers hail from all over the world. Write for a brochure or stop by shop. 8-5 Mon-Fri.

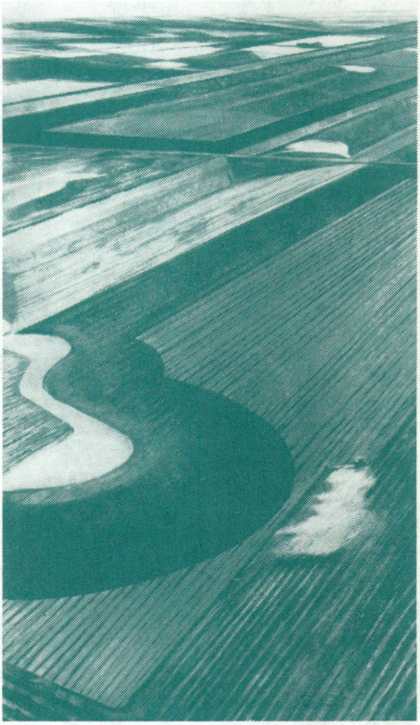

Contour Plowing (East of Pendleton), © *Liza Jones*

ENTERPRISE

4 Wallowa County Chamber of Commerce

107 S.W. First St., P.O. Box 427, Enterprise, 97828. Tel: 426-4622
Office: 8-5 Mon-Fri.
Wallowa County is a veritable treasure hiding in the northeastern corner of Oregon that even many Oregonians don't know is there. It has 3,178 square miles of rugged mountains, gentle valleys and craggy canyons. (See Northeastern Oregon Regional Notes for a description of the Eagle Cap Wilderness Area.) For those enjoying winter activities, Wallowa County has been described as a cross-country skier's and snowmobiler's paradise. Contact the Chamber of Commerce for guide services from Joseph and Enterprise on the edge of relaxing Wallowa Lake, which itself boasts fishing, camping, horseback riding and a gondola ride 3,200 vertical feet to the top of Mt. Howard at 8,200 feet.

1988 Wallowa County Area Events include:

April 28-30: Wallowa County Festival of Arts
May 30: Rotary Club Memorial Day Wallowa Valley Run-Off
July 2-4: Wallowa's Old-Fashioned 4th of July
July 2-4: Lostine Flea Market
July 4: Rotary Club 4th of July Lostine River Run
July 8-9: Wallowa County Old Time Fiddlers Contest
July 29-31: Chief Joseph Days
July 30: Rotary Club Chief Joseph Run
Aug 4-10: Wallowa County Fair
Aug 20-21: Wallowa Lake Monster Observation & Preservation Festival
Sept 10-11: Hells Canyon Mule Days
Sept 23-25: Alpenfest

5 The Bookloft—Skylight Gallery

107 E. Main, Enterprise, 97828 (across from courthouse). Tel: 426-3351
This is where local artists, people involved in the community and folks looking for a home-baked cookie and good conversation congregate. There is freshly ground and brewed coffee; the bookstore has bestsellers, magazines, Nez Perce and local history and the gallery features monthly shows of guest artists, some of whom have received fellowship awards from the Oregon Arts Commission. Visa/MC. 9:30-5:30 Mon-Fri, 10-4 Sat.

6 A Country Place on Pete's Pond

Montclair St. So., P.O. Box 459, Enterprise, 97828 (in southwest corner of Enterprise, 2 blocks south and 1½ blocks west of swimming pool). Tel: 426-3642
Ford and Marvel Petersons' place, located on a five-acre lake, faces the beautiful Wallowa Mountains. "Real home cooking," homebaked bread sandwiches, and fresh pies and cakes are served in a relaxed, homey atmosphere. Guests may eat inside, on a deck over the water, or on the lawn. There are swans to admire, wild ducks to feed, and trout to feed and pet. Gifts from Wallowa County available too. Visa/MC. 6:30 AM-8 PM daily, full-service restaurant. No reservations required.

7 Eagle Mountain Gallery

107 S.W. 1st St., Enterprise, 97828 (in the Wallowa Valley Mall). Tel: 426-4577 (also the number of the KWVR local radio station)
A gift gallery featuring Northwest artists and emphasizing bronze sculpture cast at Valley Bronze in Joseph. Pottery, prints, unusual crafts, and the "tastes and scents of Oregon," including a wine shop specializing in Oregon and Northwest wines, round out an extensive collection of tasteful gifts. Assistance in finding everything that is special in Wallowa County is available at the Wallowa County Chamber of Commerce desk located just inside the gallery. Visa/MC. 10-5 Mon-Sat.

HALFWAY

8 Birch Leaf Lodge

Go 2½ mi. northeast of Halfway to Jimtown; bear right; leave blacktop at next curve; take gravel road 2 mi. to lodge on left. Rt. 1, Box 91, Halfway, 97834. Tel: 742-2990
Each season brings something different at Dave and Maryellen Olson's 90-year-old remodeled 6-bedroom farmhouse. Convenient for jet boat or raft trips through Hells Canyon, packing with llamas in Eagle Cap Wilderness, superb fishing, and fall hunting. Barn and corral space for horses, too. Winter brings a quiet that Maryellen says "encourages cares to drop off like autumn leaves." There's a sledding hill, cross-country ski trails, woodstove, library, and large decks with great views. Available by day or week, year around. Steve Winike, resident host.

9 Clear Creek Farm Bed and Breakfast

Rt. 1, Box 138, Halfway, 97834 (go north from Halfway until pavement ends; go left to switchback and painted mailbox; go left again to farm). Tel: 742-2238
Ed and Mary Ann Carr's comfortable old farm home with several guest rooms on secluded 160 acres, with 1/4 mile wooded creek, pond for swimming, panoramic view of Idaho, upper Hells Canyon and Eagle Cap Wilderness serves B & B'ers, bikers, hikers, river floaters, snowmobilers, cross-country skiers, fishermen and hunters. Breakfasts and some dinners available. Children and some pets OK.

10 Wildflowers of Oregon

The Old Church on Main St., Halfway, 97834 (53 mi. east of Baker, near Hells Canyon). Tel: 742-6474
Sandy Kennedy received the 1985 Governor's Corporate Excellence Award for the 120 varieties of handmade wildflower wreaths, bouquets, baskets, sachets, potpourri, and northeastern Oregon gifts that she makes. She now has a beautiful new retail gift shop and gives factory tours in the Old Church. Wholesale and retail. Visa/MC. 8-5 Mon-Sat.

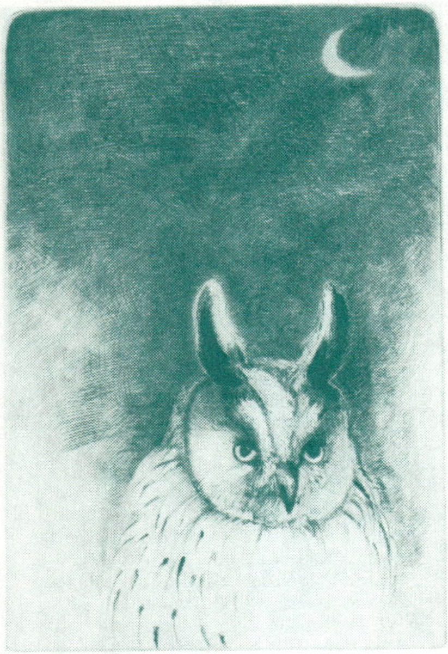

Longeared Owl, © Liza Jones

JOHN DAY

11 Grant County Chamber of Commerce

281 West Main St., John Day, 97845 (next to 1890-era white church in downtown John Day). Tel: 575-0547
Office: 9-5 Mon-Fri
Grant County has spectacular scenery, from high tree-covered mountains to sagebrush, and more in between. There's plenty of outdoor recreation year around. Ghost towns, museums, and the John Day Fossil Beds National Monument tells the story of Grant County's past. Prairie City's historic railroad depot houses a museum with ten rooms of memorabilia. The county historical museum in Canyon City has several extensive rock collections and a wealth of pioneer artifacts. The Kam Wah Chung building in John Day was once the center of the Chinese community here, and is now a fascinating museum.

1988-89 Grant County Area Events include:

1988

- May 27-28: Cinnabar Mountain Rendezvous, Mt. Vernon
- June 3-5: '62 Days Celebration, Canyon City
- July 4: Dayville 4th of July Celebration, Dayville
- July 4: Grant County 4th of July Celebration, Prairie City
- Aug 18-21: Grant County Fair, John Day
- Sept 16-17: Kam Wah Chung Days Chinese Festival, John Day

1989

- Late Jan: Snowmobile Biathlon, Lake Creek Camp

12 The Apricot Tree Country Inn and Dinner House

Rt. 1, Box 240, John Day, 97845. Tel: 575-1506
Bud and Bonnie Glimpse provide bed and breakfast accommodations and country-style dining in a delightfully decorated turn-of-the-century home. Everything is home-cooked. Their specialties are barbecued country spareribs and great steaks. Country quilts, potholders and aprons for sale. Call for dinner reservations. Visa/MC.

JOSEPH

13 Chief Joseph Band of the Nez Perce Tribe

Contact: Don Green. Tel: 432-8901
In the 1870s five chiefs of the Nez Perce Indians, including Chief Joseph, led their people in a series of battles against invading U.S. soldiers in an attempt to remain on their homeland. They were finally forced out of what is now Wallowa County and placed in exile in Kansas and Oklahoma. Later some of Chief Joseph's Band were allowed to return to Lapwai, Idaho, which became the Nez Perce Reservation. However, Chief Joseph and his family and close associates were exiled to the Colville Reservation in Nespelem, Washington, in the late 1880s.

Now those remnants of the Chief Joseph Band who have since returned to Oregon are working with Don Green, who has become the director of a program called Chief Joseph Days, to celebrate the original inhabitants of Wallowa County. The commemoration will be held July 29-31, 1988, in Joseph. Events include the Chief Joseph Rodeo Parade; a community Friendship Dinner with the Indians providing salmon and venison and the Wallowa community providing bread, salad, and dessert; and a Pow Wow in or near the Joseph High School with exhibition dancing and traditional Indian dance contests.

Descendants of some of the Nez Perce who reached Sitting Bull during the 1870s retreat, plus other remnants of the Chief Joseph Band living all over the Northwest, came back in 1987, and it is hoped more will return for future celebrations.

14 Chandlers' Bed, Bread and Trail Inn

700 S. Main (at the east end of Joseph), P.O. Box 639, Joseph, 97846.
Tel: 432-9765
Ethel and Jim Chandler offer warm hospitality and large rooms to their guests. They can accommodate families or groups. A great base for summer hiking in the Wallowas or cross-country skiing. Each of Ethel's breakfasts is different but always includes fresh fruit. Always open, reservations required.

15 Eagle Mountain Gallery/ Centennial House

No. 12 Main St., Joseph, 97846.
Tel: 432-0325
Carol-Lee and Lee Perkins operate a fine arts gallery and gift boutique in two historic, Romanesque brick buildings on Joseph's Main Street. The fine arts gallery features bronze sculpture cast at Valley Bronze in Joseph, one of the nation's finest art-casting foundries. (Tours of Valley Bronze originate from the gallery at 3:30 Mon-Fri, June-Sept, and in the winter by appointment.) Distinctive gifts centering on Oregon products abound in the Centennial House. The wine shop specializes in Oregon and Northwest wines. Wine tastings are celebrated by appointment. Visa/MC. 10-5 daily (June-Sept), 1:30-4:30 (winter, closed Wed and Sun).

16 Flying Arrow Resort

On the Powerhouse Rd. at Wallowa Lake, Rt. 1, Box 370, Joseph, 97846.
Tel: 432-2951
Since the summer of 1949 vacationers have enjoyed these charming housekeeping cottages surrounded by lawn and big trees along the Wallowa River and only a short walking distance from the lake itself. The sheets are hung out to dry in the sun so they smell good, and the staff, including receptionist Cindy Brink, were chosen for their friendly smiles. Even the deer are friendly here and come up to eat out of guests' hands. Visa/MC. Open year around.

17 Mountain Country Jam

On the Powerhouse Rd. at Wallowa Lake, Rt. 1, Box 370, Joseph, 97846.
Tel: 432-2951
Joanne Harrison's delicious homemade jam and jelly is sold nicely packaged in pine baskets and crates made by Ted Knight and King Spain. Each pack contains a folder of suggestions to take the buyer beyond toast and jam to a tangy, sweet, spicy sauce for chicken or pork. Sold at Flying Arrow Resort and Wallowa Lake Lodge. Call or write for mail-order and wholesale information. Visa/MC. 8-6 daily.

18 Wallowa Lake Lodge

At the south end of Wallowa Lake, Rt. 1, Box 320, Joseph, 97846. Tel: 432-4082
This grand old lodge, built in 1923, is undergoing extensive remodeling and will reopen May 1, 1988. Manager Joanne Harrison says, "It's going to be wonderful!" A first-class dining room will feature Northwest foods prepared by a team of young Oregon professionals. Thirty-two lodging rooms and eight cabins will be furnished with "user-friendly" antiques, and a teen lounge will replace the bar. No smoking anywhere. Visa/MC. Open May 1–Nov. 1.

LA GRANDE

19 La Grande-Union County Chamber of Commerce

1502 North Pine, P.O. Box 308, La Grande, 97850. Tel: 963-8588
Office: 9-12, 1-5 Mon-Fri
La Grande, named in honor of the area's beauty, is on the Western edge of the Grande Ronde Valley, at the foot of the Blue Mountains, on Interstate 84. The Grande Ronde Valley was once a major summer gathering place for the Nez Perce. Then the Oregon Trail came down Ladd Canyon, traversed the valley, went through what is now the southwest corner of La Grande and proceeded west over the Blue Mountains (the actual wagon tracks can still be seen). The area, which produces wheat, grass seed, livestock, and lumber products, is also rich in recreational opportunities, including hunting, fishing, hiking, golfing, camping, backpacking, river rafting, and skiing.

1988 La Grande-Union County Area Events include:

May 1-3: Raft Race/NIRA Collegiate Rodeo, La Grande
May 30: Hog Wild Days & Flea Market, Island City
June 6-11: Eastern Oregon Livestock Show, Union
June 13: 4x4 Race, Starkey
June 18: Annual World-wide Competition Timber Festival, La Grande
July 8-10: Elgin Stampede, Elgin
July 8-11: Catherine Creek Jr. Rodeo, Union
July 22-23: Blue Mt. Days, La Grande (parade, rodeo, and motorcycle rally)
Aug 3-6: Union County Fair, La Grande
Aug 20-21: Oregon Trail Days/Rendezvous, La Grande

20 Stange Manor Bed and Breakfast Inn

1612 Walnut, La Grande, 97850.
Tel: 963-2400
House tours are a popular guest activity at this gracious six-bedroom, five-and-a-half bath, 12,000-square-foot restored Georgian colonial mansion, complete with rose gardens and a ballroom with a stage in the basement. The full breakfasts are usually served by hosts Steve and Gail Hart in the elegant dining room replete with china, silver, candles, and flowers. Smoking in designated areas. Visa/MC. Open year around. Reservations required.

21 Sunflower Books

1114 Washington St., La Grande, 97850.
Tel: 963-5242
Named one of the best bookstores in the state by *Oregon Magazine*, this charming bookstore and coffee house is located in a little yellow house where Anne Stephens provides a wide selection of books, information on local events and freshly baked croissants and coffee. Visa/MC. 9:30-5:30 Mon-Sat.

PENDLETON

22 Armchair Books

39 S.W. Dorion, Pendleton, 97801 (in downtown Pendleton, across from post office). Tel: 276-7323
D'Arcy Dauble specializes in regional books and authors including travel, fiction, cookery and history. Wooden toys by local artists accompany children's books. The people who work here are knowledgeable about local events and conditions. Visa/MC. 9:30-5:30 Mon-Sat.

STATE DANCE

In 1977 the legislature declared the Square Dance to be the official State Dance. The dance is a combination of various steps and figures danced with four couples grouped in a square. The pioneer origins of the dance and the characteristic dress are deemed to reflect Oregon's heritage: the lively spirit of the dance exemplifies the friendly, free nature and enthusiasm that is part of the Oregon character.

Southeastern Oregon

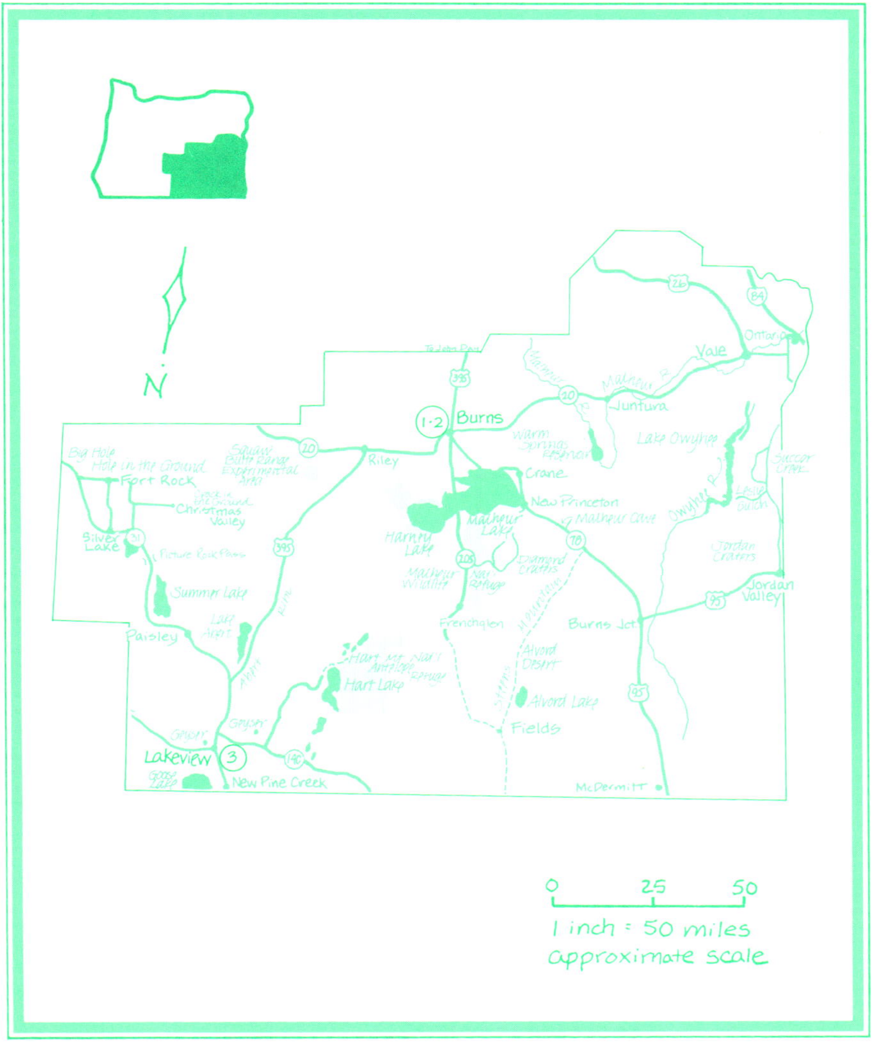

SOUTHEASTERN OREGON REGIONAL NOTES

Southeastern Oregon is a land of extremes and a land of surprises, both in terms of weather and terrain. It is a landscape created for the most part by faulting, and since so much of the area is now sparsely covered with vegetation, it is easy to get a grand perspective of how the earth is constantly moving beneath our feet. Also fascinating is how only the slightest change in exposure or rainfall is necessary to create a multitude of microclimates.

There is an Oregon Trail display at the safety rest area at **Ontario**. *The hot springs near what is now Vale on the Malheur River were a welcome discovery for weary Oregon Trail travelers. The brilliantly colored cliffs of* **Three Fingered Gulch** *and* **Painted Canyon** *at* **Owyhee Lake** *are made up of red, yellow, green, and brown volcanic rocks, and only accessible by boat or jeep. Along the lake's eastern shore, spectacular red tinted cliffs rise 1,000 feet. Farther south,* **Succor Creek Canyon** *is surrounded by purplish-brown crags.* **Leslie Gulch** *is a natural cathedral made up of highly colored rock formations.*

Malheur Lake *is a major resting and feeding stop on the* **Pacific Flyway,** *and is the focal point of the 183,000-acre* **Malheur National Wildlife Refuge** *that Theodore Roosevelt established in 1908. Ponds and crops are managed for the benefit of wildlife, and nearly 250 species have been counted on the refuge. The headquarters on the south shore of the lake includes a museum displaying nearly 200 mounted bird specimens.* **Malheur National Forest** *contains fossil beds of prehistoric plants and animals, as well as petrified wood, agates, and other semiprecious stones.*

Forty miles southeast of **Burns** *at* **Malheur Caves** *is a lava tube 1/2 mile long. The Jordan Valley area is known for its interesting lava formations, large deposits of obsidian, and* **Jordan Craters,** *some of the youngest shield volcanos in the continental U.S.*

Diamond Crater *is one of the best and most diverse basaltic features in the United States. It can be reached from Burns by traveling south on Oregon Highway 205 for about 1/2 mile beyond Milepost 40, turning left at Diamond Junction, continuing east for 7 miles, and turning left for 6 miles (following the Diamond Crater signs). No rock collecting is permitted here. Contact the B.L.M. office at 742 South Alvord Street, Burns, Oregon 97720, and ask for the self-guided tour brochure of Diamond Craters.*

The drive up the gradual slope of the west side of the massive fault block that is **Steens Mountain** *is deceptively gradual, with sagebrush, juniper, and groves of aspen. Higher up, there are Alpine wildflowers and glaciated valleys and gorges. The dry* **Alvord Lake** *and* **Alvord Desert** *can be seen a mile below on the east side of Steens Mountain. At the base of Steens Mountain Loop is the French Glen Hotel, built in 1916 by the famous local cattle baron of that time.*

Southeastern Oregon is particularly rich in **thundereggs, agates, obsidians, fossils,** *and* **petrified wood.** *There are black-banded and sheen obsidians near Burns; Pike Creek thundereggs at the north end of Alvord Desert; petrified wood, tempskya, and agates in dredging sites along many of the creeks in the Greenhorn-Bates area; basinite and wonderstone east of Burns; petrified wood, leaf prints, plume, and Paiyute jasper northeast of Burns; stinking water wood near the west end of Stinkwater Creek bridge; cinnabar diggings east of Burns; dendritic agate near the Warms Springs Reservoir junction; oolite, agate, and petrified wood at Harney Lake; red-bed thundereggs south of Harper Junction; snakeskin agate near Rome; McDermott petrified wood and agate at McDermott; thundereggs, agate, petrified wood, picture rock, and fossils at Succor Creek; agates and jasper on the shoreline at Owyhee Lake, just to mention a few of the earth's treasures that can be found in southeastern Oregon.*

The roads are rough and the directions are complicated, leading rockhounds through ranchers' gates, down Forest Service access roads, and by dilapidated old homesteads. The best thing to do is to contact the Highland Rock and Gift Shop in Burns (see Southeastern Oregon listings), where detailed instructions are given freely and maps and shovels are available.

Many **old mining ghost towns** *are to be found in the area around Greenhorn-Bates.* **Granite, Susanville, Galena, Greenhorn,** *and* **Whitney** *are a few that are worth a visit. Follow the highway and use Forest Service maps for directions.*

Geothermal activity *is evident near* **Hart Mountain,** *where a national refuge protects one of the continent's largest herds of pronghorn antelope. Information and maps indicating the best places to view the animals and other wildlife are available at* **Hart Mountain National Antelope Refuge** *head-*

quarters on the mountain's upland plateau. Four miles from the headquarters is a hot springs. Hart Mountain itself is an interesting geological attraction. Actually a massive volcanic ridge, the 8,065-foot mountain is a **study in ecological contrasts,** with its juniper and sagebrush, cool streams, green meadows, pine and aspen stands, and alkaline lakes.

An assortment of interesting geological features can be found northwest of **Lakeview** along Oregon Highway 31, which follows the historic route of an exploratory expedition led by John C. Fremont. Traveling north on U.S. Highway 395 you will pass beneath **Abert Rim,** a 30-mile-long fault scarp towering 2,000 feet above **Lake Abert.** According to geologists, it is the **largest exposed fault in North America.**

A crevice 700 feet deep called **Crack in the Ground,** almost due north of Christmas Valley, is the remnant of an ancient earthquake. Summer Lake is one of several remnants of prehistoric lakes.

Fort Rock, a state monument, is the site of an ancient volcanic crater and ocean shoreline. Indians inhabited this area more than 10,000 years ago. It is near a cave here where ancient Indian sandals dating back 10,000-13,000 years were found. **Hole in the Ground,** just west of Fort Rock, and **Big Hole,** on the opposite side of the road about 6 miles farther west, are both open craters created by steam explosions. Both are about a mile in diameter and several hundred feet deep.

Oregon has an incredible variety of **wildflowers** throughout the state. Please enjoy them, and please leave them undisturbed for others to enjoy. "A picked wildflower is a thing of beauty, but a joy for only one person for a few minutes." Some wildflowers grow in incredibly delicate environments and can take as long as seven years to bloom again.

The Nature Conservancy owns and manages a large system of natural preserves throughout the state of Oregon. Call 228-9561 or visit the conservancy's offices in Portland (see Statewide Resources section) for information about preserves the public may visit in this region.

BURNS

1 Highland Rock and Gift Shop

1316 Hines Blvd., Burns, 97720 (on Hwy. 20 and 395, 1 mi. west of Burns' Main St. across from gas station). Tel: 573-2995
Emory Clapp and his partner, Austa Carlon, take great pride in knowing about the rocks and rock formations in Harney County. It is a good rock-hounding area with thundereggs, petrified wood, fossils, jaspers, agate and the shop has excellent specimens both loose and made into bookends, pen sets, etc., plus maps and lots of information. 8-12, 12:30-5:30 Mon-Sat.

2 Frank Tuning Signs and Watercolor Studio

44 E. Monroe. Mailing address: 1840 Pierce St., Burns, 97720. Tel: 573-2435
Frank Tuning has taught art in Burns for 20 years. The whole town knows him. The West as it is now is the major subject of his own watercolors, many now in private and public collections in the U.S. and Europe. Recently his handmade wood signs and commercial art have begun to have a visual impact on Burns and surrounding communities. 10-5:30 daily, or by appointment. Calls welcome.

LAKEVIEW

3 Schminck Memorial Museum (DAR)

128 South E St., Lakeview, 97630 (½ blk. south of the courthouse). Tel: 947-3134
An unusual collection of pioneer life is located in a modest bungalow home in Lakeview. Both Mrs. Schminck's parents were of pioneer families who crossed the plains in 1845 and 1846. Established in 1936, the collection includes handmade quilts, rugs, toys, dolls and costumes, pioneers' tools, Indian artifacts and pressed glass. 1-5 Tues-Sat.

BOOTS AND WATER

Pay attention to where you are stepping, and **wear boots around horses and when walking in desert-like areas.** Boots make being stepped on or bitten less annoying.

Carry water and wear a shade hat in summer. Beer is great, but keep in mind that alcohol can dehydrate a person. 7-Up works even better than salt tablets for restoring evaporated sodium from the body. Always **tell someone where you are going** and when you plan to return.

THE LOOP

Look for this Mt. Hood Loop logo on Hwys. 26, 35 and Interstate 84.

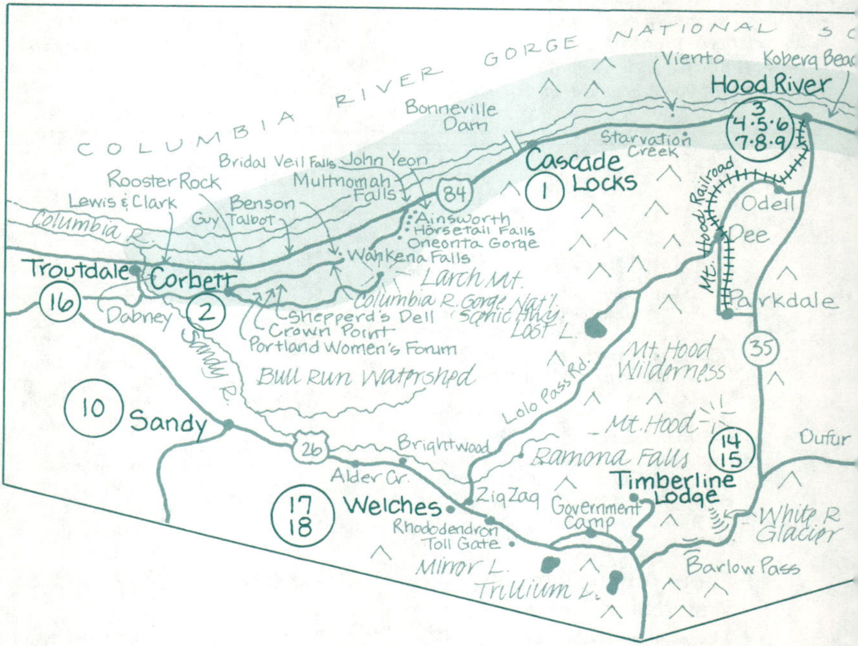

Columbia Gorge Mt Hood

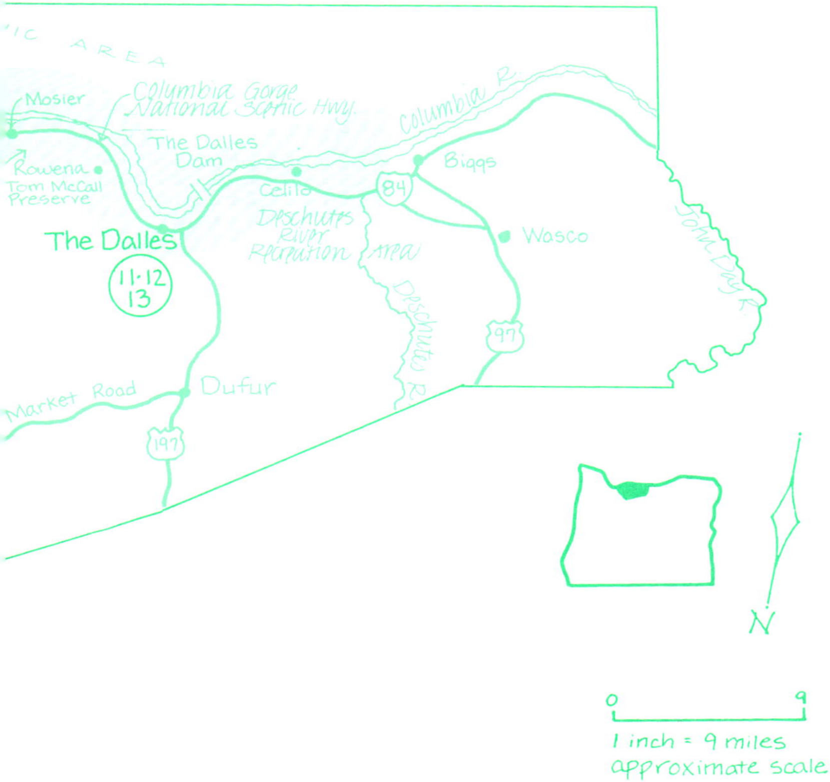

COLUMBIA GORGE-MT. HOOD LOOP REGIONAL NOTES

In the beginning, the Indians of the area called it **Wy'East.** *Later the mountain was renamed* **Mt. Hood.** *As for the* **Columbia Gorge,** *30 million years of geologic history are visible on its walls. The result of lava flows, erosion, and a massive uplift of the Cascade Range, layers of basalt and sandstone are clearly visible.*

First there was the **Columbia River.** *Then as tectonic activity pushed up the Cascade mountain range, the river cut down through the emerging mountains. Later, when the ice began to melt toward the end of the* **Pleistocene Ice Age,** *the water from the glacial melt which wanted to flow into the tributaries of the Columbia River in Idaho and Montana was blocked by ice dams in the Rockies, east of Spokane. Periodically these lakes broke through the* **ice dams,** *causing 600- to 1,000-foot floods that scoured out what is now the Columbia Gorge. The south side of the Columbia River Gorge has what might be the* **largest concentration of high waterfalls in North America,** *formed in part by these* **catastrophic floods** *of 50,000 to 13,000 years ago, that widened the valley, swept away the lower reaches of tributary streams, and left the streams falling hundreds of feet to the valley floor.*

The last and possibly **greatest catastrophic flood** *of the Columbia River Gorge occurred about 13,000 years ago. Geologists estimate that 380 cubic miles of water rushed out of the glacial lake covering modern-day Missoula, Montana, in as little as 40 hours. The flood waters reached 1,000 feet and washed over Rowena Crest viewpoint. At Crown Point, the waters reached 600 feet, then poured out to cover the Willamette Valley with a 400-foot-deep lake. The topsoil below 1,000 feet in the Gorge was scoured away, exposing underneath dramatic tilted flows of basalt, folded during the arching of the Cascade Mountains.*

In 1845, Samuel Barlow thought he had found the **end of the Oregon Trail** *at* **The Dalles.** *However, it happened to be about 100 miles away from* **Oregon City** *and the fertile Willamette Valley, his final destination. The only way to get from The Dalles to Oregon City was via one of two boats ferrying wagons down the Columbia River at very high prices. People who didn't have the cash had to forfeit cattle and other worldly goods to reach the green Willamette Valley.*

Outraged by this thievery, Barlow led his wagon party over treacherous Mt. Hood in the late fall, despite warnings of snow. Reaching only part way the first year, he left the wagons and hiked to Oregon City, where over the winter he devised a way to lower the wagons by rope over steep precipices. The rope marks on the trees can still be seen on **Mt. Hood**. *Later, he blazed a trail and, with the help of the Joel Palmer party, carved a road around the south side of Mt. Hood. While it too had its own costs (Barlow charged a toll for those who followed, unless they were widows whose husbands had been killed on the trip westward), the* **Barlow Trail** *opened up a whole new chapter in the history of the Oregon Trail. (***Tollgate Wayside** *just east of Rhododendron is the place where Barlow collected his tolls.)*

By 1925 cars traveled up and down the **Columbia River Scenic Highway,** *which by then linked Portland and The Dalles. In June of that year, Oregon State Highway 35 was completed, completing the last link of roads that circled Mt. Hood. The new loop was an improvement over the rough wagon trails of Barlow's day; yet by today's standards, it was still a challenge. For years, the route from Portland to Mt. Hood, for example, was a corduroy road made up of logs laid crosswise across the road to prevent Model T's from sticking in the mud. The loop road climbed ridges, snaked through canyons, and spanned streams on bridges that were almost as breathtaking as the surrounding scenery. One had to be a car-repair wizard to undertake those early trips. People continued to tackle the tortuous curves and many switchbacks of the loop road to experience and explore the area, however. As the roads improve, the curves continue to be straightened, and more and more of the intricate views are lost, but the thrill of experiencing the mountain and the Gorge still remains.*

Now, as one travels east and west up and down the Gorge or over the mountain, one can experience changes in the weather and environment brought about by the Cascade Mountains forming a weather block to the moisture coming in off the Pacific Ocean and the east winds blowing in from the plains. Depending on the interaction between these, the weather on Mt. Hood and in the Gorge can be quite severe, and the climate and vegetation vary greatly from east to west. The greatest change can be noticed in the areas between **Rhododendron** *and* **Barlow Pass** *on the mountain and* **Cascade Locks** *and* **The Dalles** *in the Gorge. It is in these areas, for example, where the moisture changes and firs become pines, and vice versa.*

Mt. Hood and **Mt. Hood National Forest,** *through which the loop travels, have seven living glaciers that extend to near timberline on all sides of the volcano (Mt. Hood is a volcano). For trailhead locations, maps, and fire conditions contact the Mt. Hood National Forest Supervisor's Office, 2955 N.W. Division, Gresham, Oregon 97030 (Tel: 666-0700) or the Zig Zag Ranger Station. The Mt. Hood Loop Highway crosses White River, which flows out of* **White River Glacier** *and provides an interesting view of a typical glacial stream near its source. Steam rising from the large fumaroles near the summit can be seen on many days.*

Just north and east of **Sandy** *is the* **Bull Run Watershed** *that provides all of Portland with some of the best drinking water any city can claim. Logging in the watershed is done by mule teams that wear diapers in order that the ecosystem not be disturbed, and any machinery brought into the area must come equipped with absorbent pads to protect the ground from oil drips.*

Lolo Pass Road *from Brightwood or Zigzag is a direct route around the west side of Mt. Hood. This rough road through spectacular scenery leads to Lost Lake and eventually Hood River. Lolo Pass Road, however, is closed during the winter, due to snow.* **Ramona Falls** *is an easy hike to an impressive waterfall with many cascades. The trail loops back through cool fern grottos, and the trailhead can be reached from Lolo Pass Road.*

At Rhododendron lives "Joey," who will tow your car out of a snow drift with her Mack truck should you ignore warnings to properly chain up in the winter or leave your car parked on the side of the road on which the snow plow is working that day.

The second most visited site in Oregon, **Timberline Lodge** *represents the vision that Margery Hoffman Smith and others had in the 1930s to create a tourist attraction that represented the essence of Oregon. Through the skills of local artists and craftsmen, Margery was able to have her truly regionally appropriate designs carried out, and images from the mountain itself were used to create the architectural detail and furnishings throughout the lodge. Fifty years later, the author worked with 30 more Northwest artists and craftsmen to create in the Wy'East Day Lodge a sequel to what Margery had done in the '30s. (See Columbia Gorge-Mt. Hood listings for descriptions of Timberline Lodge and Friends of Timberline.)*

Mirror Lake *is a huckleberry picker's paradise.* **Trillium Lake** *is a picturesque lake with day picnic facilities just two miles from the main road. Often a destination for cross-country skiers in the winter, it was designed by the landscape architect for Timberline Lodge as a focal point for the lodge and is the place from where much of the material to build the lodge was excavated. Barlow Pass is the highest point on the loop road, at an elevation of 4,157 feet, named after Samuel Barlow. The* **Pacific Crest Trail** *crosses here as it winds its 2,000-mile way from Mexico to Canada.*

Cloud Cap Inn, *built in 1889, is a rustic inn that served for years as the place from which many mountaineers began their ascent of Mt. Hood, and still is the place from which many begin their trek around the mountain on the Timberline trail. The inn is on the National Register of Historic Places, and while no longer open to the public, the site provides an excellent north-side view of Mt. Hood. The inn is approximately 10 miles from Oregon Highway 35. Cloud Cap Saddle Campground is open during the summer months only and offers scenic views and unspoiled high-country beauty. Like Cloud Cap Saddle Campground, Tillie Jane Campground is open during the summer months only, and is an excellent base for exploring the* **Cooper Spur area.**

Lava fields *stick up out of the pear orchards near* **Parkdale. Lost Lake,** *some 28 miles southwest of Hood River, has rustic cabins, camping, fishing, boat and canoe rentals, and swimming. In autumn, huckleberries abound, reminding us that these were once the favorite berry-picking grounds of the area's Indian tribes.*

Thousands of fruit trees cover the east slopes of Mt. Hood in the **Hood River Valleys,** *called the* **Apple Center of Oregon** *and the* **Winter Pear Capital of the World.** *The first shipment of famous Hood River apples arrived in New York in 1900. During the harvest season, amidst a profusion of fall colors, roadside fruit stands dot Oregon Highway 35. Spring brings a spectacular sight as many of the fruit trees bloom.* **Pears** *from the area have begun to be used to create a regionally distinct brandy. (See Portland listings re Clear Creek Distillery.) Recently passenger service on the Mt. Hood Railway has been restored. (See Columbia Gorge-Mt. Hood listings.)*

After a long battle and years of hard work put in by dedicated volunteers, the **Columbia Gorge National Scenic Area** *Act was signed into existence on November 17, 1986. The new law has laid a foundation for a cooperative effort to protect and enhance the scenic, cultural, and recreational resources of the Gorge while encouraging compatible economic growth and development. The temporary headquarters of the National Scenic Area are U.S.D.A. Forest Service, Columbia River Gorge National Scenic Area, Waucoma Center Suite 301, 902 Wasco Ave., Hood River, Oregon 97031 (Tel: 386-2333).*

Where Oregon Highway 35 intersects Interstate 84, one can go eastward towards **The Dalles.** *Outstanding views of the Gorge can be seen on a 9-mile stretch of the* **old cliff-side Columbia River Highway** *between* **Mosier** *and* **Rowena,** *where the 34-acre Tom McCall Preserve managed by The Nature Conservancy is a refuge for a number of native plants, many of which are endemic to the Gorge. (Access opposite viewpoint parking lot near east end of 9-mile scenic loop.)*

This plateau some 900 feet above the Columbia River is renowned for its prolific wildflower display from early spring to the middle of summer, nature trails and ponds. The Nature Conservancy owns and manages a large system of natural preserves throughout the state of Oregon. Call 228-9561 or visit the conservancy's offices in Portland (see Statewide Resources section) for information about preserves the public may visit in this region, of which the Tom McCall Reserve is one.

Oregon has an incredible variety of **wildflowers** *throughout the state. Please enjoy them, and please leave them undisturbed for others to enjoy. "A picked wildflower is a thing of beauty, but a joy for only one person for a few minutes." Some wildflowers grow in incredibly delicate environments and can take as long as seven years to bloom again.*

Where the lush, green Cascade Mountains change to the dry, sunny desert, the hillsides of The Dalles are dotted with wheatfields and 5000 acres of cherry orchards. A trading center for 10,000 years, the Columbia River brought Natives Americans here to fish for salmon, and Lewis and Clark camped here in 1805 and 1806. This was the end of the Oregon Trail until 1846 when Barlow hacked his trail over Mt. Hood.

Just past The Dalles Highway 197 loops south to Dufur, and via the **Dufur Market Road** *loops back up the east side of Mt. Hood through live oak and pine forests until it connects to Highways 35 and 26.*

To see **The Dalles Dam,** *one can stop at* **Seufert Park** *and board the free train to the visitors' center, power house, navigational locks, and fish ladders. Before the damming of the Columbia River,* **Celilo Falls** *(now Celilo Park) east of the dam was a traditional Indian fishing spot for hundreds of years. While the park is now used primarily by white men, there is nevertheless a certain, unmistakable essence here that reminds one that this place really belongs to the Native Americans who used it for so many years. Perhaps it is because the spirits of the area remain, despite the damming of the river causing the change in its character.*

Agates, jaspers, *and* **petrified woods** *are found in The Dalles Formation, which sits above the Columbia River Lava Flow. At Biggs Canyon, picture jasper is available.*

Going west from the intersection of Oregon Highway 35 and Interstate I-84 just past **Cascade Locks** *(see Columbia Gorge-Mt. Hood listings) is the Bridge of the Gods, whose name comes from an old legend about a natural land bridge that spanned the Columbia River. The story tells of its collapse during the eruption of two "warrior god" volcanoes (Mt. Adams and Mt. Hood), disputing over a third goddess volcano (Mt. St. Helens). The modern-day Bridge of the Gods is but a pragmatic solution to crossing the river.*

Eagle Creek Campground and the nearby Cascade Salmon Hatchery is the jumping off point for **Eagle Creek Trail,** *that connects to the Pacific Crest Trail on Mt. Hood. The larger pools of Eagle Creek are popular for swimming and picnicking. A short yet magical hike leads to Punchbowl Falls, that has to be seen to be believed.*

Bonneville Dam *is the oldest of four massive Army Corps of Engineer projects along the Columbia River, and is one of the most viewed attractions in Oregon. The glassed-wall visitor center on Bradford Island, an ancient Indian burial grounds, has many exhibits about the dam operations, navigational history on the Columbia River, and fish migration. When the salmon are migrating, they can be seen ascending the fish ladders.*

Several state parks are situated along a part of the existing old 24-mile **Columbia River Scenic Highway** *(U.S. Highway 30 Scenic Route), built in 1915, that begins near the Sandy River at Troutdale off Interstate 84, and ends 5 miles west of Bonneville Dam (or vice versa). It was the main highway for 30 years after its completion, and is recognized* *as an historic engineering masterpiece. Scenic attractions along the highway include impressive waterfalls, panoramic views of the Gorge, and peaceful rural surroundings. The highway is narrow, and parking and traffic congestion are problems during the summer months.*

Latourelle Falls *in* **Guy Talbot State Park** *is the second highest waterfall in the Columbia Gorge. Other nearby falls can be viewed in* **Bridal Veil**, **John Yeon**, *and* **Shepperd's Dell State Parks**. *Spectacular 620-foot Multnomah Falls is the second highest in the U.S. and the highest along the Gorge. Hikers can follow a trail to the top and watch the stream plummet into its deep pool.*

Several sections of the Columbia Gorge Trail are still complete, including two miles of trail between **Ainsworth** *and* **John Yeon State Parks**. **Angels Rest Trail** *climbs to a scenic ridge crest and then rejoins Interstate Highway 84 at* **Wahkeena Falls** *picnic site. The State Parks Division maintains other trails, ranging from short, easy, paved footpaths to strenuous hikes several miles long at the following state parks:* **Bridal Veil**, **Dabney**, **Guy Talbot**, **Seneca Falls**, **Shepperd's Dell**, **Starvation Creek**, **V. Lausman**, **Rooster Rock**, *and* **Wygant**. *At Ainsworth State Park, at the east end of the 24-mile West Loop of the original scenic highway, there are picnic sites and overnight camping.* **Horsetail Falls** *is named for its horsetail-like shape. A trail takes one to an upper cascade called* **Ponytail Falls**. *Additional trail information is available from Oregon State Parks and the Mt. Hood National Forest Supervisor's office at 2955 N.W. Division, Gresham, Oregon 97030 (666-0700).*

At **Oneonta Gorge** *during summer, one can walk upstream on the river bed to explore the cool, narrow gorge that ends in a refreshing waterfall. This is a* **U.S. Forest Service Botanical Area** *treasured for the rare ferns, mosses, lichens and hepatics clinging to its sheer walls. Over 50 species of wildflowers, flowering trees and shrubs thrive in the always cool, protected and moist environment.*

Vista House *(see Columbia Gorge-Mt. Hood listings) at* **Crown Point** *was built in 1918 as a memorial to Oregon's pioneers. At 725 feet above the river, it provides a spectacular view of the Columbia Gorge. The Vista House is accessible via U.S. Highway 30 Scenic Route, i.e., the Columbia Gorge Scenic Highway. Original Italian stone work still lines the highway, including a segment at Crown Point. A 14-mile side trip on the* **Larch Mountain** *Road results in a picnic site with an impressive view of the surrounding Cascade peaks.*

The **Portland Women's Forum Park** *has a panoramic view of the Gorge with Crown Point and Vista House to the east and Rooster Rock to the north. The* **state park** *at* **Rooster Rock** *is an excellent spot for swimming and boating on the Columbia River. At* **Benson State Park** *there are two lakes that make it a picturesque day-use park.* **Lewis and Clark State Park**, *at the mouth of the Sandy River, is a popular spot also.*

There are boat ramps to the Columbia River at Benson (Dalton Point), Mayer, and Rooster Rock State Parks. There is a boat ramp to the Sandy River at Lewis and Clark State Park, and there is a boat basin and docks at Rooster Rock State Park.

The **Amtrack Pioneer** *follows the banks of the Columbia through the Gorge and can be boarded eastbound in Portland with time to enjoy the sternwheeler at Cascade Locks and catch the westbound train back to Portland. Or it can be taken on to Hood River, The Dalles, and points east.*

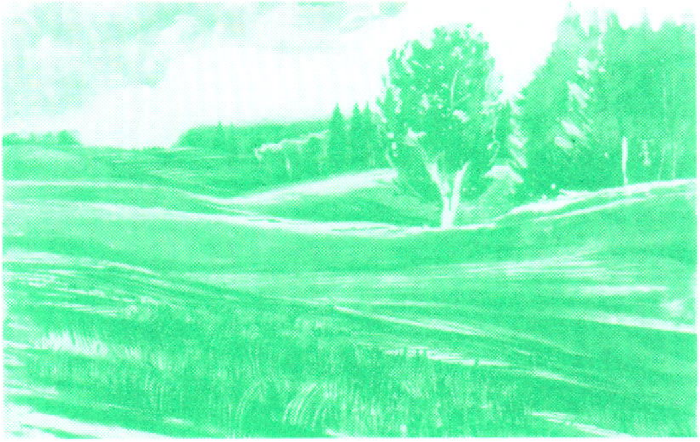

Pasture Lands (Hood River), © Liza Jones

CASCADE LOCKS

1 The Port of Cascade Locks/ Sternwheeler "Columbia Gorge"

P.O. Box 307, Cascade Locks, 97014.
Tel: 374-8427
Named for the navigational locks built here that allowed river traffic to bypass a dangerous "cascade" of rapids. Until the locks' completion in 1896, boats were portaged overland. When the Bonneville Dam was built, the rapids were submerged, rendering the locks obsolete. The former canal locks are now used by Indians for their traditional dip net fishing. Known as Marine Park, the site also has two visitors museums, one of which is housed in the former home of the lock tender, and the Port of Cascade Locks Visitors Center that houses the ticket office for the sternwheeler "Columbia Gorge" and where there are photographs and displays about river travel of the past. "The Oregon Pony," the Northwest's first steam locomotive, is also on display there.
This 599-passenger sternwheeler is moored at the east end of Marine Park and makes several excursions daily, plus weekend dinner cruises, on the Columbia River from mid-June through September. The balance of the year it is moored in Portland where it does waterfront tours. Private charters and group discounts available. Daily from Cascade Locks (June-Sept); Sat, Sun from Portland (Oct-May). Visa/MC/AmEx.
1988 Cascade Locks Events include:
June 17-19: Sternwheeler Days

CORBETT

2 Vista House Gallery and Gifts

At Crown Point State Park on Historic Columbia River Hwy., east of Troutdale and west of Multnomah Falls, P.O. Box 204, Corbett, 97019. Tel: 695-2230
The shop in this national historic landmark sells handcrafted artwork from the Columbia River Gorge, in addition to books about the gorge, film, and postcards. Folk art demonstrations every weekend. Operated by local residents interested in restoring the building. Proceeds are used to restore Vista House and provide local employment and interpretation of the gorge. Visa/MC. 10-6 daily (May 1-Oct 15).

HOOD RIVER

3 The Coffee Spot

12 Oak St., Hood River, 97031.
Tel: 386-1772
City councilmen, port commissioners, and Forest Service executives enjoy the relaxed atmosphere as much as do the toddlers of young mothers allowing themselves a coffee break at this delicatessen/coffee house. With a reputation for excellence at very affordable prices, the Coffee Spot offers deli sandwiches, imaginative house specialties, beer, wine, fresh-ground coffee and espresso drinks. All desserts, soups, salads, and dinner specials are handmade on the premises, or about town, with fine, quality ingredients. Visa/MC. 8-5:30 Mon-Fri, 9-4 Sat. Closed Sun. Extended summer hours. Java Hour with half-priced coffees 3-5 PM. Check the schedule for live folk music.

4 Columbia Art Gallery

207 Second, Hood River, 97031.
Tel: 386-4512
Established in 1975, this not-for-profit community arts organization provides a sales outlet for regional and local artists with an emphasis on art and contemporary crafts from the Columbia Gorge region. Nine exhibitions and a Christmas show annually. Musical and some drama performances also. Write or call for updated schedules. Some of the gallery's programs have received support from the Oregon Arts Commission. Visa/MC/ AmEx. 10-4 Tues-Sat.

5 Columbia Gorge Hotel

4000 Westcliff Dr., Hood River, 97031 (Exit 62 off I-84, just west of Hood River and right on the Columbia River).
Tel: 800-826-4027 (in-state), 800-345-1921 (out-of-state)
No two of the 46 guest rooms are alike in this completely restored inn built by a lumber magnate in 1921. Overnight guests are served a complimentary "World Famous Farm Breakfast"™. Dining room specializes in Northwest cuisine, including fresh Columbia River salmon, dry-aged eastern prime beef and Columbia Gorge Apple Torte Flambé. Visa/MC/AmEx/Diners. Daily year around.

6 Hackett House Bed and Breakfast

922 State St., Hood River, 97031.
Tel: 386-1014
A classic 1903 three-story Dutch Colonial home near downtown Hood River, Hackett House offers guests a choice of rooms which share a common bath. The hearty "Buckaroo Breakfast" may be enjoyed in the spacious country kitchen, the sunny dining room, or on the sundeck. Guests are invited to enjoy the living room for relaxing, music, or browsing in the library. Smoking on porch. AmEx. Open year around.

7 Hood River Brewery Co./ White Cap Brew Pub

506 Columbia St., Hood River, 97031,
Tel: 386-2281
Their "Full Sail Golden Ale" was chosen as winner of "Oregon Beer of the Year" in 1987. White Cap Brew Pub has "two great views: of the Columbia River and of brewers making a great Oregon ale." Also available are nachos and beer sausage plus seltzers made with Hood River spring water, and an assortment of regional wines. Hood River Brewery will soon have an expanded line of specialty beers. Open daily afternoons and evenings (summer), 4-9 PM Thurs-Sat (winter).

8 Mt. Hood Railroad

110 Railroad Ave., Hood River, 97031 (Hood River City Center Exit from I-84; turn south onto 2nd, left onto Cascade, and left into Depot parking area).
Tel: 386-3556
This 82-year-old freight train now offers passenger service April through October. The 22-mile line runs from the Columbia River at Hood River to Parkdale in the foothills of Mt. Hood. Passengers view rivers, forests, and fruit orchards, stopping at lumber mills and fruit-packing houses. View of Mt. Adams and Mt. Hood punctuate the experience. Visa/MC. Weekend service April, May, and Oct and Tues-Sun service June-Sept. Call or write for schedule.

9 Three Rivers Winery

275 Country Club Rd., Hood River, 97031 (located at West Hood River next to freeway; take Exit 62 and turn immediately onto Country Club Rd. just south of freeway). Tel: 386-5453
The four varieties of table wines are made from grapes harvested from several Columbia Gorge vineyards. Wines are available to taste in a beautifully converted turn-of-the-century home. Owner and winemaker is Bill Swain, who had years of experience in California's Napa Valley before choosing the Columbia Gorge as a location for his own winery. Picnic facilities next to nearby creek. Visa/MC/ AmEx. 11-6 Mon-Sat, 1-5 Sun (April-Dec); 11-6 Fri-Sat, 1-5 Sun, and during the week by chance (Jan-March).

SANDY

10 Wasson Bros. Winery

41901 Hwy. 26, Sandy, 97055.
Tel: 668-3124
The Wasson brothers have a wine for everyone: Pinot Noir, White Riesling, Gewurztraminer, Loganberry, Raspberry, Blackberry, Bing Cherry and Rhubarb. They also have wine and beer making supplies for the home winemakers. Tasting room and tours. 10-5 daily.

LISTEN TO THE MOUNTAIN

Some savvy skiers and hikers have said, "If you get a funny feeling saying 'be careful,' it's the mountain telling you to watch out." Pay attention to your feelings. **Do not attempt to climb Mt. Hood or any other mountain (especially those with glaciers) without an expert guide.** *And always* **tell someone where you are going** *and when you plan to return. While the Mt. Hood Ski Patrol (the first in the country to be chartered) and Oregon Mountain Rescue do a fantastic job, there are many who have not been rescued to tell their tales.*

THE DALLES

11 Dobré Deli and Bed and Breakfast

308 E. Fourth, The Dalles, 97058 (from I-84 take City Center exit). Tel: 298-8239
Jan Mlnarik's Dobré Deli offers atmosphere in downtown The Dalles. Jan makes homemade salads, crockpot soups, sandwiches, espresso, and delicious desserts. She has outside seating, Northwest wines and imported beers, and can do group catering or create box lunches. Also operates a local bed and breakfast home. Visa/MC. 8-8 Mon-Fri, 9-5 Sat (June-Aug), 8-7 Mon-Fri, 9-5 Sat (Sept-May).

12 Muirhead Canning Co.

5267 Mill Creek Rd., The Dalles, 97058. Tel: 298-1660
Canners of "tree-ripened" fruit in the heart of Oregon's fruit growing country. Family-owned operation since 1946. Delivery to homes in the Northwest at close of canning season (Nov and early Dec). Tours of cannery available during canning season. Fruits and vegetables canned in sugar syrups, diet pack or water pack, without preservatives or coloring. Gift packs available. 8:30-5 Mon-Sat during canning season (July-Nov). Call or write for brochure, price list, delivery route and/or appointment between Dec and June.

13 Williams House Inn Bed and Breakfast

608 W. 6th St., The Dalles, 97058. Tel: 296-2889
Listed on the National Register of Historic Places, this large, gracious 1899 Victorian home occupies its own wooded hilltop with groomed, green grounds. The two upstairs rooms with balconies and shared bath and the three-room, main-floor master suite all have good desks, reading lamps, TV's, and telephone jacks. Breakfasts are prepared by Don and Barbara Williams, who delight in sharing their knowledge of the area. Air-conditioned. Visa/MC. Open year around.

TIMBERLINE

14 Timberline Lodge and Wy'East Day Lodge

Timberline, 97028 (on the south side of Mt. Hood at 6000 ft. elevation). Tel: 226-7979 (toll free from Portland), 800-452-1335 (from elsewhere in Oregon), 272-3311 (out-of-state)
A National Historic Landmark, Timberline Lodge is a magnificent wood and stone structure housing a full-service hotel and convention center. The new Wy'East Day Lodge is a day use facility for skiers and sightseers. This all-season resort offers winter and summer skiing, scheduled summer events, forest service presentations, alpine walks and glacier mountaineering.

15 Friends of Timberline

Timberline, Oregon 97028. Tel: 226-7979 (toll free from Portland), or 272-3311
Craftsmen of the 1930s built Timberline Lodge and all its furnishings (tables, chairs, lamps, rugs, curtains, beds, iron work, handcarved newel posts, et al.) on the slopes of Mt. Hood in Mt. Hood National Forest. Craftsmen of the 1980s built all the furnishings for the new Wy'East Day Lodge (tables, chairs, benches, store cases, ski racks, signs, tapestries, glass room divider, photo mural, concrete containers, exterior sculpture, et al.) Friends of Timberline, the not-for-profit organization that is the caretaker of these objects that make Timberline and Oregon unique, recently constructed a museum on the first floor of Timberline Lodge.

TROUTDALE

16 Trailblazer Fruit Products, Inc.

22815 N.E. Sandy Blvd., Troutdale, 97060. Tel: 666-6680
In 1903 the Townsend family began growing raspberries. In the early 1800s the Walls family "trailblazed" their way to Oregon, bringing family recipes for jams and syrups. In 1984 the two families joined operations to provide consumers with Oregon-grown, hand-filled jams, fillings, and syrups. Gift shop has Oregon-made specialty food products. Write or call for mail order (wholesale and retail) brochure. Visa/MC. 8-4:30 Mon-Fri.

WELCHES/WEMME

17 Mt. Hood Recreation Association

P.O. Box 342, Welches, 97067.
Tel: 622-3101, ext. 1600

The association promotes the entire area as "One Mountain For All Seasons." The communities from Alder Creek to Mt. Hood Meadows provide the support system for Mt. Hood's ski areas. There are cabins and motel rooms for rent here as well as restaurants, a laundromat, grocery stores, specialty gift shops, and a 27-hole golf course. Call for more information on area events and activities.

1988 Mt. Hood Area Events include:

June 3-4: Golden Rose Ski Classic, Timberline

June 12: Rose Festival Golf Team Championship, Rippling River Resort

July 10: "Preservation Hall Jazz Band" Alpine Concert, Rippling River Resort

July 11 & 22: Oregon PGA Senior Pro-Am Golf Tournaments, Rippling River Resort

Aug 13: Chili Cookoff, Timberline Lodge

Aug 22-24: Mt. Hood Loop Classic Bicycle Race (three-day race including criterium at Rippling River Resort, circuit race in Gresham, 130-mile race around Mt. Hood Loop, and time trial from Government Camp to Timberline Lodge)

Aug 28: "Lionel Hampton" (evening performance), Alpine Concert, Rippling River Resort

Sept 3-5: Labor Day Wine & Craft Fair; Swiss Weekend, Timberline Lodge

Sept 5: "John Hartford/Hot Rise" Alpine Concert, Rippling River Resort (more Alpine Concerts will be added to schedule)

Oct 8-9: Timberline Classical Music Weekend, Timberline Lodge

Oct (call for dates): Wild Gourmet Mushroom Festival, Rippling River Resort (clinics, cooking competition, exhibits, and hunts, all involving the proper use of mushrooms)

Oct 18-19: Pro-Pro-Am Invitational Golf Tournament, Rippling River Resort

18 The Store (Natural Foods and Café)

Look for Carrot Banner on south side of Hwy. 26 near Wemme, Box 226, Welches, 97067. Tel: 622-3130

Will Frank's Café and General Store is where local folks, backpackers, bicyclists and others looking for fresh, pure food, home cooking and great gifts can stock up. Will's world-famous lunch box collection provides a backdrop for the varied menu and exchange of local information that creates an ambience of comfortable camaraderie. Over 21 imported beers and many regional fine wines now available by bottle or glass. Visa/MC. Open until 8 PM daily.

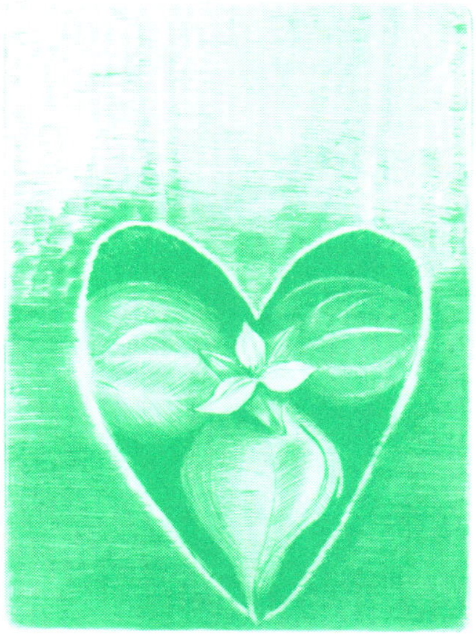

Trillium Valentine, © *Liza Jones*

Central

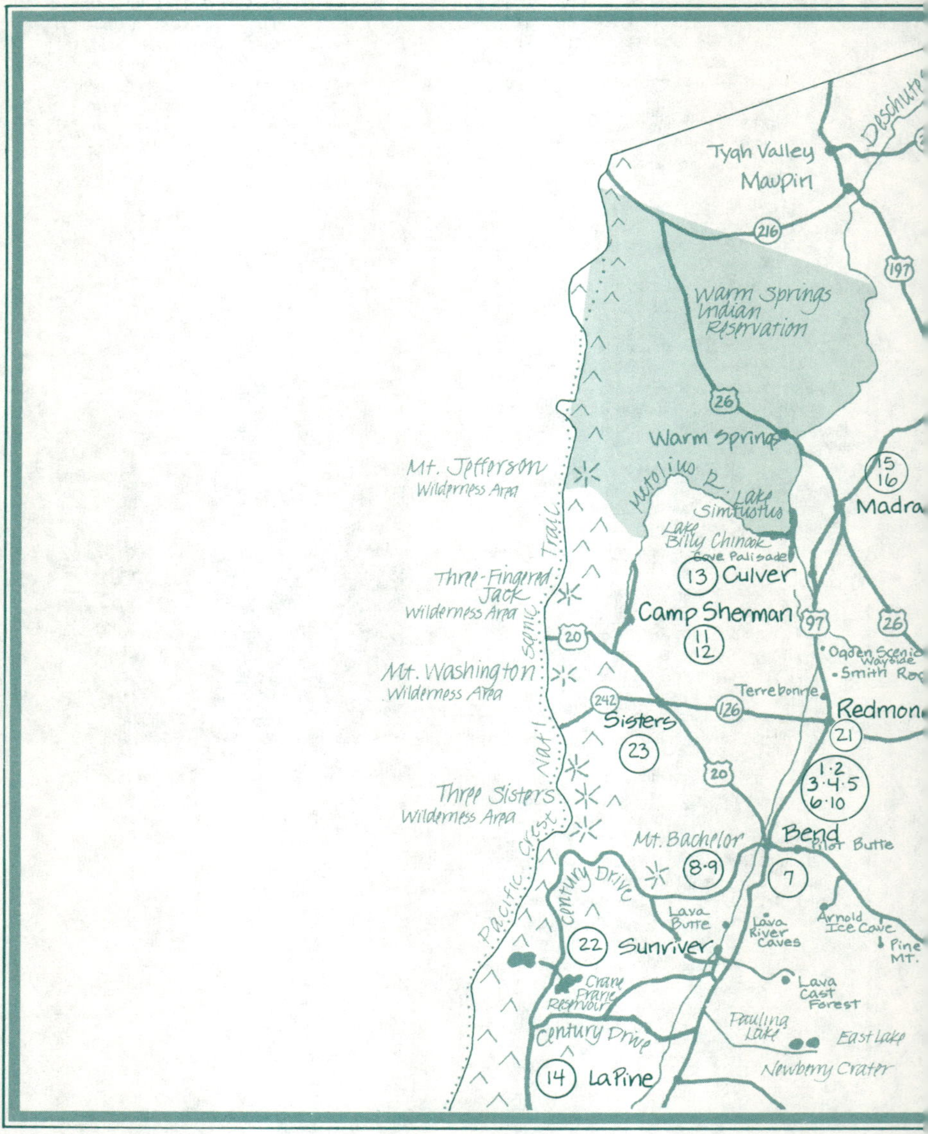

Deschute
Tygh Valley
Maupin
216
197
Warm Springs Indian Reservation
26
Warm Springs
Metolius R.
Lake Simtustus
Mt. Jefferson Wilderness Area
15 16
Madra
Lake Billy Chinook
Cove Palisade
13 Culver
Three-Fingered Jack Wilderness Area
Camp Sherman
11 12
97
26
20
Ogden Scenic Wayside
Smith Ro
Mt. Washington Wilderness Area
Pacific Crest Nat'l Scenic Trail
242
Terrebonne
126
Redmon
Sisters
21
23
20
1·2 3·4·5 6·10
Three Sisters Wilderness Area
Bend
Pilot Butte
Mt. Bachelor
8·9
7
Century Drive
Lava Butte
Lava River Caves
Arnold Ice Cave
Pine MT.
22 Sunriver
Crane Prairie Reservoir
Lava Cast Forest
Century Drive
Paulina Lake
East Lake
Newberry Crater
14 LaPine

Oregon

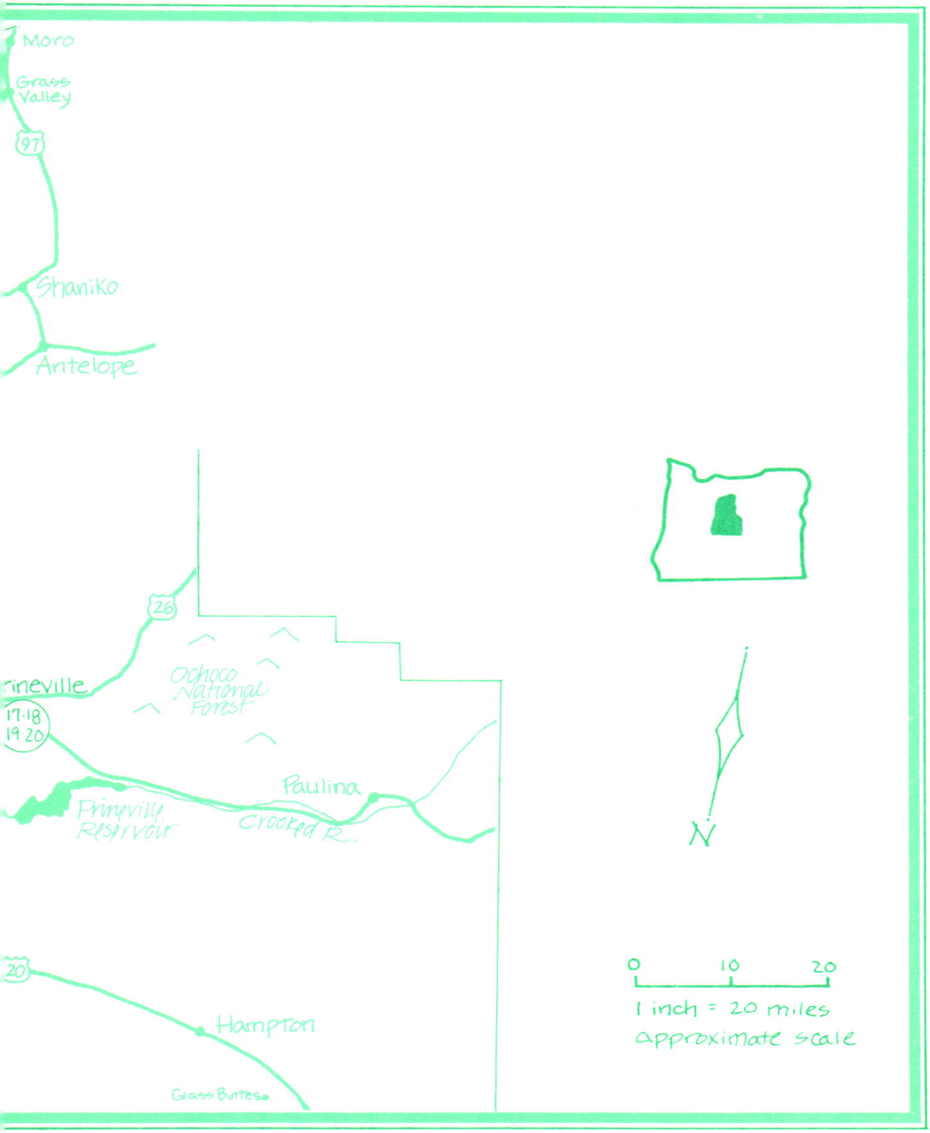

Moro
Grass Valley
97
Shaniko
Antelope
26
rineville
17·18
19·20
Ochoco National Forest
Paulina
Prineville Reservoir
Crooked R.
20
Hampton
Glass Buttes
N
0
10
20
1 inch = 20 miles
approximate scale

CENTRAL OREGON REGIONAL NOTES

The snow-covered peaks of Mt. Hood, Mt. Jefferson, Mt. Bachelor, Broken Top (Three-Fingered Jack), Mt. Washington, and the Three Sisters (from north to south), poking through the **Cascade Mountain range** *on the western horizon of Central Oregon, can often be seen holding back the rain clouds bearing Pacific Ocean moisture. Hence, it is more often sunny than not in Central Oregon. These were once active volcanoes. Some, like Mt. Hood, still emit steam, and no one knows when one might erupt again. A good way to tell the difference between active and inactive volcanoes is to look at their shapes. If symmetrical and cone-shaped, a volcano probably has been active since the last ice age and is very likely alive and capable of erupting again. If it is craggy, carved, and eroded by glaciers, it has not been active since the last ice age and is more likely to be extinct. The entire Central Oregon area has many traces of volcanic activity and is a reminder that human beings' presence on the earth in terms of geologic activity and time is relatively insignificant.*

A few miles east of Terrebonne is **Smith Rock State Park,** *where multicolored volcanic rock formations rise above the Crooked River Canyon. Smith Rock State Park has excellent climbing walls (for experienced climbers only) and a primitive camp. At* **Peter Skene Ogden Scenic Wayside,** *U.S. Highway 97 crosses this deep canyon. Just east of Prineville,* **Stein's Pillar** *pokes 350 feet up out of the Ochoco National Forest. Nearby, on Oregon Highway 126 is* **one of the world's largest stands of western juniper. Lake Billy Chinook** *and* **Lake Simtustus** *are the result of the damming of the* **Deschutes, Metolius,** *and* **Crooked Rivers** *into two reservoirs. The narrow, steep-sided, rock-rimmed, basaltic canyon walls of Lake Sintustus that can now be seen by boat are amazing geologic wonders, complete with balancing rocks. The experience one can have here, near the little community of Culver, is one of Oregon's best-kept secrets.*

Below the Pelton Dam, the **Deschutes River** *is designated a* **State Scenic Waterway** *all the way north to the Columbia River, and is recognized as one of Oregon's premier white-water attractions. Deschutes River State Park has an Oregon Trail display, and Indians still fish the river with great nets.* **Warm Springs Indian Reservation** *operates a multimillion-dollar resort that mysteriously was not touched by a raging range fire that destroyed everything around it to within a few feet in the spring of 1985. Wild horses from the reservation are featured at the all-Indian rodeo at Tygh Valley every May.*

Pine Mountain Observatory, *35 miles east of Bend off Highway 20 at the summit of 6,395-foot-high Pine Mountain, is one of the most active small-medium research observatories in the nation, and is the only full-time professional observatory in the Northwestern states. It is a unit of the University of Oregon Physics Department, and has three Cassegrain reflector telescopes, diameters 32," 24," and 15." Pine Mountain research projects have been devoted to various kinds of binary stars (including "black-hole" binaries), planets, magnetic and pulsating stars, and the Sun and sunspots. A new project has to do with searching for planets around nearby stars.*

Just east of Bend is **Pilot Butte,** *a lone cinder cone. There are unobstructed views of Central Oregon and the Cascade Mountains from its 511-foot height.*

South of Bend on U.S. Highway 97, in the **Deschutes National Forest,** *there is the* **Lava Lands Visitors Center** *at the base of* **Lava Butte,** *a 500-foot cinder cone that is one of the many miniature volcanos that hurled ashes and cinders over the fields to the north and east. A lava flow poured out of its base and dammed the ancient Deschutes River within the last 2,000 years. Walking trails lead through a moon-like landscape of lava fields immediately outside the center, and a paved road winds to the top of the butte, where there is a small observatory building containing an outstanding collection of accurately labeled volcanic rocks and panoramic paintings identifying the Cascade volcanoes along the horizon.*

At **Lava River Caves State Park, Lava River Tunnel,** *a nearly 1-mile-long lava tube, is 50 feet wide and 35 feet high, and is one of the largest of its kind.* **Lava Cast Forest Geological Area** *contains molds of many pine trees that were engulfed by slow-moving lava some 6,000 years ago.*

Newberry Crater, *the source of the lava flows that created the Lava River Cave tubes and the Lava Cast Forest, is a giant caldera divided into two parts by cinder and pumice cones; each segment is occupied by a lake, and* **one of the world's largest glassy flows of obsidian** *is present in the caldera. Although the least visible, Newberry volcano is probably the largest and most extraordinary of all the volcanoes in the Oregon Cascades.*

It does not make much of a landmark because it is so broad and its flanks' slope so gentle that it makes only a very subtle outline against the sky. The only way to appreciate its unusual geology is to take the side road east from U.S. Highway 97 to Paulina and East Lake, which are right in the collapsed floor of the caldera. (See Roadside Geology of Oregon, *reference page 3, for more detailed information on this and other geologic features around Oregon.)*

There are a number of **ice caves** *in the area (see map). They are not leftovers from previous ice ages but rather exist wherever caves in fairly cold climates breathe through vertical openings. Ice accumulations filling lava caves often make them quite beautiful.*

The **Willamette National Forest,** *which straddles the Cascade Mountains to the east, is limited to horse and foot travel in some parts, including the* **Three Sisters** *and* **Diamond Peak Wilderness Areas,** *that have extensive volcanic formations. For trailhead locations, maps, and fire conditions contact the Willamette National Forest Supervisor's Office, Federal Building, 211 E. 7th Ave. (P.O. Box 10607), Eugene, Oregon 97440 (Tel: 687-6522).*

Century Drive, *otherwise known as Cascade Lakes Highway Drive or Oregon Highway 46, is an enchanting loop drive through the* **Deschutes National Forest** *east of Bend—119 miles long if one includes the 22.8-mile segment back to Bend on Highway 97 from the south. For trailhead locations, maps, and fire conditions contact the Deschutes National Forest Supervisor's Office, 1645 Hwy. 20E, Bend, Oregon 97701 (Tel: 382-6922). It passes by alpine lakes and meadows, an* **osprey management area** *at* **Crane Prairie,** *and numerous old and rustic resorts, and is the access to many hiking trails in the Sisters Wilderness Area.*

For hikers and climbers, there are trails at E. R. Corbett and Smith Rock State Parks. There are boat ramps at Ochoco Lake and Prineville Reservoir State Parks. There are a marina, boat ramps, and dock at Cove Palisades State Park. Group picnic facilities are available at Tumalo State Park. Group tent facilities at Cove Palisades and Tumalo State Parks, and club camping at La Pine, Prineville Reservoir, and Cove Palisades State Parks.

The area around **Sisters** *is especially well suited for* **llamas.** *A number of people have started breeding them in the past decade, making llama treks into the adjacent national forests popular.*

From huge springs at the base of Black Butte in Camp Sherman, flow the **headwaters** *of the* **Metolius River.** *The Sam Johnson family, who owned these headwaters, dedicated them to the State of Oregon a few years ago in order that the public could experience the cold, clear, clean water bubbling out of the earth.* **Wizard Falls,** *just downstream from the headwaters, is one of Oregon's most park-like fish hatcheries.*

The **Ashwood area** *northeast of Madras is composed mostly of "pay diggings" sites on private property for* **petrified woods, agate, thunder eggs, jaspers,** *etc. Stop at Richardson's Recreational Ranch. (See Central Oregon listings for more information.)*

There are numerous **mining locations** *under mining claims around* **Prineville** *maintained by the Prineville-Crook County Chamber of Commerce. These claims provide free diggings to the noncommercial rock hound. Stop at Elkins' Gemstones for samples and details. (See Central Oregon listings.)*

Jasper thunder eggs are found at White Fir and White Rock Springs; carnelian cores have been found near White Rock Springs; moss dendritic agate and angelwing are found at Eagle Rock, southeast of Prineville; Bear Creek petrified wood is found at Bear Creek, south of Prineville; at Maury Mountain there are red, green, and yellow moss agates; Crooked River white, pink, green, and dendritic limb casts can be found near Paulina; wood replacement in jaspers and agates can be found at Hampton Butte—the color varies from green, brown, black, to white. For more details on where to find digging sites, contact Richardson's Recreational Ranch (Central Oregon listings); Elkins Gemstones (Central Oregon listings); or Highland Rock and Gift Shop (Southeastern Oregon listings), that publishes "The Rockhound's Map of Oregon," from which much of the rockhounding information was taken.

Oregon has an incredible variety of **wildflowers** *throughout the state. Please enjoy them, and please leave them undisturbed for others to enjoy. "A picked wildflower is a thing of beauty, but a joy for only one person for a few minutes." Some wildflowers grow in incredibly delicate environments and can take as long as seven years to bloom again.*

See Statewide Resources section regarding The Nature Conservancy's preserves in this area that the public may visit.

BEND

1 Charles A. Blakeslee—Photography

61649 S.E. Fargo Lane, Bend, 97702.
Tel: 389-8825
Charles Blakeslee specializes in photographing the rural life of Oregon and the wilderness of the Pacific Northwest in color and black and white. All prints can be custom framed. Scenic photographic note cards available. Studio and gallery open by appointment only. Charles' work can also be seen at the Blue Sky Gallery in Bend.

2 Blue Sky Gallery

147 Minnesota Ave., Bend, 97701.
Tel: 388-1877
Featured works by Central Oregon and Northwest artists include watercolors, pottery, fine wood crafts, jewelry, photographs, metal and wood sculpture, weaving, and other fine arts and contemporary crafts. Also represented are limited edition prints by national artists. The gallery's Custom Framing Center offers the full range of framing services and specializes in creative mat designs and conservation framing. Visa/MC/AmEx. 10-5:30 Mon-Sat.

3 Blue Spruce Pottery

61021 S. Hwy. 97, Bend, 97702 (on the west side of Hwy. 97, just south of Bend proper). Tel: 389-7745
Michael and Michele Gwinup produce a full line of functional and decorative stoneware in their studio next to their gallery. They also carry a variety of pottery produced by several regional artists, which includes raku, porcelain, and wood-fired pottery. The public is welcome to watch potters working in their studio. Visa/MC. 10-5:30 Mon-Sat, 12-5 Sun.

4 Cascade Festival of Music

842 N.W. Wall St. #6, Bend, 97701 (Performances held in Drake Park).
Tel: 382-8381
A week-long festival of concerts held June 17-26 in 1988 in Bend's Drake Park alongside the Deschutes River: classical, pops and jazz, with a special Children's Concert, at very affordable prices. There is also daily free entertainment in Drake Park, a Champagne Brunch and Concert atop Mt. Bachelor (June 20), and Orchestra a la Carte (June 25). Call for tickets and 1989 dates. Visa/MC.

5 Frame Design and Sunbird Gallery

836 N.W. Wall St., Bend, 97701.
Tel: 389-9196
Sandra and Steve Miller provide museum-quality framing and restoration of prints, photographs, and paintings. Their gallery features posters, art prints, and works of carefully chosen Oregon artists and craftspeople, including Pacific Northwest Native American art. Some of the artists represented have received Fellowship Awards from the Oregon Arts Commission and the National Endowment for the Arts. Visa/MC/Discover. 10-5:30 Tues-Sat.

6 The Guest House at The Farm Antiques

20020 Glen Vista Rd., Bend, 97701 (2 mi. north of Bend, off O. B. Riley Rd.).
Tel: 382-8565
This small, very private log house comes complete with a wood stove and a mountain view from the covered porch. Furnished by The Farm Antiques, just down the lane, the house sleeps four comfortably, and up to eight in a pinch. The kitchen is completely equipped and the makings for a farm-fresh breakfast are provided daily. Children and pets welcome. Pasture for horses too. Visa/MC. Open year around. Reservations required.

7 The High Desert Museum

59800 S. Hwy. 97, Bend, 97702 (6 mi. south of Bend on Hwy. 97). Tel: 382-4754
A "living" museum specializing in the cultural and natural history of the arid, intermountain Northwest, which includes two-thirds of Oregon. There are live animal exhibits (both indoor and outdoor) featuring river otters, porcupines, reptiles, and birds of prey, plus pioneer and Native American historical exhibits, Western art, artifacts, Nature Store, and visitor information center. Visa/MC. 9-5 daily (April 1-Sept 30), 9-4 daily (Oct 1-March 31, except Thanksgiving, Christmas, New Year's Day).

8 **The Inn of the Seventh Mountain**

7 mi. west of Bend on Century Dr., P.O. Box 1207, Bend, 97709. Tel: 382-8711 or 800-452-6810 (in-state toll free)
Guests can enjoy whitewater rafting or canoe float trips on the Deschutes River or horseback riding along the banks from the inn's stable. Winter brings outdoor ice skating and horse-drawn sleigh rides. This is a full-service resort in the Deschutes National Forest setting, featuring three restaurants, nightly rates, and activity package rentals. Closest lodging to Mt. Bachelor ski area. All major credit cards accepted. Open year around.

9 **Mt. Bachelor Ski and Summer Resort**

335 S.W. Century Dr., P.O. Box 1031, Bend, 97709. Tel: 382-2442
Mt. Bachelor is the largest ski and summer resort in the Pacific Northwest, with ten chairlifts and 3,100 feet of "vertical." Winter activities include skiing, sleigh rides, Nordic skiing, and special events. Summer activities include chairlift rides, mountain bike rentals, special events, summer camps for all ages, and summer skiing, usually until the end of June. All major credit cards accepted. Call or write for more information.

10 **Sun Fruits of Sunriver®**

Bend River Mall, 3078 N. Hwy. 97, Bend, 97701. Tel: 388-3232
After two-and-a-half years in Sunriver, Betty Marshall has moved her fancy fruit, nut, and gourmet food shop to larger quarters in Bend. Oregon food products and wines combine with unique in-shop chocolate-dipped specialties in the creation of fancy gift packs and custom-designed basket arrangements. A mail order catalog is available. UPS shipments go out daily. Visa/MC. 10-9 Mon-Fri, 10-6 Sat, 12-5 Sun.

CARRY A HAT

Fact: **One loses 70% of his body heat from the top of his head.** *By taking off and putting on a wool stocking hat one can regulate one's body temperature. Keep one in your pocket at all times of the year.*

Wool: Wool dries from the inside out *and helps keep a person warm even when wet.*

CAMP SHERMAN

11 **Lake Creek Lodge**

Camp Sherman (3½ mi. north of Hwy. 20 on Camp Sherman Rd., 1½ mi. before Camp Sherman). Mailing address: Star Rt. 1, Sisters, 97759. Tel: 595-6331
Originally a summer-only guest resort, the lodge was built in the early 1900s. Lake Creek flows through the 60-acre property. There are pine-paneled cabins with screened porches, some with stone fireplaces; home-cooked meals in the main lodge in the summer; a swimming pool; tennis and children's privately stocked trout pond. Diana Pepperling is the lodge's manager and Blanche Williams the "super cook." Off-season and workshop rates available. 9 AM-10 PM daily.

12 **Metolius Inn Bed and Breakfast**

3.5 mi. north on Camp Sherman Rd. (Forest Service Rd. #1419) from Hwy. 20 intersection, P.O. Box 642, Camp Sherman, 97730. Tel: 595-6445 or 549-7441
Metolius Inn is bordered by forests, meadows, and mountains. Near the quaint western town of Sisters, the area also offers fishing, hiking, trailriding, skiing, boating, swimming, and golfing. The inn provides two large guest rooms, king-sized beds, private baths and patios. The "common room" has a cozy fireplace, TV, small library, and games. Complimentary wine, full breakfasts with fresh-baked pastries. Picnic lunches available. Smoking in patio areas only. No children or pets. Visa/MC. Open year around.

CULVER

13 **Old Courthouse Gift Shop**

511 First St., P.O. Box 198, Culver, 97734. Tel: 546-8641
"You'll find upon entering, a world full of talent and imagination. The talent is all local. Central Oregon local. All items are handcrafted by a friend or neighbor with lots of Tender Loving Care. Come, enjoy a journey back in time," says Barbara Frazier, whose shop is in the courthouse built circa 1914-1917. Visa/MC. 10-5 Tues-Sat.

LA PINE

14 Russell Industries, Inc.—Forest Furniture

51636 Pengra-Huntington Rd. (1 blk. off Hyw. 97), P.O. Box 323, La Pine, 97739. Tel: 536-2229 or 389-2289

The scale here is immense. Marvin and Marilyn's forest furniture workshop makes incredible furniture from dead Ponderosa Pine that Marvin carefully hauls out of the forest. The etchings of the pine beetles that lived in the dead trees add character to his massive furniture. Large, unforgettable display. Custom work available also. 8-4:30 Mon-Sat.

MADRAS

15 City of Madras

City Hall: 416 6th St., Madras, 97741. Tel: 475-2344

Office: 8-5 Mon-Fri.

Chamber of Commerce: 366 5th St., P.O. Box 770, Madras, 97741. Tel: 475-2350

Madras, first settled in the late 1800s, and the "Peppermint Capital of the World," offers its 2250 residents and its visitors 300 days of sunshine a year. With the Cove Palisades State Park in its back yard, camping, swimming, fishing, skiing, jet skiing, hiking, and houseboating abound on Lake Billy Chinook. Haystack Reservoir is ideal for windsurfing and bass fishing. Hunters, rockhounds, and whitewater rafters will find many opportunities. The Madras Airport has the second longest runway in Oregon. An art gallery, the Jefferson County Museum, historical buildings, and the County Seat are all located here too.

1988-89 Madras Area Events include:

1988

April 9-10: Sports & Recreation Show
May 13-14: Fancy Foods & Wine Festival & Rodeo
June 15-19: Good Sams Samboree
June 24-26: Pi-ume-sha Treaty Days
July 2-9: All Rockhound Pow Wow
July 4: Sparklers 4th of July
July 17: Pioneer Picnic
Aug 10-14: Jefferson County Fair
Oct 15-16: St. Pat's Cowdeo (kids' rodeo)
Nov 26: Geo. Wilson Memorial Run
Dec 3: Craftsman Bazaar

1989

TBA: Central Oregon Farm Fair
TBA: Sports & Recreation Show

16 Richardson's Recreational Ranch, Ltd.

Gateway Rt. Box 440, Madras, 97741 (11 mi. north of Madras on U.S. 97, go east to ranch office). Tel: 475-2680

The Richardson family supplements its cattle-ranch business with recreational offerings including camping, photography and rockhounding. They own and operate the Priday thunderegg beds and visitors can dig every day (weather permitting). Their rock shop includes such other Oregon materials as moss agate, Oregon sunset and rainbow agate. Visa/MC. Daylight until dark daily.

PRINEVILLE

17 Baldwin Inn Bed and Breakfast

126 W. First St., Prineville, 97754. Tel: 447-5758

Innkeepers Sandy and Wayne Demaris have recreated the spirit of "Grandma's house" that "echoes the refinements of an earlier era" in Prineville's largest and finest historical home. Built by Thomas Baldwin, founder of Prineville's first bank, the house was placed on the National Register in 1987. Now carefully restored, with three guest rooms, music and reading rooms, parlor, gardens, and private meeting rooms. Farm-fresh breakfasts. Also available for wedding services. Visa/MC.

18 Elkins Gem Stones

833 S. Main, Prineville, 97754. Tel: 447-5547

Judy Elkins specializes in thundereggs (the state rock), fossils, agates, crystal specimens and custom silverwork using one-of-a-kind stones. She and her family have been a fund of information on local rockhounding areas since 1959. 8-6 daily (summer), 8-5 Mon, Tues, Thurs, Fri, Sat (winter).

19 Odyssey Fibers

295 West Third, Prineville, 97754. Tel: 447-1424

Liz Currier is a natural fiber artist producing handspun yarns, handwoven yardage, garments and wall hangings. She also sells supplies and High Desert Wheat Weavings in her shop, and does work on commission. Call or write for more information. 9:30-5 Tues-Fri, 10:30-5 Sat.

20 Victoria's Vintage Sewing and Doll House

970 N. Harwood St., Prineville, 97754. Tel: 447-4606
Victoria Glazebrook is a woman of many talents. She calls herself a "vintage dressmaker" but also makes dolls of fine porcelain, with the 18-inch "Gibson Girl" a favorite. She also scales down patterns from the 1800s-1900s to create miniature dresses for 11½-inch fashion dolls. A family collection from 1911 is on display now. 5 AM-6 PM Mon-Fri.

REDMOND

21 Wickman Hill Gallery

525 S.W. Sixth St., Redmond, 97756 (in the Nendels New Redmond Hotel complex). Tel: 923-5208
Wickman Hill Gallery is an owner/artist gallery showcasing the oil and pastel work of Susan Wickman and the clay, glass, and metal work of Linda Gilmore Hill. Monthly "theme exhibits" highlight the work of many fine Central Oregon artists. The gallery also has an art rental plan for corporate offices and personal residences. Visa/MC. 11-6 Wed-Sat, 10-2 Sun. Other times by appointment.

SUNRIVER

22 Sunriver Lodge and Resort

Sunriver, 97707. Tel: 593-1221, 800-452-6874 (in-state), 800-547-3922 (out-of-state)
Surrounded by the Deschutes National Forest with mountains, pines, and meadows, and Central Oregon hospitality, Sunriver offers year-around canoeing, rafting, and fishing on the Deschutes River, miles of bike trails and horseback trail rides, tennis, and two championship golf courses. The nature center has activities for nature lovers. When the snow falls, there's Nordic skiing and ice skating (plus downhill skiing at Mt. Bachelor). Sunriver Music Festival, in its 11th year in 1988, is held every August, and monthly art shows and a three-week juried exhibition are held in the main lodge in February. All major credit cards accepted. Open year around.

SISTERS

23 Sisters Chamber of Commerce

P.O. Box 476, Sisters, 97759. Tel: 549-0251 (to verify times of events)
A few years ago a local lumber company offered to pay a stipend to any Sisters merchant who would refurbish the front of his business in a turn-of-the-century western style. It worked. Now the town is charming and because the townspeople participated themselves they have adopted zoning laws to maintain the integrity of the concept.

1988-89 Sisters Area Events include:

1988

April 2: John Craig Nordic Race/ Spring Festival
May 7: John McAdams Memorial Run/Merchants' Crazy Days
June 9-11: Sisters Rodeo
1st Sats of July-Sept: Sisters Saturday Market (all handcrafted items)
July 3-5: Round-up of Gems
July 4: Old West 4th of July Celebration
July 9: Sisters Outdoor Quilt Show (only outdoor quilt show in U.S.)
July TBA: Centennial Celebration for Sisters Post Office (a week-long event)
Oct 8: Harvest Festival
Dec 3: Christmas Festivities with Old-fashioned Parade

1989

Last Sat of Feb: Sisters Casino Night (Old West gambling with scrip, at Hotel Sisters)

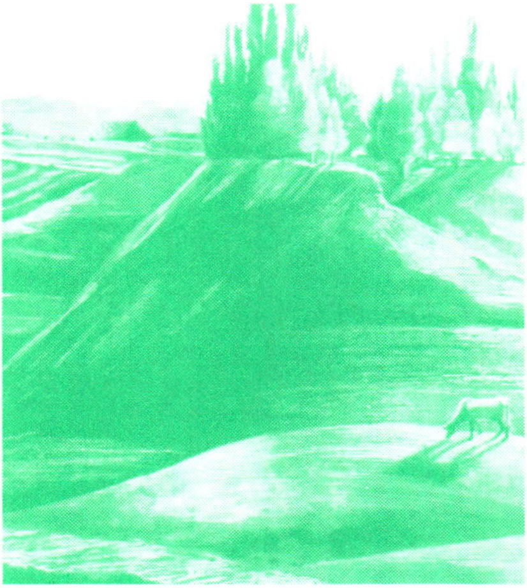

Red Hills (Deschutes), © Liza Jones

Index

Readers' Suggestions

Your comments about the success of this year's guide and suggestions for future editions are always welcome . . . and often used. Many suggestions regarding previous editions have been incorporated into this year's guide.

This is a grassroots, **self-help project** initiated by the Oregon Arts Commission in 1984 and now totally **supported by the participants themselves** in order to let the world know of the products and services they provide. **If this guide helped you find a participant, please tell him.**

If you know of people, products, places, services or events that are not included this year, but **who you feel should be encouraged to participate in future editions** of the guide, **please (1) tell them and (2) let us know who they are.**

The Regional Notes are just that. They usually do not include things that communities say about themselves in their own listings. They are mostly about natural or other phenomena that could not describe themselves, e.g. a sand dune. Suggestions of things you think should be included to give people a better understanding of Oregon as a distinct place unto itself are welcome.

TO ORDER ADDITIONAL GUIDES

Send $8.45 (includes postage and handling) to **Where to Find the Oregon in Oregon**, 7277 S.W. Barnes Rd., Portland, Oregon 97225. (Bulk orders require less postage and handling. Call or write us for wholesale and retail bulk prices.) Tel: 292-4549

Your name ____________________

Street ____________________

City ____________________ State ____________ Zip code ____________

Number of guides requested ____________ Check in the amount of ____________ enclosed.

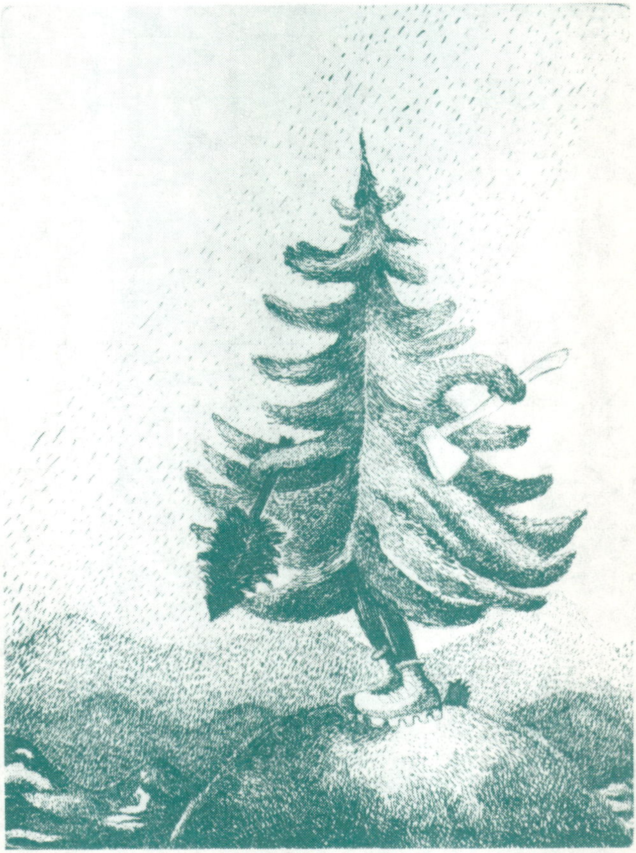

"Oregon, My Oregon," © *Liza Jones*